POLITICS

AND

PERFORMANCE

Theatre, Poetry and Song
in Southern Africa

EDITED BY LIZ GUNNER

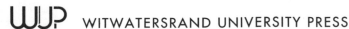 WITWATERSRAND UNIVERSITY PRESS

Witwatersrand University Press
1 Jan Smuts Avenue
Johannesburg
2001
South Africa

ISBN 1 86814 214 0

First published 1994

Typeset by The Natal Witness Printing and Publishing Company (Pty) Ltd

Printed and bound by CTP Book Printers, Cape

The following articles have been reprinted with the permission of the *Journal of Southern African Studies*:

Towards Popular Theatre in South Africa; Apartheid and the Political Imagination in Black South African Theatre; Trends in Zimbabwean Theatre Since 1980; Backstage on the Frontline: Iluba Elimnyama — a Bulawayo Theatre Collective; Traditions of Poetry in Natal; Reflections on a Cultural Day of Artists and Workers on 16 April 1989; Marotholi Travelling Theatre: Towards an Alternative Perspective of Development; Theatre for Development in Zimbabwe: An Urban Project; Mental Colonisation or Catharsis? Theatre, Democracy and Cultural Struggle from Rhodesia to Zimbabwe; Patronage, the State and Ideology in Zambian Theatre and Interview: Gcina Mhlophe.

Certain inconsistencies in the form of the notes throughout the book are due to the fact that several of the contributions are drawn directly from the originals published in the *Journal of Southern African Studies* 16 (2), June 1990.

BK4702

PN2984 POL

POLITICS
AND
PERFORMANCE

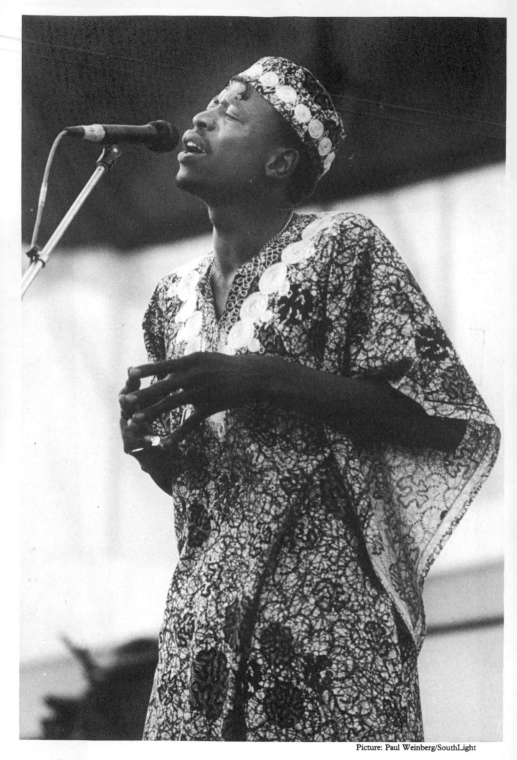

Mzwakhe Mbuli, the 'People's Poet' in action at a rally held at FNB Stadium, Johannesburg in November 1989 to celebrate the release from prison of eight ANC leaders

Contributors

TYRONE AUGUST is editor of the Johannesburg-based *Learn and Teach* magazine and before that was cultural editor of the newspaper *New Nation*.

STEPHEN CHIFUNYISE worked for many years in theatre in Zambia and after Zimbabwe's independence took up a post in Zimbabwe's Department of Youth and Culture. He is a playwright and a leading figure in theatre and the media in Zimbabwe.

MOREBLESSINGS CHITAURO teaches Shona language and literature in the Department of African Languages and Literatures at the University of Zimbabwe. Her main fields of interest are gender and literacy. She is currently studying at the University of Florida.

STEWART CREHAN has worked in theatre departments at the Universities of Zambia and Swaziland and now teaches in the English Department at the University of Transkei.

CALEB DUBE of the Department of African Languages and Literature at the University of Zimbabwe is currently working on a doctorate on music and popular culture at Northwestern University.

PAUL GREADY is a Leverhulme Research Fellow in the Department of African Literature, University of the Witwatersrand. He is working on autobiography in South Africa.

LIZ GUNNER teaches African literature in the Department of African Languages and Cultures at the School of Oriental and African Studies, London University. Her main field of interest is performance culture in Southern Africa.

ALI HLONGWANE is a director and actor and has worked for a number of years with the Soyikwa Theatre Company and with the FUBA (Federated Union of Black Artists) Arts Centre in Johannesburg.

DEBORAH JAMES has written on music and popular culture in South Africa and teaches in the Department of Social Anthropology at the University of the Witwatersrand.

PREBEN KAARSHOLM is Director of the Institute for Development Studies at the University of Roskilde, Denmark and has written extensively on politics and popular culture in Southern Africa.

ROBERT MSHENGU KAVANAGH (Robert McLaren) is Head of the Department of Theatre Arts at the University of Zimbabwe and is widely known as an actor, critic and director in South Africa, Ethiopia and Zimbabwe.

ZAKES MDA is a writer, painter and musician who has worked extensively with development theatre in Lesotho. He taught for seven years at the National University of Lesotho and has recently completed a year as a Research Fellow in the Yale Southern African Fellowship. He is currently Visiting Professor of Literature at the University of Vermont.

BHEKIZIZWE PETERSON teaches in the African Literature Department at the University of the Witwatersrand. He writes extensively on culture and politics in South Africa and has for some years been active in theatre projects with youth.

ARI SITAS was a member of the Junction Avenue Theatre Company in Johannesburg until he moved to Natal where he is in the Department of Sociology at the University of Natal, Durban. He has been involved with worker culture for several years.

IAN STEADMAN is Dean of the Faculty of Arts at the University of the Witwatersrand and former Head of the university's School of Dramatic Art. He has written widely on theatre in South Africa.

Contents

Introduction: The Struggle for Space

LIZ GUNNER

Theatre, poetry and song all feature in this collection of essays, reports and personal experience on the topic of Politics and Performance in Southern Africa. This volume will have its life in a very different context — particularly in South African terms — from the earlier collection on which it is based.[1] In South Africa many of the barriers of apartheid legislation have fallen and the old form of government is set to disappear. Much, however, remains to be resolved and the crisis of legitimacy has been replaced by a crisis of identity which has allowed space for intense debate and the flowering of new creative work by those with their eyes fixed on a post-apartheid culture. It has also, though, seen an intensified mobilisation of ethnicity and its cultural manifestations on behalf of a spurious national destiny.

Commentators on music and popular culture such as Veit Erlmann and David Coplan, constantly point to the fluidity of cultural identity in South Africa. The shifting boundaries that Erlmann mentions in regard to black and white culture, rural and urban music, and popular and élite hegemonic culture are frequently inferred in the studies included here. Yet, as Rob Nixon has recently stated, the very porousness of such boundaries and cultural identities has forced the architects of ethnicity towards a kind of 'ethnogeneticism' in their desperate and destructive efforts to make cultural differences inbred and inviolate.[2]

There are no such discourses of difference resonating from the pages of this book. However, these essays engage with other interlocking debates relating to empowerment, space, voice, identity, nationalism and gender. There is also an urgent sense that performance culture has, and still does, engage with the political sphere at a number of levels. There is very little indication from these essays that culture and politics have their own autonomous spheres. Indeed, the content of a number of papers reminds us that the richness and complexity of a great deal of South African resistance culture was far too simplistically dismissed by Albie Sachs in his controversial paper Preparing Ourselves for Freedom.[3]

Another message that comes from this volume is that in the South

African, and indeed the wider, regional context, print culture, that of the written word, must concede equality with the multiple other ways of 'writing the nation', namely performance based forms which have long co-existed with but not been accorded the same status as print. And here the theme of voice and empowerment, which comes up again and again in this volume, is central. The constant crossing of the print/performance boundary is now an established feature of work by artists such as Mzwakhe Mbuli, the worker poets A T Qabula, Gladman Ngubo, as well as by Lesego Rampalakeng, Sandile Dikene and new rap groups active in Cape Town. These latest examples of performance culture need to be seen as linked to the resilient and on-going making of culture by those with no recognised voice and no respected place in the older order of things.

Unscripted, performed words have a long and honourable place in the making of Southern African culture. One example of this is described in the article by Deborah James on women's migrant performance, *Basadi ba baeng*/Visiting Women. The Sotho lyrics which so crucially shape this emergent form, and largely hold its identity, show the 'past in the present'[4] yet can undergo a continual process of recomposition and reinterpretation. They are not, for those who use them, scripted lyrics. Nor, in the lives and careers of the Zimbabwean singers discussed by Moreblessings Chitauro, Caleb Dube and Liz Gunner in their article Song, Story and Nation, is it the script of the songs that mattered most but rather the sound coming over radio waves, on a cassette, or live, and staying in people's memories and their consciousness. In much of the theatre discussed here, both from South Africa and Zimbabwe there has been no written script at all.

Stewart Crehan's richly informative essay on Zambian theatre points to the negative feelings of a number of Zambian playwrights towards producing a written script because 'their interest is in the *performance*, not in the play as something to be read, studied or appreciated as literature'. Thus while writers such as J M Coetzee, Etienne van Heerden, Chenjerai Hove and Tsitsi Dangarembga are part of the brilliant mosaic of Southern African culture, those written forms must, in the African context, coexist and interact with the other myriad forms of performance culture which are constantly being produced and reworked and are part of indigenous discourse.

The role of audience is one that has been consistently under-explored in the discussion of culture and its production in South Africa.[5] It is, though, a crucial component in the making of culture 'from below' rather than its imposition 'from the top down'. The active, dialogic role of audience relates to the broader issues of voice and space which are present in this collection and is addressed most directly by Gcina Mhlophe in her interview with Tyrone August, and in the articles by Paul Gready and Ari Sitas. For Mhlophe, the narrow constraints of protest theatre were, by the late eighties, becoming suffocating and she turned her energies elsewhere — to storytelling, 'thinking it would be a part-time thing'. Instead it grew to a company of fifteen performers, called *Zanendaba*, and the close presence, demands, preferences of her fairly diverse audiences, clearly played a crucial part in her development of this form.

Such forms, like the African languages in which they are usually couched, need to play an important role in the culture of the South Africa of the future.

Audience has also been an instrumental force in the making of new cultural space by what Ari Sitas has elsewhere referred to as a combination of 'creativity and mobilisation'.[6] Worker poetry and worker theatre, based largely in Natal, have demonstrated a new kind of empowerment and shifting of identities — both showing the sham behind any 'ethnogenetic' approach to 'Zulu culture'. A crucial factor in the shaping of both the poetry and the theatre has been the role of audience as an 'interpretive community'.[7] And as Paul Gready points out in his searching and innovative paper on worker theatre as autobiography, Political Autobiography in Search of Liberation, the role of audience has been crucial in the formulation of identity for this new form and this new process of autobiography in South Africa. Acknowledging the importance of mobilisation, Gready refers to the Aims and Principles of the Durban Workers Cultural Local as playing the role of a paradigmatic autobiographical text standing behind the autobiographical practice, and he calls it 'one of the many documents including the Freedom Charter which attempt to write a country into being'. He shows the tensions of the diverse subject positions which emerge as one voice and one autobiography and concludes by suggesting the importance of autobiography — related in this case to worker theatre — in emancipatory politics.

Although none of the essays here deals directly with the role of the print media, radio or television, in those areas, too, the question of voice, space and audience is crucial. As Malcolm Purkey pointed out recently in a hard-hitting paper on representation and the media in post-apartheid South Africa, 'The voices that have been hidden by apartheid and oppression must be heard in their own accents, ideolects, concerns and content. They must tell the stories of our country that the apartheid state has tried to keep hidden for so long.'[8] This too is part of the process of autobiography on a national scale as *self*-definition which Gready sees as moving beyond the confines of the printed page and the usual confines of the genre.

The writing in of the self in terms of gender and performance is also central to the presentations of women and performance in the essays by Deborah James and Chitauro, Dube and Gunner. James describes how women who migrated to the Rand from a number of Northern Sotho-speaking areas in the Northern Transvaal made use of, and in subtle ways subverted and changed to suit their own needs, the men's genre known as *kiba*. She points out that it is often the freer, marginalised and unofficial genres that become the basis for transformed cultural forms for both men and women in an urban or migrant context. In this instance, whereas men made use of dance and instruments — mainly pipes and drums — women made use of lyrics (as well as dance, instruments and sometimes dramatic sketches). In doing so they gave themselves greater freedom to improvise and comment, to make links with the past, and to create an identity for themselves in a way that they were not previously able to do.

Unlike the women of Phokeng with whom Belinda Bozzoli and Mmantho Nkotsoe worked, whose stories are centred in the fixed points between Phokeng and the Rand[9], the migrant women who use *kiba* come from a variety of rural places with no built in urban networks. The makers of *kiba* form their unity through performance of the new genre in the city. The trajectory of belonging, for them, goes from the city back to a re-imaged past, rather than moving from the countryside to the city. In the paper on Zimbabwean performers, women are shown as having to redefine their place in urban space, attempting to write themselves into the script of a nation which preferred to see them as outcasts, prostitutes but not makers of culture in the city. The paper focuses on the lives and careers of three singers — Dorothy Masuka, Susan Mapfumo and Stella Chiweshe — whose 'stories' and songs cover a period of close to fifty years. The ambiguous relation between woman and nation is also explored in this paper which throws up questions which are germane to the whole of the Southern African region about the place of women in the discourse of nationalism.

Language is another component of the discussion on identity with which the papers engage. A number of the essays in the collection, particularly Ian Steadman's and Bheki Peterson's on theatre, demonstrate the intermeshing of cultures and languages in South Africa as part of a many-layered discourse of resistance. Their work substantiates Martin Orkin's claim that theatre, more than any other art form in South Africa, has been able to challenge the discourse of domination by drawing on a variety of alternatives and by exploiting the relation of language to the operation of power in South Africa.[10]

What is also striking is the multi-lingual nature of the cultural terrain of the Southern African region covered by the essays in this book. The position of English in the region, in terms of social practice, is that of one of many languages and unless this is actively — rather than passively — recognised there is a danger, as Ngugi has constantly warned, that the élite and the masses will become irreparably divided. Thus, although the language used in these articles is English it is often a language that is acting as intermediary for another language with its own arteries of relations to history, power, gender relations and so on. There is a distinct sense in the discussions that English co-exists with, but by no means dominates the broad articulation of culture in the southern part of the continent. In every article, whether the discussion is of theatre, poetry or song, what we are being shown is a multiple existence of languages.

There is, in the countries of Southern Africa, a 'brilliant chaos of languages' and these pages give some sense of that. Often English and Shona, or English and Zulu, Xhosa or Sotho feature in a single performance under discussion. The plays about which Zakes Mda writes when he relates the work of the Maratholi Travelling Theatre in Lesotho were performed largely in Southern Sotho; the women's hostel play process described by Robert McLaren (R Mshengu Kavanagh) took place largely in Shona; those discussed by Stephen Chifunyise and Preben Kaarsholm cover English, Ndebele, Shona and often more than one of these in a single play; some of the plays discussed by Steadman and Peterson are in English and others are not; the same co-existence of languages marks the Cultural Day described by Ali Hlongwane; the trajectory of poetry followed by Sitas moves through various kinds of English to Zulu. What these pages repeatedly show is the way in which various forms of drama either avoid or break through the encasing of English and exploit both the intimate and public oratorical devices of the indigenous African languages. Yet, as Gcina Mhlophe points out, in South African theatre there is still sometimes the sense that African languages are not respected in plays — they are used sometimes as second best, or to make the least important points, the humorous asides, the bawdy jokes. They need a wider space than that, she states.

The contributions in this book also cut through the usual urban-rural divide that has been present in much that has been written on culture and verbal and written art. Theatre, the papers here emphasise, is currently a potent expressive vehicle in both the urban and rural contexts in Southern Africa. It is an empowering agency which can give people a new sense of control over their own lives. Zakes Mda describes how, through enactment and dialogue, rural people can come to have a new sense of social control. Nor is this necessarily cut off from a wider social situation in which the rural poor are often denied a voice. The two can interrelate, and Mda's second example of a theatre for development situation in action highlights how a common problem relating to land can be resolved and the power of a corrupt chief curtailed. The paper bears out his statement in his new, longer study of development theatre that 'of all these functions, the most important is that theatre for development gives the periphery access to the production and distribution of messages'.[11] But is this enough? Robert McLaren's succinct and disturbing piece on urban theatre for development in Zimbabwe describes both the difficulties and the rewards of development theatre work with women hostel-dwellers in the Matapi Hostels in Mbare, a high-density suburb of Harare. Both Mda and McLaren are aware of the dangers of this kind of theatre as a panacea rather than a long-term solution. For McLaren, the options at first seemed to be to go neither for reformism nor for revolution but to see this as participatory theatre in which the articulation of specific problems (in this case rooted in urban poverty) leads to dialogue with the authorities. His postscript, written in the austerity of the new lean days of Zimbabwe's Economic Structural Adjustment Programme (ESAP), with its sharpened problems of poverty and long term unemployment, undercuts his earlier conclusion. In reconsidering the long-term validity of theatre for development, he comes to the following bleak conclusion:

> Such a system [in which people are either unemployed or when employed are not paid enough to ensure a decent livelihood] has to be revolutionised and for a theatre that promotes such exigency the only genuine basis for development is revolution. The theatre worker must ultimately make a choice — theatre for development to make a bad system easier to put up with or theatre for development as a revolutionary bid to transform that system in the interests of those who suffer at its hands.

Community theatre, alongside theatre for development, is also a vibrant art form in Zimbabwe, one which again cuts through urban and rural boundaries and which can make space for gender issues. Evie Globerman provides a brief insight into the working of a particular community theatre group, *Iluba Elimnyama*, in Bulawayo. She shows how actors tackled the usual silence on issues relating to women and the city by shaping a play around the problems of pregnancy and single mothers. Such work, her article suggests, can shape gender discourse at a public, even a national level through legislation and can change the course of people's lives. Older patriarchal relations can also be gnawed away at, thus 'deep-seated problems of difference in the treatment of sons and daughters' are touched on although not, in Globerman's view, adequately treated in the play *Impilo-le* (That's life!)

The question of state control and its relation to theatre features in the papers by Kaarsholm, Chifunyise and Crehan and also in Bheki Peterson's paper. Stephen Chifunyise's paper provides an insight into the vitality of a variety of theatre groups, attempting to use theatre as an expressive social and political form, the use of theatre not as élite culture, or as the property of the dominant culture, but as a new form of people's culture. This is clearly a vital part of the reconstruction of independence. The distance between this and colonial theatre is emphasised by Chifunyise and is also explored by Preben Kaarsholm. The latter outlines the way in which colonial theatre was used as an instrument of cultural dominance which was itself part of a wider hegemony of social and political power set to exclude African cultural forms and counter discourses. Both writers stress the importance of experimenting with and developing new forms of theatre, and mention the new performance modes which began to take shape in the guerrilla camps during the war of liberation.

Kaarsholm's paper draws on interviews with those who had firsthand knowledge of the kind of experimentation that was in operation in the camps, often with very young participants. It was there that oral forms were used, sometimes in conjunction with western theatrical modes, and there emerged the sense of the possibility of new forms blending orature, dance and drama.[12] These new forms were then taken into the independence era and formed part of a confident new culture which has come into existence alongside the older colonial forms. There is, though, a sharp difference between the viewpoints of Chifunyise and Kaarsholm over the role of theatre in independent Zimbabwe and more generally, of the role of theatre in articulating ideological aims in a post-liberation situation. Chifunyise is prepared for theatre to focus singlemindedly on emphasising the goals of the new society, to conscientise, to heighten awareness of a restructured social order. Kaarsholm, on the other hand, sees this as a dangerously repressive and limiting use of theatre. This debate points to the central issue of control, and of self-censorship in particular historical situations where, in order to rectify the dominance of the past, there is an emphasis on new aims, new ideas and a consensus not to criticise but rather to use theatre as a crucial means of conscientisation in a new social order.

Stewart Crehan's paper on Patronage, the State and Ideology in Zambian Theatre presents a rich and detailed critique of Zambian theatre and focuses on the development of certain trends in Zambia and in particular on the negative, deadening influence of a benevolent state patronage. Crehan presents us with an ironic contradiction in the history of Zambian theatre: the country's theatre artists called for state intervention and this began by being progressive. However, after 1980 it became more repressive than supportive, reflecting the state's need to control the ideological sphere.

Crehan also explores the actual and potential role of popular theatre in Zambian culture. The subversive and at times satirical uses of traditional dances such as *Fwemba, M'ganda and Nyau* during colonial times could, he argues, have been the beginnings of a new and important synthesis in terms of form and dynamic social comment. The uses to which such dances were put by the nationalists could have been the beginnings of a new dramatic mode overriding the gulf between popular and élitist forms. The very lack of such a synthesis, Crehan argues, reflects the absence of any real struggle for social transformation and the absence of any post-independent alliance between the petty-bourgeoisie and the masses. Instead of any synthesis, the two forms of popular and scripted performance exist uneasily side by side with the differences between Bemba and English, conceived of in terms of register, further separating the two types of theatre.

Peterson's article on Apartheid and the Political Imagination in Black South African Theatre also addresses the issue of state attempts to control culture and the direction of black theatre in South Africa. In his historical overview of black theatre initiatives Peterson outlines the shifts in attitudes to theatre by the African élites of H I E Dhlomo's time, and the key move away from regarding theatre as a morally uplifting part of high culture to seeing it as a vehicle for the expression of a burgeoning nationalism. Having outlined the measures to control theatre, Peterson moves to a stimulating discussion of the key contribution of Gibson Kente to South African theatre. He acknowledges Kente's brilliance in using township popular culture, its slangs, fashions and topical issues, and his use of evocative, melodramatic spectacle. Kente's *Too Late*, unlike the other plays discussed, turns its back on political action and 'gestures to the capacity in all of us to do good as the most feasible solution'. Finally Peterson challenges the simplistic politics of black theatre and its chauvinistic inability to make an imaginative space for women as agents and participants in the kinds of transformation imaged in the drama.

Ian Steadman, like Peterson, focuses on the role of the Black

Consciousness movement of the seventies in liberating black theatre and making it a key element in the popular political consciousness of the time. He sets out to explore what he calls the adversary tradition in black South African theatre, its inability at first to achieve any consonance with a popular audience, or to achieve what Raymond Williams calls 'a structure of feeling'. Only with the advent of Black Consciousness, Steadman argues, did the adversarial form of theatre also become a popular one within which, in theatrical terms, a vision of political liberation could be articulated. Steadman, like Peterson, regards Kente's popular style as crucial, pushing theatre performers into exploring new techniques such as chanted responses, emotive music, unison speaking. Theatre was 'no longer self-conscious literary expressions but performed images of black anger and resistance'. It was also — and here there are fascinating links with the later worker theatre discussed by Paul Gready — a collaborative tradition, rather than the earlier one of single, solitary creativity. He suggests, finally, that the popular theatre of the nineties may take on new forms — trade union theatre, community theatre and cabaret. Whatever it may be there is, he claims, no fixed, final relationship between the adversary and popular tradition, rather a constant redefining of the two.

Steadman and Sitas, like Peterson and to an extent, Gready, are concerned with the relation of a work of performance to a broader structure of feeling which represents a large popular consciousness. Sitas, however, has a specific regional concern, namely with Natal and with traditions of poetry in Natal. He sets the present rich array of trade union poets within a linked progression of resistance poetry, beginning with the work of Dhlomo, through Mazisi Kunene and on to Mafika Gwala. He makes a case, as does this volume as a whole, for placing performance culture in a more central role if any real social and political transformation is to be achieved in Southern Africa. Sitas argues that whereas oral poetry has remained close to the experience of those who have moved as workers between rural and urban culture, 'the scripted sign' moved its users towards the more remote English literary tradition which a poet such as Dhlomo first accepted and then rejected as he moved to a more nationalist and radical position. Sitas claims a vision from within 'the contents of everyday oppression and violence' as central to the popular poetry which expresses a new cultural identity, focusing on the workers' struggle but set in the old poetic language. There are though, he argues, crucial commonalities of experience between the scripted and the new oral tradition — in terms of their combination of the themes of hope, violence and death and their defiance and determination to create new ways of understanding and of perceiving both the present and the past.

The energies that have produced the many strands of culture in South Africa and in the Southern African region described in these pages are rich and wonderful and also often combative and challenging. The essays and the voices that follow give some sense of that wealth. They also demonstrate, I believe, the necessity always of relating performance to politics.

1 *Journal of Southern African Studies* 16 February 1990. Special Issue on Performance and Popular Culture. Liz Gunner (ed).

2 For instance, Veit Erlmann, *African Stars: Studies in Black South African Performance*, University of Chicago Press: Chicago (1991); David Coplan, Performance, Self-Definition and Social Experience in the Oral Poetry of Sotho Migrant Mineworkers *African Studies Review* 29(1), 1986, pp 29-40; Rob Nixon, Of Balkans and Bantustans: 'Ethnic Cleansing' and the Crisis in National Legitimation, *Transition*, June 1993.

3 The text is reproduced in Ingrid de Kock and Karen Press (eds), *Spring is Rebellious: Arguments about Cultural Freedom by Albie Sachs and Respondents*. Cape Town, Buchu Books, 1990.

4 A phrase used by James from Leroy Vail and Landeg White's *Power and the Praise Poem: Southern African Voices in History*. Charlottville: University of Virginia Press; London, James Currey, 1991.

5 David Coplan's work, particularly that on *lifela*, is something of an honourable exception to this.

6 See his The Sachs Debate: A Philistine's Response in *Spring is Rebellious*, pp 91-8.

7 See Steve Kromberg, The Role of Audience in the Emergence of Worker Poetry. In *New Wine in Old Bottles: Oral Tradition and Innovation*, E Sienart, N Bell and M Lewis (eds), ODRC, University of Natal, Durban. 1992, pp 180-203 and The Problem of Audience: A Study of Durban Worker Poetry, Master's Dissertation, University of the Witwatersrand, 1993.

8 Malcolm Purkey, Twenty-Something Inches Square: Landscape, Mind and Representation. Paper read at the Southern Spaces Conferences on Land, Representation and Identity in South African and Australian Literature held at the School of Oriental and African Studies, London University, 4 to 6 June 1993.

9 Belinda Bozzoli with Mmantho Nkotsoe, *Women of Phokeng: Consciousness, Life Strategy and Migrancy in South Africa 1900-1983*. Johannesburg: Ravan, 1991.

10 Martin Orkin, *Drama and the South African State*. Manchester: Manchester University Press; Johannesburg: Witwatersrand University Press, 1991.

11 Zakes Mda, *When People Play People: Development Communication Through Theatre*, London: Zed Books; Johannesburg: Witwatersrand University Press, 1993.

12 Similar theatre sketches were used by MK fighters in the ANC camps in Angola and have yet to be discussed at any length.

Towards popular theatre in South Africa

IAN STEADMAN

Theatre and Popular Performance in South Africa

During the eighties South African scholars focused increasingly upon the political significance of theatre in a rapidly changing society. Much of their work produced insights into the strategies of theatre practitioners who were attempting to define new identities in South African cultural life, and their analyses of the work of these practitioners often illuminated the political determinants of specific plays and performances.[1] This essay attempts to argue the relevance of broad themes and ideological issues which arise from such analyses. I will show how questions of race and class, as they feature in the work of theatre practitioners, have produced contradictions in the creation of popular performance based on a notion of resistance to dominant cultural practices. I take my cue from Tom Lodge's assertion[2] that while his own work on black politics in South Africa elucidates one terrain of resistance, there are other areas of social life which need to be investigated. The theatre is one such domain.

Central to this investigation is the relationship between an oppositional cultural aesthetic and popular performance. There have been assumptions that performance opposed to the dominant received tradition informed by apartheid culture is necessarily popular, while performance located within the dominant tradition simply exhibits the elitist concerns of a marginalised minority. Specifically, the term 'popular' has been used to refer to the ways in which members of a majority oppressed group use literature and performance to conscientise audiences in relation to a broad vision of structural change in society.[3] This usage of the term has come to ignore the notion of box-office appeal (which, it is argued, is inextricably tied to marketing strategies based on access to media and capital), and is aligned with experiments in Latin America and elsewhere in which popular performance was produced by the intervention of radical intellectuals. This argument has also been extended to provide a critique of how 'people's' entertainment, despite enjoying box-office success, frequently shows people contributing to their own oppression. It is suggested by supporters of this view that there is a necessary distinction to be made between 'popular' and 'people's' culture, the latter being produced by and addressed to the oppressed people in any society, often domesticating them in a conservative way, and precluding any real interrogation of the structural causes of their oppression.

Part of the aim of this paper is to expose some of the contradictions of these notions. I prefer to describe developments in oppositional work as part of an 'adversary tradition'[4] which has seldom achieved popular status. On the other hand, work which has achieved popular status, while it has only occasionally articulated a genuinely oppositional aesthetic, often opens 'a window onto popular consciousness'.[5] I am particularly interested in those writers and theatre practitioners who have the notion of structural change in society in mind, but whose work shows the contradictions referred to here. Their attempts to reach a popular audience have failed for various reasons, some of which I touch upon in this essay.

No study of these issues can ignore Karin Barber's excellent overview of the field of popular arts in Africa.[6] Barber's model adapts a conventional Western tripartite classification of the arts as (a) folk/traditional, (b) popular or (c) elite, but incorporates important aspects of syncretism, urbanisation and rapid social change. One major aspect of her study is particularly relevant in the present South African context, and that is her discussion of popular art not in relation to its origins but in relation to the interests it serves. Although Barber discusses many other aspects of popular arts, it is this aspect alone which informs this study, because inextricably linked to it is the notion of an adversarial theatre which purports to serve the needs of the majority of 'the people' in South Africa.

The growth and development of an adversary idea of South African theatre must be analysed against a background of repressive legislation and hegemonic co-option. While access to media and capital ensured that for decades a dominant tradition of theatre was established, the activities of theatre practitioners creating work in opposition went largely unrecorded. Analysis of examples of this work — with a focus upon the features of *performance* which they embrace — provides useful insights into the ways in which performance is inscribed with value systems which might not immediately be apparent to the textual scholar.[7] The study of performance is the study of a complex, multi-dimensional cultural practice. Frequently, the focus of an analysis is a printed text, but that text is merely the residue of an event, the edited version of creative processes. Any analysis of such a text must be sensitive to the complexities of performance which are inscribed therein, complexities in which surplus meanings are produced and often subvert the meanings intended for the reader of the printed text.

There has been no more articulate theoretician of this problem than Raymond Williams, and much of the theoretical framework of what I have to say is attributable to his unrivalled achievement in going beyond contemporary preconceptions and habits of thought in two major ways. Firstly, he has theorised the nature of dramatic action in ways which have distinguished the study of performance from the study of dramatic literature.[8] Secondly, he has demonstrated how the lessons to be learnt from such theorisation are of value not only to the scholar in the arts and humanities, but equally to the social scientist.[9] In the second of these two achievements, Williams's work demonstrates his concern not only with the qualities of a work of art which define its irreducible individuality, but also '...the continuity of experience from a particular work, through its particular form, to its recognition as a general form, and then the relation of this general form to a period.'[10] This continuity of experience he calls a 'structure of feeling'.

Williams's notion of a structure of feeling is not without difficulty. Crude expression of it might give rise to a simplistic reflection theory, and there are problems in merely importing his ideas into the southern African context.[11] Nevertheless, it is significant that numerous commentators on popular arts use analogous expressions in talking about the ways in which popular artists 'touch a chord' or articulate 'something' which is related to the 'needs' or 'aspirations' or 'feelings' of their audiences.[12] Furthermore, in a study of theatre in South Africa there is a useful insight to be gained by referring to Williams's expression. The failure of writers and theatre practitioners of the adversary tradition to articulate a 'structure of feeling' in their work commensurate with the needs and aspirations of their audiences has frequently marginalised them. Conversely practitioners who have succeeded in such articulation have created works which have enjoyed great popularity, even when their themes have been, in the opinion of radical intellectuals, politically conservative. This essay argues the general case that until the seventies the essential factor which determined attempts by dramatists of the adversarial tradition to establish connections between the structure of feeling in the creative work and the structure of feeling in the envisaged audience was their concern with race. The essential factor inhibiting these attempts was their class and their ideological position. In addition the failure by artists of the adversary tradition to take cognisance of the relations between race and class explained why their theatre was marginalised in cultural struggle and never found a popular audience. The inhibiting factors become less prominent in the seventies, leading to the emergence of forms of performance conceived not merely as ends in the struggle for social and political freedom,. but as a means of achieving these goals. This change in conception becomes, in that decade, the defining characteristic of a theatre both adversarial and popular.

Race, class and black consciousness theatre

The notion of an adversary idea of the theatre derives from my sense of how theatrical performance in South Africa has expressed oppositions to hegemony in ways directly parallel to political developments. In opposition, however, to much of the scholarship on theatre in the eighties, I do not locate these oppositions entirely within a perspective which sees class as the determining factor in describing different types of creative work. Following Chantal Mouffe,[13] I prefer to view the creative practitioners of South African theatre as being inscribed in a multiplicity of social relations ranging from relations of production to relations of race, sex, vicinity, language and religion. Unlike some commentators, I argue that the practitioners of theatre have many subject positions. The playwrights I study might well be inscribed in relations of production as workers or petit-bourgeois intellectuals, but they are also either male or female, white or black, Zulu or English. As Mouffe argues:

> A person's subjectivity is not constructed only on the basis of his or her position in the relations of production. Furthermore, each social position, each subject position, is itself the locus of multiple possible constructions, according to the different discourses that can construct that position. Thus, the subjectivity of a given social agent is always precariously and provisionally fixed or, to use the Lacanian term, sutured at the intersection of various discourses.[14]

These observations are especially pertinent in studying the growth and development of what has been called 'black theatre' in South Africa.[15]

The growth and development of the Black Consciousness Movement in South Africa prompted many significant developments in theatre. A study of developments in drama related to this phenomenon provides an interesting example of structures of feeling at work. It can be argued that black consciousness enabled the practitioners of black theatre to create a 'structure of feeling' within their plays and performances commensurate with the larger mythology of blackness prevailing amongst audiences during the groundswell of consciousness-raising in the formative years of the Black Consciousness Movement. Prior to the articulation of black consciousness principles in the seventies, on the other hand, it can be argued that the absence of such a mythology for theatre audiences meant that the notion of a structure of feeling as Williams envisaged it was seldom realised in the work of South African playwrights. Black consciousness, in short, gave black theatre an identity. In order to arrive at such an argument, however, it is necessary to trace some background.

The history and development of black theatre in South Africa has only comparatively recently been documented in any significant detail.[16] There is consensus regarding a number of milestones in that history. One of those milestones is the publication in 1936 of the first play in English by a black South African. Herbert Dhlomo's *The Girl Who Killed to Save: Nongqause the Liberator* has been described by numerous commentators as a play which demonstrates its author's 'assimilation'[17] into middle-class European cultural norms. It is in many ways the weakest of Dhlomo's plays. Yet as an example of mission literature, as the first play by a black South African in English, and as a play which exemplifies liberal middle-class black writing under a system of tutelage and co-option, it serves as a good example of the ways in which black middle-class dramatists were frustrated in their attempts to articulate progressive arguments in dramatic form. Dhlomo's own subsequent development shows that to characterise all of his writing by reference to this play is a distortion. Later plays and poems reveal a writer more mature and more politically and socially aware than this play reveals. His career shows a clear pattern of movement away from tutelage to a rejection of the patronising attitudes of liberal whites (a movement parallel to his own active involvement in ANC politics). Nevertheless, because this first play stands at the forefront of our adversary tradition, and because Dhlomo has been called 'the pioneer of modern black drama in South Africa',[18] discussion is justified — if only to map the terrain for an argument about the obstacles to be overcome in the search for an adversarial theatre that would also be popular.

The plot of the play follows very closely the version of events reported historically in various letters from the Gaika Commissioner of the eastern Cape Province, Charles Brownlee, and his wife, leading up to the famous cattle-killing of 1857.[19] The action of the play begins in that year. The young Nongqause already commands the respect of Kreli, the paramount chief of the AmaXhosa, and thousands of her people. Prompted by her witchdoctor uncle, Mhlakaza, she claims to have talked to the spirits of the ancestors, who promise to return and help the AmaXhosa defeat the English settlers of the eastern Cape. They will only do this, however, if the AmaXhosa destroy their cattle and crops in sacrifice. After Nongqause's claims are publicised, the sacrifice is undertaken by many tribes. The first scene of the play shows Kreli visiting Nongqause, who pretends to have a dream in which the prophecy is repeated. Kreli is sufficiently convinced to send word to the recalcitrant tribes, telling them to obey the commands of the ancestors and to sacrifice their crops and cattle. Prompted by the superstitions of Mhlakaza, the craze soon spreads amongst the various tribes, and cattle and crops are destroyed. The characters of the Gaika Commissioner and his wife are introduced to provide the playwright with the opportunity for descriptive exposition, and to allow Dhlomo to argue relations between tribal custom and modernisation. The action then leaps forward a few months. In a Xhosa home, Christian missionaries help the starving Xhosa victims of the prophecy. Nongqause's dreams have been proven false: superstition and outdated tribal customs have led to the destruction of the nation.

The play has been severely criticised for its sentimentality and because it inscribes the values of Dhlomo's petit-bourgeois Christian missionary education, but there are other dimensions of the play which make it a little more sophisticated than this. Dhlomo has presented the action in such a way as to show that the tragic events have some positive end: although the nation has been virtually destroyed, the AmaXhosa will be able to reject their superstitious tribal customs and begin to modernise. He was not merely writing another historical drama, but dramatising an attitude which perfectly tied in with his essay 'Native Policy in South Africa', written in 1930, in which he stated: '....the tribalism which so many people desire to protect and prolong, must be broken down at all costs and hazards.   It is one of the most formidable foes to Bantu progress ...'[20]

Dhlomo's play is fundamentally a demonstration of these critical attitudes. Certainly, the style and language of the play demonstrate the idiom of its author's class and ideology, as Couzens has argued[21] — but what is more interesting for present purposes is the play's structure of feeling. For it is not so much a conflict between benevolent missionaries and superstitious pagans, as between progressive modernism and retrogressive tribalism. But, as Williams suggests, there is always a discernible relation between a 'structure of feeling' and its effective conventions, and in this play there is a disjunction in the relation between Dhlomo's search for an idea of African drama and the conventions he uses to dramatise his vision. The conventions are mechanically received from an imperfectly-remembered imported tradition. It is not simply a matter of Dhlomo 'assimilating' a western model of middle-class drama, for the model of western drama that Dhlomo might have had in mind simply did not exist, except in his own dislocated impressions of lines, characters and situations from sentimental melodramas and school plays.

Dhlomo only imperfectly understood the models of English middle-class drama as exemplified by writers like Granville-Barker, otherwise he might have turned them to good effect.[22] Similarly, he was unable fully to exploit, in his dramatic writing, the interest he so often professed in indigenous performance forms (about which he wrote critically).[23] There is, in the play, no organic relation between Dhlomo's social consciousness and the conventions which he selects to purvey that consciousness dramatically. Through the persistence of old habits, he is unable to create a 'controlling illuminating form',[24] to find techniques which would become the new conventions of a new kind of drama, a drama which expressed for a contemporary audience a view of African history and legend, and in dramatic discourse organically related to that view. The tensions between the form and vision of the play are apparent from a number of examples one could select from the text. To choose but one:

MRS BROWNLEE: (Aside) When duty calls love is sacrificed. When duty calls life is endangered...
BROWNLEE: Thank God I have the noble wife I have.
MRS BROWNLEE: (Tears in her eyes, and running into his open arms) Oh! Charles!
BROWNLEE: (Emotional) Darling! (They embrace. Silence long and profound.)
[Scene Three)]

Dhlomo's mission education, the received conventions of literature which he embraced, and his very conception of drama as literature rather than theatrical action, lead to what has been described as 'a somewhat narrow, and even elitist conception of literature as a particular kind of elevated utterance'.[25] The criticisms of the play which have been made by numerous scholars can be recast by reference to the notion of a 'structure of feeling'. Distanced from middle-class whites by racial discrimination and from working-class blacks by status discrimination, Dhlomo was — in this play — unable to articulate a dramatic discourse which would reach either. There is, throughout the play, a disparity between action and writing. Dhlomo had learned the accepted rules in dramatic writing, but those rules were the expression of a 'structure of feeling' more attuned to Dhlomo's middle-class Christian mentors. The audience he wished to reach remained beyond reach because Dhlomo's dramaturgy remained circumscribed by his different class and ideological interests.

One way for the dramatist to solve the problem of this kind of disjunction is to work with a theatre company, but to make that possible one needs audiences. The theatre as a social institution in South Africa at the time did not make it possible for Dhlomo in any significant way to explore his vision collaboratively with audiences and practitioners in order to achieve the formal changes necessary — the new relations between speech and action, which would be authentic responses to the changing 'structure of feeling' which Dhlomo tried to articulate. It is also known that Dhlomo did not much care for such a collaborative approach.[26]

This was despite numerous attempts by Dhlomo to investigate indigenous African dramatic forms and conventions in order to articulate contemporary ideas about freedom and oppression. Commentators have illustrated Dhlomo's significant achievements in a number of areas, and have gone so far as to suggest that Dhlomo is a forerunner of a characteristic style of poetry which emerged in the seventies in Soweto.[27] It is clear, in fact, that the Dhlomo of *The Girl Who Killed to Save* is a very different writer from the Dhlomo of the forties, when he did more than enough to contradict the accusation that he was a co-opted middle class African writer assimilated to the European model. It is also clear that by the forties Dhlomo was moving away from the ideological embrace of tutelage, evident in the quaint and stilted language and structure of the early play, and beginning to embrace an ideal of black nationalism more attuned to contemporary political developments. This brought him closer to creating in his work a 'structure of feeling' consonant with the interests of a popular audience. The later plays of Dhlomo frequently demonstrate this, while nevertheless still demonstrating that he remained unable to open a window on popular consciousness in quite the same manner as the seventies generation of writers and theatre practitioners would be able to. Later Dhlomo plays like *The Pass* demonstrate far more clearly a writer in touch with urban political realities, capable of dialogue stripped of literary self-consciousness, and rooted in a more clearly defined political vision. The trouble is that even this play preceded the political moment which might have given it a 'structure of feeling' linked to a broader popular political consciousness. It was left to Gibson Kente, writing at that later political moment, to reproduce the last line of Dhlomo's play: 'How long, O Lord, how long!'[28] and redefine it as the cornerstone of a structure of feeling which made theatre, in the formative period of black consciousness, a popular medium for the articulation of political aspirations.

Herbert Dhlomo's *The Girl who Killed to Save* was the first play by a black South African to be published in English. *The Rhythm of Violence* by Lewis Nkosi has been claimed as the second.[29] Both Dhlomo and Nkosi are important figures in the development of black South African drama, not merely because they wrote the first and second black plays to be published in English, but also because their respective plays reveal much about changes in black social consciousness prior to the emergence of the Black Consciousness Movement. More symbolically, what distinguishes Nkosi's play from Dhlomo's is the crisis of Sharpeville. If Sharpeville did indeed represent a turning point in African nationalism 'when protest finally hardened into resistance',[30] Nkosi's play was a timely index of the process.[31]

The Rhythm of Violence appeared within four years of Sharpeville. The theme is made clear by the title and context: after the Sharpeville shootings, a rhythm of violence was to enter the political arena. The play anticipates in some respects what we know as black consciousness theatre, but with significant differences. It deals with major issues in the political life of South Africans in the early sixties. The plot can be simply outlined. The action occurs in Johannesburg. Act One in three scenes shows Piet and Jan, two armed South African policemen, nervously watching an African political meeting just before sunset. They discuss their reactionary attitudes to black political activism and joke about the attempts of black people to bring about political change in South Africa. Act Two opens later that evening in 'a dingy basement clubroom which serves as headquarters of a group of left-wing university students'. Black and white students of the University of the Witwatersrand, dominated by Gama, a militant activist, are waiting for the midnight explosion of a bomb they have placed beneath the city hall. The bomb is timed to explode during a National Party political meeting. During the four scenes of this Act the group of students becomes increasingly nervous and drink flows easily as they talk about political change and inter-racial conflict in South Africa. Gama's brother Tula and a white Afrikaans girl by the name of Sarie (who does not yet know about the bomb) are drawn closer together, the playwright depicting them as innocent pawns in a political game. The climax of the Act is reached with the news, just minutes before midnight, that Sarie's father is attending the political meeting at the city hall in order to tender his resignation from the National Party, which he has come to reject. Tula, in an attempt to save the girl's father, rushes to the city hall. Act Three opens an hour later at 'the charred ruins of what had been the city hall'. Jan and Piet, the two policemen, discover Sarie weeping over the body of Tula. When they discover that he is the brother of Gama, who is well known to them as a political activist, they arrest her on suspicion of conspiracy.

More in touch with rising political militancy on the Witwatersrand than the Dhlomo of *The Girl who Killed to Save*, and arguably more in touch with the nuances of dramatic language rooted in a consciousness of proletarian politics,[32] Nkosi was able to create a 'structure of feeling' in the play related to the racial issues of the time, although, as we shall see, in discourse laden with contradictions. Nkosi's play was effectively marginalised, not only by the censorship machinery of the state but also by a dramaturgical approach attributable to its author's class and ideological location. Like Dhlomo — though arguably less so — Nkosi was caught in a situation where the way in which theatre was institutionalised precluded a free collaborative process of playmaking which might have led to a genuinely popular performance before audiences whose aspirations were depicted in the play.[33] Such opportunities might have allowed for the creation of a dramatic form and discourse more relevant and appropriate — and more authentic — in the context of the political life of the Witwatersrand which is the fabric of the play. The text which Nkosi wrote, however, is something else. Nkosi was unable to establish in *The Rhythm of Violence* a 'structure of feeling' commensurate with the political vision expressed through the play. There remains a disjunction between the vision of the writer and the forms and conventions in which he tries to express that vision. These forms and conventions are interesting indices of Nkosi's attitudes towards race and politics in the South Africa of the sixties.

The ways in which Nkosi promulgates a vision of black liberation are somewhat fettered by class and ideological constraints. These are manifested in the text through language usage, characterisation, and through such idiolectical signals as gender attitudes. A few very brief examples illustrate this. We read in one stage direction:

> Tula advances from the confusion of the crowd; they come face to face with each other. Momentarily, their eyes meet and the girl's eyes fall to her feet. Tula puts out his hand. The girl takes it, and they hold on to each other a bit longer than is necessary, as if they've struck quick sympathy with each other.
> TULA: Hello!
> SARIE: Hello!
> TULA: May I get you anything to drink?
> SARIE: (shyly) If you have gin, I'll have a gin and tonic.
> [Act Two, Scene Two]

> Tula, predictably, majors in fine arts. As Sarie inspects his work she says: 'It's beautiful. It's very gentle. Now I understand a lot of things about you.'

She is quickly drawn to him, and Nkosi places them with the noise of the party behind them:

> (Kneeling down, facing each other in the foreground of the stage.)

SARIE: You know what I like about you?
TULA: No. What?
SARIE: You seem to be very sincere about everything you're doing ... You know something, too? You're very gentle! I mean, a woman can tell these things very quickly. When a man is gentle, a woman can feel it immediately.
[Act Two, Scene Three]

Such dialogue is not merely the product of the characters' naïveté, for it permeates the whole play, and there are numerous instances where women express these sentiments. Sarie says (Act Two, Scene Four) 'I am a woman, so [sic] my optimism is boundless'. Lili is slapped on the bottom by Gama, which action is enough to drive her to 'pummel him with her fists' before he pulls her roughly to him and she then 'seems to melt in his arms as he kisses her' (Act Two, Scene Three). Kitty, who elsewhere exhibits an air of independent maturity and aloofness, says that 'Men are such beasts' (Act Two, Scene Two). All the women — members of the 'Left Students Association' at the University of the Witwatersrand and therefore presumably at least slightly enlightened in such matters (!) — are represented as being grossly subservient to men and often downright silly. It is, of course, part of Nkosi's intention to characterise Gama as egotistical and chauvinistic, and to contrast him with Tula, but there is no mistaking the common factor in his characterisation of the women in the play. The dominant discourse in the play is patriarchal, and fairly typically, chauvinistic.[34]

Throughout, the text reads as a self-consciously literary artefact by a writer with an eye on publication rather than performance. The most obvious feature of the dramaturgy of Nkosi's play is this self-conscious literariness. Nkosi has elsewhere[35] presented a critique of other writers in these very terms. An essay by him entitled *Toward a new African theatre*[36] is instructive in this regard. Here he criticises the model of African theatre which borrows from Europe 'indiscriminately whatever forms come from our former colonial masters'[37] and elsewhere he says that permeating the 'entire effort' of African art is 'a European presence'.[38] All these observations are directly applicable to his own play.

It is instructive to focus briefly on some of the problems of race and class which Nkosi faced and about which he has written. Nkosi has attempted to explain the difficulties faced by the black writer by reference to the matrix of problems of race and class:

It is true that because of the obvious reasons, black South Africans did not produce an elite which was alienated from the black masses or even from the conditions of everyday life under which our people laboured. In South Africa

we were saved from the emergence of a Black Bourgeoisie by the levelling effect
of apartheid ... the life of the educated class is as insecure as those [sic] of the
illiterate and semi-literate masses of our people.[39]

In an obvious political sense imposed by the policy of apartheid, there is
a germ of truth in what Nkosi says here. Clearly, however, the 'levelling
effect' does not work quite so simply. There most certainly was a 'Black
Bourgeoisie' at the time Nkosi wrote this. And he was firmly located
within it in a way which circumscribed his writing.

Nkosi often generalises black experience in this way. *The Rhythm of
Violence* is fraught with the results of such generalisation. Elsewhere, he
has endeavoured to articulate a slightly more sophisticated position. At a
conference of African writers of English literature in Kampala in 1962,
organised by the Mbari Writers' Club of Nigeria and the Congress for
Cultural Freedom,[40] and attended by writers like Chinua Achebe, Alex la
Guma, Bob Leshoai, Bloke Modisane, Es'kia Mphahlele and Wole
Soyinka, Nkosi came to the realisation that:

ultimately, what linked various African peoples on the continent was the nature
and depth of colonial experience; and this was the final irony. Colonialism had
not only delivered them unto themselves, but had delivered them unto each
other, had provided them, so to speak, with a common language and an African
consciousness; for out of rejection had come an affirmation.[41]

Nkosi began, he argues, to understand the real implications of being
'black' :

I took my colour quite for granted. I discovered my Africanness the day I
learned that I was not only black but non-white ... In that small prefix put
before the word white I saw the entire burden and consequence of European
colonialism ...[42]

In his essay 'Black Power or Souls of Black Writers'[43] Nkosi discovers and
affirms a forceful consciousness not of African but of *black* power. Nkosi
did not enjoy this revelation at a youthful age as would the practitioners
of black consciousness theatre in the seventies. His play is not imbued
with the 'coherent vision' which, he later argues, younger Africans were
beginning to realise towards the end of the sixties. The 'New Africans', as
he calls them, are not present in *The Rhythm of Violence*. His play
preceded by half a decade the articulation of the black consciousness
philosophy which would underpin plays of the seventies. This is not to
say that there was always an *absence* of the kind of social and political

consciousness that would characterise the Black Consciousness Movement of the seventies. The ideological precedents for black consciousness existed not only in negritude in Africa, in black power in the USA, and in black nationalism elsewhere in the Third World, but also in the historical roots of African nationalism in South Africa — and Nkosi was certainly aware of the implications.[44] But the ideological concerns of *The Rhythm of Violence* are not those of black consciousness. The very notion of political liberation through multiracialism which lies at the centre of the play illustrates this. The play argues that racism is something which is perpetrated by the state and which can be overcome by personal relationships — but in the play this is only possible because the black students have been incorporated into white middle class culture and function in their relationships as equals. The very attitude that racism can be overcome on the individual level is fraught with problems (quite apart from the liberal-humanist rhetoric that such attitudes utilise). The play does not engage with the reality of racism and oppression at *all* levels of society. This problem of content is analogous to the problem of form. The 'structure of feeling' of the play, provided by Nkosi's vision of political liberation, is articulated within the received formal categories of an imported tradition of dramatic writing.

Black consciousness in performance

It is instructive to turn now to the theatre of the seventies, both to extend the critique of Nkosi's play and to continue the search for a theatre both popular and adversarial. I do not intend to undertake a detailed analysis of one of the seventies black consciousness plays here.[45] Even a broad description of the plays and poetry of the Black Consciousness Movement shows that theatre practitioners, taking advantage of a broadly shared mythology of blackness provided by the Movement, were able to create plays which were part of a consonance with popular consciousness — although there were still many problems.

Black Consciousness in the seventies never enjoyed homogeneity. It embraced various strands of conflicting arguments. Nevertheless, the Movement of the seventies provided a context within which theatre practitioners could articulate their vision of political liberation, and do so by creating a 'structure of feeling' in harmony with the growing political conscientisation of their audience. One of the first differences between their vision and that of Nkosi relates to the notion of multiracialism. The first precondition of a liberated society for the early advocates of black consciousness was a rejection of a role for whites in black liberation, and the severing of links with the multiracial accommodationist option represented by the students who feature in Nkosi's play. The Black Consciousness Movement was often ahistorical, often blind to a class analysis of society, and it often romanticised the past in attempting to recover it from colonisation. Nevertheless it presented an important challenge to dominant ideological constructions, it engaged in rapid consciousness-raising and politicisation of black people, and it did more to Africanise theatre in South Africa than Dhlomo or Nkosi. This influence is still being felt in many ways today. There were limitations in black consciousness theatre, but it did articulate a direction for many theatre practitioners, and it did so by offering a view of transcendence based on a shared mythology of blackness, however circumscribed.

For practitioners of this theatre, it was not the specific argument about black liberation that was important — that was often flawed — but the process of developing the argument. Through a shared 'structure of feeling' concerned with black solidarity, with resistance, and with political liberation, many arguments, however defective, were able to be articulated on the basis of a commonality of discourse with audiences. The rhetoric was agreed upon. So was the common enemy.

What such activities managed to accomplish was a rejection of the liberal-humanist rhetoric of Nkosi and Dhlomo in favour of more militant, more clearly defined political arguments. Theatre practitioners located their arguments within the political aspirations of their audiences in ways that Nkosi could never manage. Black theatre became a consciously articulated cultural counterpart of the movement towards political liberation. The theatre was given an identity. One spokesman[46] talked about a 'new approach in theatre' emerging in Soweto which was given an 'identity basis' through black consciousness. He described black theatre in terms of a 'black sub-culture (which) will act as a counter-culture', leading eventually to an authentic national culture. Such grandiose notions were only possible in the context of a growing political and cultural movement which shared the rhetoric.

What was most important was the way in which these ideas were implemented. The practical creation of theatrical performance during this period was something which enabled theatre practitioners to overcome many of the obstacles not overcome by Dhlomo or Nkosi. In groups like TECON (Theatre Council of Natal) and PET (People's Experimental Theatre), plays were created in workshop. Scripts were reshaped and recreated collaboratively and were seldom the products of the individual artist at his or her desk. With the conscious intention of breaking received norms and conventions in order to shape a radical political message, theatre practitioners created highly polemical works. Scene three of PET's workshopped *Shanti* , a typical black consciousness play originally scripted by Mthuli Shezi,[47] demonstrates the conscious didacticism intended by the creators of the play. Stage directions have one of the central characters, Koos, boldly standing centre stage facing the audience during this scene, saying: 'I am Black. Black like my mother. Black like the sufferers. Black like the continent.'

Shouting slogans and issuing proclamations, the characters in the play frequently address the audience in this way. *Shanti* might well be subject to charges of the same class and ideological disjunctions as those exhibited by the plays of Dhlomo and Nkosi, in that the governing consciousness of the play is one of an educated sector of the black bourgeoisie, but it differs from the earlier plays in that it was conceived in *performance* terms as a dynamic representation of black consciousness principles in presentational[48] didactic form. Unconcerned with literary finesse, but rather with slogans of political resistance underpinned by theatrical performance, it communicated simply, directly, and dynamically.

Nkosi's play might well have flourished in this different context.[49] To illustrate the role that theatre played at this time, one only has to note that of the five organisations which were charged in the notorious Treason Trial of 1975, two — PET and the TECON — were theatre groups. A perusal of the texts might surprise the reader in this regard, because they are frequently quite trite. But the ways in which they functioned in performance were clearly of some concern to the state, which alleged that they were subversive.

There are many details of formal construction which reveal important distinctions between the plays of the seventies and those of an earlier generation. Nkosi imported American rhythms into his play, and his play is very reminiscent of a particular American genre of the time.[50] The black consciousness theatre practitioners were also influenced by such factors, but the collaborative process of workshop theatre served to ensure that such influences were at least assimilated in a practice of rehearsal based on a search for new forms. Mothobi Mutloatse states the position thus:

> We are involved in and consumed by an exciting experimental art form that I can only call, to coin a phrase, 'proemdra': Prose, Poem and Drama in one! ... We are going to pee, spit and shit on literary convention before we are through; we are going to kick and pull and push and drag literature into the form we prefer. We are going to experiment and probe and not give a damn what the critics have to say. Because we are in search of our true selves — undergoing self-discovery as a people.[51]

Nkosi's imported formal conventions and his multiracialism were thus overtaken by different attitudes to form and content. I am not arguing that use of traditional forms and local music necessarily makes a play more popular than one which draws on other borrowed conventions. Syncretism is an essential element in the definition of popular theatre in South Africa. What I am proposing is that an important element in communicating through popular performance is the use of the audience's own forms and conventions, however syncretised through contact with imported and urbanised forms and conventions, in order to give authenticity to that communication and thereby play a role in both expressing and constituting popular consciousness. In a different context, David Coplan comments:

> When the cast of *King Kong* had their professional dreams shattered in London by criticism that asked 'Why don't you do something African, something of your own?', the shock was felt deeply in different ways throughout Johannesburg's African community ... a struggle began to regain control of African performing arts for the urban community: to promote self-awareness, cooperative unity, and the positive self-identity of 'Black Consciousness'.[52]

The extraordinary popularity of Gibson Kente's 'township musicals' in the seventies, the popularly-supported and critically acclaimed collaborative work of Athol Fugard, John Kani and Winston Ntshona from 1970 to 1976, and the growing popular interest in the experimental workshop theatre of Workshop '71, were primarily attributable to their success in creating a type of syncretic performance which drew on many different influences but which were crystallised in the processes of rehearsal. Building upon this, the seventies produced a crop of theatre directors and performers who dedicated their energies to articulating a local identity in rapidly evolving local formal conventions.

All these influential practitioners — even Fugard, for a short period before he abandoned the workshop process in favour of the convention of the writer producing drama at his desk — were influential in prompting black consciousness practitioners to experiment and innovate in the rehearsal process in an attempt to create syncretic performance. More significantly, despite the fact that Gibson Kente's popular township musicals were frequently criticised by black consciousness student leaders as being vacuous escapist entertainment out of step with growing black political awareness, Kente continued to attract ever-growing numbers of supporters and this introduced an important debate about the notion of popular political theatre. Kente certainly responded to criticism by making his plays of the early seventies more directly political in orientation. Conversely, however, his critics receded in the face of his enormous popularity. Terence Ranger, in a different context, offers reasons why this might be so: '...we have to look at the informal, the festive, the apparently escapist, in order to see evidence of real experience and real response.'[53]

The dismissal of Kente by radical intellectuals who accuse him of perpetrating false consciousness, reinforcing stereotypes, and being frivolous, points to a major contradiction in interpretations of popular culture. We should remember Barber's important point that: 'Through popular art, expression is given to what people may not have known they had in common'.[54]

Also important is the fact that whatever radical intellectuals might think of Kente's moderate political stance, his audiences, in a climate of oppression and growing resistance, responded favourably to his work. Instead of imposing one's own response, we need to understand their responses. These were to both the syncretic entertainment value and those elements in his plays — however sugar-coated — that related directly to their own lives. For Kente, in creating sentimental musical entertainment about life in the township, could not help rooting his plays in the problems of unemployment, alcoholism, alienation, and all the other consequences of political oppression. If Kente's intended themes were somewhat moderate in their politics, his audiences perceived from the substance of the plays a 'structure of feeling' consonant with the rising tide of political resistance. Kente opened a window on popular consciousness through the medium of spectacular dance, acting and singing. It was, in short, performance which broke the mould that had contained writers like Dhlomo and Nkosi. For no matter how bourgeois in conception many of the seventies plays were, the ways in which they functioned in performance to a large extent helped the practitioners overcome the problem of elitist discourse. This is clear from the texts not only of black consciousness plays, but of poetry as well. At political meetings, rallies and cultural functions, artists presented 'performance poetry'. Not only was this one way of avoiding censorship (it being more difficult to ban an ephemeral performance than a text), but the dynamism of the communication ensured that the text was merely the residue of often quite different and spectacular meanings. The artists were less concerned with the literary nuances of their work, than with the opportunities provided by theatrical performance to explore new forms and techniques. Literature in performance broke down the rules and constraints imposed by publishing conventions. Instead, there emerged a concern with a communal approach to creativity. The lived experience of literature in performance was a far richer one than that captured in textual form, because of the added dimensions of participation from audiences in the form of chanted responses to signals from the stage, emotive music, unison speaking, a metonymical rather than metaphorical construction, and language which worked as utterance rather than statement. This sense of performance means that there was a different dynamism in the performance of black consciousness theatre, a dynamism which was in many ways still operative in South African theatre at the end of the eighties. One commentator has observed of poetry, and the comments may be seen as directly applicable to the theatre: '... the characteristics of oral transmission would seem to suit the requirements of political poetry. For example, the 'covert' qualities of poetry may be brought to the fore by the nature of the performance, by the stress on words and phrases, by the tone of voice, and by gestures.'[55]

In the poems and plays of the Black Consciousness Movement it is important to distinguish between the texts and performances in this way. The petty-bourgeois radical intellectuals who spearheaded the literary and dramatic movement could not help reproducing in their literary works the ideological distance between themselves and the 'black mass' which they so often claimed to represent.[56] But an analysis of the texts in performance indicates something entirely different. Performance of these pieces brings them into more accessible relationships with audiences, transforming mere intellectual statement into dynamic utterance. These pieces were, furthermore, performed quite presentationally, in a simple and direct way, in an effort to establish the didactic relationship with the audience. The more distanced, removed and representational approach of Nkosi and Dhlomo signals quite different performance values. In their different approach the black consciousness theatre practitioners were further strengthening the link with the audience. As utterance, the words are no longer self-conscious literary expressions, but performed images of black anger and resistance. The words have a robust materiality — they don't just communicate meanings, they embody them. Phrases and exclamations like 'arise!', 'stand up!', 'now is the time!' are all dynamically supported in performance by the gestures and movements which had entered the popular vocabulary of communication about liberation. Not the text, but the signifying actions accompanying the text, create the desired effects.

The workshop techniques of Fugard, Kani and Ntshona, of the black consciousness theatre groups, of groups like Workshop '71, The Company, and the Junction Avenue Theatre Company, enabled them to create performances which rapidly captured the imaginations of audiences and identified their work as uniquely South African. Characterising all the new work were formal innovations like episodic structures, quick shifts of scene and tempo, oral narrative, music and street rhythms, jazz, and factory work-rhythms. These were the results of collaborative creativity. Identification occurred not just at the level of content but also at the level of form. There is obvious resonance in the words of Raymond Williams: 'Here, undoubtedly, is the point of growth of any drama of our century: to go where reality is being formed, at work, in the streets, in assemblies, and to engage at those points with the human needs to which the actions relate.'[57]

Despite the fact that much of this work was created in the struggle with state repression, with a lack of capital and with little or no access to media and marketing facilities, it signalled the maturation of the adversary tradition into popular South African performance. This tradition, by the seventies, stood in sharp contrast to the activities of state-subsidised theatre, evidenced in the opulent palaces which were erected from the late seventies into the eighties as monuments to marginalised white culture.

Conclusion: The Contradictions of Popular Theatre

In the above exploration of kinds of adversary theatre beginning with Dhlomo, and moving to Nkosi, I have given only the briefest account of the historical context in which such a theatre is set. Yet even without a wealth of historical detail what is clear is the double disadvantage experienced by black dramatists in the decades leading up to the emergence of the Black Consciousness Movement. First they were intellectuals and writers without access to significant audiences for whom they could create a recognisable 'structure of feeling'. Second, and related to this, they constructed plays at their desks rather than in the rehearsal room. Even on those rare occasions when they were involved in the processes of theatrical production — as both Dhlomo and Nkosi were[58] — the involvement was minimal and without access to the theatrical possibilities which were to prevail from the seventies. Furthermore, they had to work virtually in isolation, with a few colleagues, whereas the practitioners of the seventies were able to relate their work to the concerns of a movement which saw culture as a means of resistance. For a popular performance to emerge it was essential that the individual intellectual writer at his desk leave the study for rehearsal-room encounters with actors. This process has extended into the eighties: the preponderance of plays made through the collaborative processes of 'workshop' theatre can be seen as analogous to the emergence of progressive action based on a

mass democratic movement in South African politics. There are, however,
uncomfortable contradictions that have emerged from this new form of
resistance theatre, and these relate to the sometimes problematic link
between performers and audience. The adversary tradition established as
the dominant face of South African theatre in the eighties, was
immediately marketed abroad. Not a year passed in the eighties without
South African theatre featuring prominently in some international festival
of theatre. The corollary of this is that theatre practitioners in South
Africa, when creating new works, have one eye on the international scene.
Oppositional theatre seems increasingly to seek an international rather
than a local audience. One strategy of the South African government in
an era of so-called 'reform', is being seen to allow oppositional theatre to
tour abroad. This creates an impression of freedom of expression which
has surprised foreign audiences.[59] It also points to contradictions in the
notion of a popular theatre which claims to be oppositional. For if Gibson
Kente's popular township musicals are criticised for being escapist and
insufficiently politicised, it might be argued that at least he represents a
theatre which is made out of the struggles of the people and consumed by
the people. Theatre for the export market, however, is made out of the
struggles of the people but not consumed by the people. Such theatre
might be viewed as an instrument of ruling class hegemony exactly as
perceived by Gramsci. Furthermore, such theatre can sometimes lead to a
rupture of links with the real primary audience within the country. And in
this way the 'structure of feeling' is not strengthened but broken. For the
image of South African culture prepared for outsiders is highly selective
and often reinforces the very stereotypes that it seeks to undermine.[60]

New forms of theatre are, in fact, emerging which may well escape the
seductive pressure of conforming to an external and simplified image of
struggle. A different kind of adversary theatre is being forged in trade
union and community theatre, in cabaret, and in various forms of dance
theatre. Perhaps these will be the focal points of popular theatre in the
nineties. At present, the image of South African theatre, as it has been
marketed abroad with enormous critical and commercial success, and as it
is purveyed in local theatres, is an image rooted in the adversary tradition
as crystallised by black consciousness theatre and refined by non-racial
progressive groups in the seventies. Plays like *Woza Albert!*, *Bopha!*,
Asinamali, and *Sarafina* have marketed political struggle and resistance
abroad in the current images of South African politics: the freedom song,
the *toyi-toyi* dance and the burning-tyre 'necklace'.

The major difficulty facing the new theatre practitioners, however, is
that oppositional theatre in a changing society needs also to be constantly

changing. There is an ever-present danger that the adversarial work will become trapped within once dynamic but soon static formulae — especially if the work is made for an export market, where such formulae have been the basis of spectacular success amongst foreign audiences. Once adversarial theatre becomes popular, it needs constantly to re-examine and redefine itself and its relationship to popular consciousness as that popular consciousness changes. If it fails to do so, it becomes established as part of the dominant order which it once opposed.

t. Fanon.

1 See especially Coplan, D. *In Township Tonight: South Africa's Black City Music and Theatre.* Johannesburg: Ravan Press, 1985; Kavanagh, R. *Theatre and Cultural Struggle in South Africa,* London: Zed Books, 1985; Sole, K. Black Literature and Performance: Some notes on Class and Populism. In *South African Labour Bulletin* 9(8), 1984, pp. 54-76; Steadman, I. Drama and Social Consciousness: Themes in Black Theatre on the Witwatersrand until 1984, unpublished Doctoral Thesis, University of the Witwatersrand, 1985; von Kotze, A. *Organise & Act: The Natal Workers Theatre Movement* 1983-1987, Durban: Culture and Working Life Publications, University of Natal, 1988; Tomaselli, K. The Semiotics of Alternative Theatre in South Africa. *Critical Arts* 2(1), 1981, pp. 14-33; amongst numerous others.

2 Lodge, T. *Black Politics in South Africa since 1945.* Johannesburg: Ravan Press, 1983, p. ix.

3 See Kidd, R. Folk Media, Popular Theatre, and Conflicting Strategies for Social Change in the Third World, pp. 280-301. In Kidd, R. & Colletta, N. (eds.), *Tradition for Development: Indigenous Structures and Folk Media in non-formal Education.* Bonn: German Foundation for International Development, and International Council for Adult Education, 1981, especially p. 281. See also, for a critique of this notion of 'popular', Barber, K. Radical Conservatism in Yoruba Popular Plays. In Breitinger, E. & Sander, R. (eds.), *Bayreuth African Studies Series* 7, 1986, pp. 5-32.

4 'Adversary tradition' is a phrase used by Susan Sontag in her essay on Artaud in *Antonin Artaud: Selected Writings.* New York: Farrar, Strauss and Giroux, 1976, P. xliii.

5 Barber, K. op. cit. p. 6.

6 Barber, K. Popular Arts in Africa. In *African Studies Review,* 30 (3), September 1987, pp. 1-78.

7 See, as examples, various essays in the special issue of *Critical Arts,* 4 (3), entitled Black Performance Revisited.

8 Williams, R. *Drama in Performance.* Harmondsworth: Pelican Books. 1972.

9 Williams, R. *Drama from Ibsen to Brecht.* Harmondsworth: Pelican Books. 1976.

10 Williams, R. 1976, p. 9.

11 See, for example, Said, E.W. *The World, the Text, and the Critic.* London: Faber & Faber, 1984, esp. pp. 226-247, for a discussion of what he calls 'Travelling Theory'.

12 See, for example, Barber's comment (1987, p. 39) that '(the new form) should appeal to the audience by corresponding to something in their own experience or desires' — which seems perfectly analogous to the whole notion of a structure of feeling in a work of art corresponding with a structure of feeling in an audience.

13 Mouffe, C. Hegemony and New Political Subjects: Toward a New Concept of Democracy, trans. S. Gray, pp. : 89-101. In Nelson, C. & Grossberg. L. (eds.), *Marxism and the Interpretation of Culture.* London: MacMillan Education, 1988. Mouffe argues on pp. 89-90 that she opposes classical Marxism's 'class reductionism'

and affirms instead 'multiple subject positions corresponding both to the different social relations in which the individual is inserted and to the discourses that constitute these relations. There is no reason to privilege, a priori, a 'class' position as the origin of the articulation of subjectivity.'

14 Mouffe, op. cit. p. 91.

15 The term 'black theatre' has obvious difficulties, and it is interesting to note that most commentators on oppositional theatre have experienced other problems of nomenclature related to issues of race and class. See, for example, the debate about 'working class culture' in *South African Labour Bulletin* vols. 9 (1984) and 10 (1985), and about 'black' theatre in *Critical Arts* 4(3), 1988.

16 Apart from studies already cited, *Critical Arts: A Journal for Cultural Studies*, Durban: Centre for Contemporary Cultural Studies of the University of Natal, has produced two issues on the subject: vol. 2 (1) 1981 and vol. 4 (3) 1988.

17 Graham-White, A. The *Drama of Black Africa*. New York: Samuel French, 1974, p. 17, says that the play 'seems to be one of the most thorough examples of the assimilation of the occupier's culture'. Graham-White is referring here to Frantz Fanon's suggestion, in Fanon, F. *The Wretched of the Earth*, Harmondsworth, 1967, p. 179, that before the colonised writer reaches a stage of creating truly indigenous literature, an initial period of assimilation has to be undergone. See also Coplan 1985, op. cit . for the same kind of comment on Dhlomo.

18 Visser, N. & Couzens, T. (eds.) *H.I.E. Dhlomo: Collected Works*. Johannesburg: Ravan Press, 1985, p xv. They also inform us (p. xii) that he wrote 24 plays and that 9 survived. Those 9 are published in their collection.

19 The letters are reproduced in Chalmers, J. *Tiyo Soga: A Page of South African Mission Work*. Grahamstown: James Kay, 1877, pp. 108-129).

20 The essay is reprinted in Visser, N. (ed.), *Literary Theory and Criticism of H.I.E. Dhlomo*, published as a separate issue of *English in Africa* , 4(2), 1977.

21 Couzens has written extensively on Dhlomo. His major work is Couzens, T. *The New African: A Study of the Life and Work of H.I.E. Dhlomo*. Johannesburg: Ravan Press, 1985.

22 A point for which I am indebted to Liz Gunner.

23 In an essay entitled 'Why Study Tribal Dramatic Forms?', written in 1939 (and reprinted in Visser, N. ed. op. cit.), Dhlomo argues that a search for 'archaical art forms' must be based on an attempt to write about contemporary matters.

24 Williams, R. 1976, p. 395.

25 Visser and Couzens, op. cit. p. xiii. They go on to argue that his work reflects 'an apparent need to prove his credentials, as it were, to an English-speaking audience', and describe the plays generally by saying that many of them move 'towards a novelising mode with long set pieces'.

26 Visser and Couzens op. cit. p. xiii quote Dhlomo's own pronouncements on the subject: he 'wrote repeatedly that African playwrights should attempt to write 'literary drama' rather than 'acting plays'.'

27 Chapman, M. Soweto Poetry: Socio-literary phenomenon of the Seventies. In Malan, C. (ed.) *Race and Literature* , Pinetown: Owen Burgess, 1987, p. 178.

28 Kente, G. *Too Late*. In *South African People's Plays* ed. Kavanagh, R. London: Heinemann, 1981.

29 Zell, H. & Silver, H. *A Reader's Guide to African Literature*. London: Heinemann, 1972, p. 162.

30 Lodge, T. op. cit. 1983, p. 225.

31 Nkosi has commented in Nkosi, L. *Home and Exile*. London: Longman Group, 1965, p. 8: 'The fifties were important to us as a decade because finally they spelled out the end of one kind of South Africa and foreshadowed the beginning of another. Sharpeville was the culmination of a political turmoil during a decade in which it was still possible in South Africa to pretend to the viability of extra-parliamentary opposition.'

32 Nkosi was actively involved in the intellectual life of the Witwatersrand in 1960. On the eve of the Sharpeville shootings in March 1960, he lectured prophetically to students of the University of the Witwatersrand: 'I believe that the first crisis will be political and it is going to occur within the next few weeks — possibly on Monday — and the people who may be creating the first crisis for 1960 are members of the Pan Africanist Congress ... whether the campaign they are going to launch will be successful or not doesn't matter. Some action is going to be taken and this will bring us all closer to a crisis.' (Nkosi, L. op. cit. 1965, pp. 8-9.)

33 This is not to suggest that Nkosi was never involved in such a collaborative process, but rather that the involvement was minimal compared to the ways in which theatre was created in the seventies. Nkosi's collaboration on Fugard's *No-Good Friday* is well known, but any interrogation of that text will show that the collaborative processes did not extend far enough to break down the literariness of this early work of Fugard, about which both Fugard and Nkosi have been critical. See Kavanagh, op. cit. for a discussion of the language of this play.

34 This is a feature of much of black theatre even in the eighties.

35 Nkosi, L. 1965, op. cit.

36 Ibid. pp. 108-114.

37 Ibid. p. 110.

38 Ibid. p. 47.

39 Ibid. p. 45.

40 See Manganyi, N. *Exiles and Homecomings: A Biography of Es'kia Mphahlele*, Johannesburg: Ravan Press, 1983, pp. 211-213.

41 Nkosi, L. op. cit. p. 117.

42 Ibid. pp. 44-45.

43 Ibid. pp. 91-107.

44 He once reviewed the beginning of these precedents with reference to Pixley ka Izaka Seme's notion of a 'level of consciousness'. (Ibid. p. 98).

45 See both Kavanagh and Steadman, op. cit. for analyses of Black Consciousness theatre of the seventies.

46 Pascal Gwala in *South African Outlook*, August 1973, p. 131-133.

47 The play is published in Kavanagh, R. (ed.) *South African People's Plays*, London: Heinemann, 1981.

48 See Barber, 1987, pp. 45-7, for a discussion of the presentational style of Yoruba popular theatre.

49 The sheer volume of work in theatre might have ensured this. The journal *Black Review* carried frequent discussions of the extraordinary level of energy which was being created in theatre at the time: 'Like a powerful subversive organisation this spontaneous outburst of real Black creativity is slowly seething through the entire Black community. Perhaps it will be posterity that will recapture the growing spirit of Black determination and Black creativity.' (*Black Review* 1973 p. 111.)

50 The play in many ways emulates *Dutchman* by Leroi Jones, utilising an American Black Power discourse even in its stage directions.

51 Mutloatse, M. *Forced Landing*. Johannesburg: Ravan Press, 1980, p. 5.

52 Coplan, op. cit. p. 210.

53 Ranger, T. *Dance and Society in Eastern Africa* 1890-1970. London: Heinemann, p. 3.

54 Barber, K. 1987 p. 48.

55 Emmett, A. Oral, Political and Communal Aspects of Township Poetry in the Mid-Seventies, *English in Africa* 6 (1), 1979, pp. 72-81. P. 74.

56 Maishe Maponya, in his play *The Hungry Earth* (1981) frequently invokes the notion of 'the people' of Africa as a seamless, unified group. This is typical of other playwrights as well. See, for example, the plays of Matsemela Manaka.

57 Williams, op. cit . 1972, p. 184.

58 Dhlomo was a founder member of the Bantu Dramatic Society in the Thirties, but for

a discussion of the Eurocentric nature of this group see Steadman, op. cit. Nkosi was also involved in collaborative rehearsal work with Fugard and other intellectuals in Sophiatown, but these never extended into his own playwriting efforts.

59 See Steadman, I. The Other Face. *Index on Censorship* 14 (1), 1985. London. pp. 26-28.

60 See Vandenbroucke, R. South African Blacksploitation, *Yale/Theatre* 8 (1), 1976, pp.78-81 for an analysis of how South African theatre marketed abroad entrenches the racial stereotype.

Apartheid and the Political Imagination in Black South African Theatre

BHEKIZIZWE PETERSON

The historical predominance of coercion as the base of hegemony in the South African social formation has marked out the social terrain as a key area for contestation between the state and its radical oppositions. Cultural practices have featured prominently in these resultant conflicts because of their potential to give meaning to individuals' experiences of social processes and transformations. Black theatre has addressed itself, as part of the projects initiated by radical oppositional movements, to the negation of the state's myths about South African history and society by presenting alternate historical narratives and hopes. The locations of conflict between black performance and the government have shifted historically and the changing nature and terrain of struggle can be seen in the contents of plays, and in the ways in which black performance is organised. The first part of the paper examines the political uses theatre has been put to in South Africa between 1948 and 1988. It will also attempt to tease out the social relations specific to the area of performance production. The second part of this study is a critical presentation of the politics and historical content of four plays that are representative of popular black performance, excluding workers' theatre.[1]

Black Performance and Social Conflicts

The introduction of Africans to formal theatre in South Africa is largely due to missionary activities. Faced with serious social limitations, especially the different cultural backgrounds, worldviews and languages of Africans, missionaries realised that performance could help overcome these constraints. Performance demands for its success the harnessing of all of one's senses, be they visual, mental, oral, physical or sensual. These human attributes are transformed during performance into cultural codes of representation, rhetoric and reception. Performance, then, is potentially more accessible than other forms of signification such as writing. A Chief

Inspector of Native Schools, Dr C.T. Loram, acknowledged as much in an introduction to an article entitled 'Education Through the Drama':

> Learning by doing is one of the wisest educational maxims we have. It is founded on the right psychology because when we make use of the eye and tongue and hand, these several activities make our understanding of the thing better. It is for this reason that we have action songs for infants and practical work in science, agriculture or woodwork for older students.[2]

The Reverend Father Bernard Huss was one of the earliest, and most influential pioneers of the social and pedagogical uses of theatre. Huss was based at St Francis College, Mariannhill, for seventeen years and it was while at St Francis that he experimented with theatre in a sustained manner, drawing national attention. The dramas performed at St Francis under the direction of Huss spanned a range of theatrical styles and contents. The three types that seem to have predominated were medieval morality plays, secular European comedies and dramatisations of Zulu oral narratives. The earliest recorded performances at St Francis took place in 1904 when African students staged *Joseph in Egypt*.[3]

The pedagogic appeal of performance for missionaries and liberal whites was that it seemed amenable to the transmission of Christian and 'civilised' ideals and values. Furthermore, theatre could be locked into their political and social projects. The stock themes of Theatre-in-Education in mission schools were those of repentance, character training, habits of industry, diligence, thrift and obedience. A corresponding racism soon crept into the practice of performance so that apart from transmitting ideas of progress, theatre became a tool with which to challenge the 'limited' intellectual capacities of Africans: 'The difficult gulf between the concrete and the abstract, which the African finds so hard to step over, can be bridged by drama'.[4] In the Witwatersrand towns, theatre was extolled by whites and members of the African elite as a 'healthy' and 'morally improving' entertainment unlike the 'sensational recreations of bioscopes and dance halls'.[5]

But theatre also became an important activity in the cultural practices of elite Africans from the Twenties. The use of theatre by members of the African elite was characterised by a range of socio-political ambivalences and tensions. The complex ways in which Africans appropriated and reformulated the forms and contents of theatre can be gleaned in the initiatives of the Bantu Dramatic Society and in the critical and dramatic literature of H.I.E. Dhlomo.[6] The Bantu Dramatic Society was formed in July 1932. At its inception the Society remarked that while it would present

European plays, 'the aim of the Bantu Dramatic Society is to encourage Bantu playwrights and to develop African dramatic and operatic art'.[7] Despite this supposed bias towards developing African drama, the first productions mounted by the Society were from the European dramatic tradition, the first being Oliver Goldsmith's *She Stoops to Conquer* in 1933. The initial preference for European plays reflected the liberal hegemony inscribed into the Society and its members. European plays embodied in their content, forms and even in the way criticism has conventionally described them, *a way of life* that members of the middle class aspired to. It is also likely that the lack of scripted African plays was a contributory factor because of an ideological bias towards the literary as opposed to the improvisational nature of traditional performance.[8]

These kinds of attitudes would seem to suggest a thorough assimilation of the ideas and values inculcated at mission schools and expounded by liberal whites. In many respects this is true but the struggles the Society experienced in their attempts to mount productions must have, on the other hand, emphasised the disadvantaged social positions that Society members occupied. The Society had to contend with social constraints such as the lack of performance venues, transport, financial support and rehearsal time because of the need for Society members to be in full-time employment. As Miss Elsie Solomon realised during her stint of directing the Society's production of *Lady Windermere's Fan*, working with Africans had its 'peculiar difficulties'.

> One of the main difficulties has been that of rehearsing ... our greatest trouble has been the curfew. Rehearsals have usually begun at about 8 pm, but all the actors had to leave at 9.30 pm and what can one do in one-and-a-half hours? For the three performances we have arranged for all the actors to be given special passes ...[9]

It can be appreciated then that the Bantu Dramatic Society operated under very restrictive social circumstances, which, coupled with the increasing segregationist policies pursued by the Pact Government, must account for their move towards nationalist themes. The plays of Dhlomo performed by the Society, especially his historical plays, show important shifts in his ideology and aesthetics. Although still informed by Christian and liberal ideas, *Dingane*, *Cetshwayo* and *Moshoeshoe* show a transition towards a militant nationalism which starts to articulate the need for self-awareness and self-determination. The availability of Dhlomo's mature plays reveal that the Society's initiatives were radical, despite class contradictions, and clearly fell far short of the 'innocent' and 'wholesome' recreation desired by Huss and white liberals.

The parliamentary ascendancy of the National Party in 1948 and its implementation of apartheid were to have an important bearing on the social and political experiences of blacks. The social formation which informed black cultural practices in the post-1948 period, though essentially having a longer historical inheritance, was very particular in its development of political oppression, economic exploitation and social segregation. The government was acutely concerned with the role that cultural practices could fulfil in *negotiating* social conflicts and, more importantly, in how the 'creative arts' could embody, symbolise, transmit and provide the demonstrative rationale to support its national policies. The state felt the need to construct 'a framework in which the arts could be performed' and which set up the religious, social and political boundaries within which to regulate cultural work.[10]

The framework for the arts had the articulation of Christian Nationalism as its operative axis. A range of institutions, formal and informal, were set up and linked with local, regional and central administrative structures. In 1960 a conference was held to deliberate on the 'promotion of the arts'. Delegates included Mr. B.J. Vorster, the then Deputy Minister of Education, Arts and Science and later Prime Minister.[11] Censorship legislation crystallised in the Publications and Entertainments Act of 1963 and its administrative body, the Publications Control Board. The government's promotion of the arts included an attempt to dislocate cultural practices from social struggles and to market them instead as universal and trans-historical 'civilising forces'. Patronage of the arts became the barometer with which to measure South Africa's level of 'civilisation', and the state's and capital's commitment to 'social responsibility' programmes.

However, the social origins and locations of performance spaces, their quantity and quality, reveal the partisan nature of the state's role in cultural development and its attempts to regulate cultural practices. There are at least 49 theatres nationally and all of them are located in areas which are officially designated as white. These theatres are controlled by white managements although some, like the Market Theatre, have blacks as patrons and in administrative positions. The majority of theatres were built by provincial councils as cultural metaphors of South African history. The Nico Malan, in Cape Town, and the Pretoria State Theatre, completed at a cost of R46.5 million, correspond with the 10th and 20th anniversary celebrations of the Republic. The Johannesburg Civic Theatre is a reminder of 50 years of Union, and the Etienne Rousseau Theatre was donated to Sasolburg by Sasol on the latter's 25th anniversary.

Windybrow Theatre in Hillbrow is a product of Johannesburg's centenary celebrations, while the Johannesburg Art Gallery received a face-lift courtesy of the centenary celebrations. The history represented by these venues is only one view of South African history, one that diarises the triumphs of the current government and capital.

There is, on the other hand, no single theatre in any township in South Africa. A theatre complex was supposed to have been built in Jabulani, Soweto, in 1969 though and, according to a newspaper report, ministerial approval had already been granted, yet it never materialised.[12] The theatre was to be called the Will Carr Theatre, after a Mr W.J.P. Carr, in recognition of his contribution to the development of African townships as manager of the Johannesburg Non-European Affairs Department. Production plans included the staging of 'ambitious productions' by private enterprise as well as ballet, opera, plays and musicals. There are only two rudimentary theatres under black control in the Witwatersrand area, the Dhlomo Theatre (closed in 1983 by the authorities as a 'fire hazard') and the Funda Centre Experimental Space. Black performance in the townships generally takes place in local community and church halls and cinemas. These venues are literally empty spaces, or all-purpose venues if you prefer, with no stage facilities. The paucity of performance venues is the result of the state's policy that black cultural practices had to be catered for by their respective racial or ethnic administrations. Since urban Africans were regarded, in accordance with Verwoerdian ideology, as temporary sojourners en route, hopefully, to their respective ethnic homelands, no encouragement was to be given that would contradict this eventuality. The government's policy on the political status of urban Africans obviously contradicts its refrain, then and now, of 'separate but equal' facilities. Access to city-based theatres was controlled through the application of the Group Areas Act and the official segregation of performers, venues and audiences in 1965.

Prior to 1965 most black performance initiatives were mounted under the banner of Union Artists, a company formed in 1955 and composed of black and white members. The Sixties saw the demise of Union Artists and the development of productions which were to a significant degree under the initiative and control of blacks. This was in part a response to the unequal power relations that existed between black and white members of multiracial groups. The increase in independent productions was, paradoxically, given a measure of stimulus by the government's segregation policies which, in a sense, advocated independent productions for black audiences. Important trailblazers of independent initiatives were Ben Masinga's *Back in Your Own Back Yard* (1962), Sam Mhangwane's

Crime Does Not Pay (1963), *Unfaithful Woman* (1964) and Gibson Kente's post-1966 work starting with *Sikhalo*, produced in 1966.

By 1972 a significant amount of black performance was operating under the Black Consciousness Movement. This development found structural expression in the formation of MDALI (Music, Drama, Arts and Literature Institute) in Soweto and, on a national level, in the formation of the South African Black Theatre Union (SABTU). In the Seventies black consciousness took on board a number of themes including black initiative, self-definition, determination and liberation. A significant cultural focus ran through all these objectives, and cultural practices were accorded a prominent political role within the movement. The rest of the decade and the Eighties have seen the appearance of innovative and committed individuals and groups. The growth of non-racial and worker groups, especially the Cultural Desks and Cultural Locals established by the UDF and COSATU, has significantly expanded and, at times, reformulated the debates and practices of black performance. The performance groups have consistently engaged with each other in complex ways, both supportive and contradictory. They have fed off each other in terms of the pool of performers available, the logistics of performance and even with regard to content, aesthetics and strategies.

The political pronouncements of black theatre elicited popular responses from the black communities because from the Seventies black communities have been receptive to and experiencing radical interventions. The plays were performed for township audiences and frequently they formed part of the cultural rhetoric and spectacle of political rallies. Furthermore, the social organisation of black performance has, in certain respects, contradicted the policies of the state. Independent productions, and those organised on the principles of black consciousness, emphasised black initiative, control, and trans-ethnic solidarity as preconditions for the attainment of liberation. The ethics of nonracialism, on the other hand, have challenged the state's insistence on racial divisions as the basis for social organisation; cultural contact and exchange across racial classifications is seen as a process which could facilitate the construction of a nonracial society.

The state responded to black performance by trying to control access to venues. In Soweto the West Rand Administration Board (WRAB), set up its own Cultural Section in 1975. Duties of the Cultural Section included the collection, reading and viewing of scripts and plays before they were cleared for performance in WRAB controlled venues.[13] The head of the Cultural Section, H. Pieterse, even attempted to stage a production of *Shaka*, written and directed by himself.[14] Plays which were performed at church-owned venues were still subject to the controls of legislation, censorship laws, and, from 1985, emergency regulations. The state's suppression of black political opposition has always affected the radical sections of black performance. Bannings, exile, and treason charges, for instance, have also exercised a stifling impact on creative persons and organisations. At the SASO/BPC treason trial of 1975 the accused were also charged with conspiring to 'make, produce, publish or distribute subversive and anti-white utterances, writings, poems, plays and/or dramas'.[15]

There have been more indirect ways in which the state and capital, via various individuals and organisations, have attempted to influence black performance. The most prevalent attempts at control have been the staging of collaborative productions involving blacks and white artists or entrepreneurs. The productions which were 'influential' were those which had a degree of 'authenticity' because they made use of black initiative, traditional themes and cultural forms. The most noteworthy of such productions were *Dingaka* (1962), *uMabatha* (1973), *Meropa* which was tellingly retitled *KwaZulu* (1973), *Ipi Tombi* (1975) and *King Africa* (1987). The privileging of traditional African culture in these productions is meant to celebrate some organic tribal past now lost or under threat from the evils of the city. The ahistorical narrative of these plays implicitly gestures towards the modern 'homelands' as reincarnations of tribal society. The illustration of 'traditional' cultural practices is nothing but an attempt to titillate Eurocentric minds with various forms of 'African exoticisms' while the depiction of great chiefs differs little from standard representations of the noble savage.

The politics and power relations that are operative in collaborative productions can be seen in a project mounted by the Native Affairs Department of the Johannesburg City Council in 1972. The Native Affairs Department commissioned Doreen Lamb to 'assist' in the development of black performance in Soweto. Lamb worked with a group of twelve performers for eighteen months at the end of which they performed a play that she had written, *The Frightened Lady*. Apart from 'teaching' acting, stage-craft, and 'correct' pronunciation, Lamb impressed upon the actors that 'politics do not belong in the theatre, social evils yes' because 'the minute you drag politics into theatre, it falls apart'.[16] *The Frightened Lady* was based on the theft of a diamond ring at a function held at the Malawian ambassador's residence in Pretoria. The culprits turn out to be well-respected members of the Soweto elite — so much for their social responsibility and, given the rise of black consciousness, their political activism!

The interventions of white philanthropy *à la* Doreen Lamb, the processes of censorship and the suppression of black political opposition, especially in the period 1975–1980, effectively undermined the relationship between black theatre and township audiences. Radical performances became sporadic in the aftermath of June 1976.[17] The end of the Seventies saw an increased migration of black performers to theatres located in the city centres. The multiracial operations of the Market Theatre, established in 1976, accelerated this process. The migration to city-based ventures was initially held in check by the government's prohibitions of mixed casts and audiences. Public performances and venues, with the exception of cinemas, were officially desegregated in 1978.

The years after 1978 saw the 'liberalisation' of the arts as part of the state's new discourse of 'reform' and 'effective government'.[18] We can detect the new slants of meanings in the government's discourse by comparing the terms of reference of two commissions on the performing arts: the Niemand Commission, appointed 1975 and tabled in 1977, and the Schutte Commission, appointed 1981 and tabled in 1984. In the Niemand Commission references to 'the population of South Africa' are used as being synonymous with whites as in 'the cultural needs of the two language groups concerned,' meaning white English and Afrikaans speakers.[19] By contrast parts of the Schutte Commission are radical in their reformulations, as when it departs from orthodox Verwoerdian premises, but it does not overturn the central tenets of apartheid. Classic keywords in this reformulated discourse include the promotion of the arts 'among all population groups', a concern for the 'other indigenous languages of South Africa' and 'every member of South Africa's heterogeneous community'.[20]

The processes that went into the government's struggle to elicit a broader base of consent were loaded with profound tensions in the need to maintain control while addressing the prerogatives of conflicting audiences as far as possible. In the area of cultural production this juggling-act found expression in the application of the Publications Act from 1980, two years after its second amendment in 1978. What is striking about the application of the Publications Act from 1980 is the fairly sophisticated understanding of the workings of cultural processes, especially with regard to their consumption and codes of signification. There is an emphasis on understanding the centrality of socio-political variables in determining the shifting historical meanings of cultural products and their consumption. There is, in other words, a shift from an 'absolutist approach', in terms of censorship, to a preference for *situational* assessments.[21]

The issues considered in the assessment of literature and performance include: the intelligibility of the work, that is, are its codes of signification 'above' the intelligibility of the 'common person'? Is the work based on sentiments or codes (example, a clenched fist) 'which had through frequent use lost any of the inflammatory effect which it might earlier have had' and how accessible is the work in terms of price, admission, location and manner of performance or distribution?[22] These kinds of considerations coupled with attitudes of 'tolerance', such as the notion that 'the expression of grievances often acts as a safety valve for pent-up feelings', partially explain why radical performances have been tolerated in city-based theatres.[23] Where creative works are judged as being 'undesirable' and accessible to a larger audience than the 'sophisticated minority', their outreach is regulated through the use of age and place restrictions. 'Protest Plays' have on occasion been restricted to 'experimental theatres' such as the Market Theatre. The state's ambivalent appreciation of the arts is aptly illustrated in a speech by the then Minister of National Education and now State President, Mr F.W. de Klerk:

> Our artists, just like any other important group, must be given a fair opportunity to perform their chosen task and to make their own contribution. Truly creative individuals must be able to develop fully and the arts must be allowed to play their legitimate role in society. And this must take place within the realities and the many restrictions within which the State performs its functions in South Africa.[24]

The attempts of the state to tread a thin political line have been strained by developments in oppositional politics and theatre in the Eighties. The resurgence of unrest since 1983, the year of the formation of the United Democratic Front, has led black theatre, again, to make increasing visits to the terrain of political rallies. This development seriously undermines the censors' abilities to gloss their role with 'tolerant' or 'reformist' qualities. It has also revealed the different layers of censorship operating, by provoking the recent attack on 'resistance art' by the Minister of Home Affairs, Stoffel Botha.[25] The 'tolerant' application of the Publications Act is constantly undermined by the application of the emergency regulations and by the activities of bodies such as WRAB. These three distinct bodies of censorship are not necessarily accountable to each other, with the result that uniform decisions are more the exception than the rule. It must also be noted that the control and power exercised by newspaper critics, academics, theatre managements and publicity agencies are equally crucial in circumscribing and censoring black performance that is deemed inappropriate. This is achieved not only by hostile reactions but, more effectively, through selections of what is worthy of promotion and what is to be banished by maintaining a silence about it.

Stages of Resistance: Black Performance 1973–1986

Black performance initiatives from the Seventies represent a response and challenge to the apartheid policies of the South African government. The representation of history has been an important preoccupation of black performance. The themes of oppression and exploitation in South Africa have been the major concern of black performance. The most frequent depictions have been those of pass arrests, the humiliation experienced at the medical examinations conducted at the labour bureaux, petty bureaucracy, police violence, prison conditions, examples of racial discrimination, the struggles of migrant workers, conditions in the hostel compounds, and the breakdown of moral and cultural values in the townships. Although questions of class and economy are always latent if not explicitly stated in black theatre, they are rarely explored prominently.

Few plays limit themselves to the presentation of one major theme. As if to indicate their social character, the dramas record events in the manner of tabloids, moving from one headline to the next. The expansive nature of the content treated is reproduced by the similarly expansive nature of the aesthetic premises and codes of representation utilised. Forms as diverse as dialogue and mime, song and tableau, sounds and dance, are combined into a striking and aesthetically appealing total performance. The language used is equally syncretic and in a single performance it can shift from indigenous languages to Afrikaans and English or to a mixture of all of them in township slang.

While black theatre primarily explores the struggles informing the current political climate, there are also representations of the past because of the general perception that 'calling back on the past' is a precondition for 'the forging of the future'.[26] The simultaneity of past and present, history and struggle, is culturally embodied in the passing on of narratives of the struggle from one generation to the next:

> Oupa with his calabash enjoying the beer, and *the tone of his voice always blending with the ancestors*. Telling stories taught us how to live. How to survive the grips of Piet Retief and fight for liberation ... I will tell stories to my children. I will let them sit around the fire like we did during our times with Oupa.[27]

The need to construct trans-historical continuities and to embark on projects of cultural retrieval is informed by the search for the causal origins of colonial conquest and the current crisis, when 'the gourds (were) ... broken'[28] and 'how the honey went bitter'.[29] Playwrights are, consequently, committed to negating Eurocentric utterances on African history and to advancing the modern correlative struggles for psychological and social liberation.[30] Consequently representations of what is in many ways an enigmatic past are further strained by the need to view that past through the political and ideological demands of the current political struggles. For one, the processes of constructing pride and control over *self*, given the presence of racially charged myths, tends to call for the adoption of a heroic mode of narration. But how does one narrate in a heroic mode a 'journey' that, after all, ensued with the defeat of African societies? It is in trying to confront this paradox that Credo Mutwa's *uNosilimela*, first performed in 1973, and Maishe Maponya's *The Hungry Earth*, first performed in 1979, resort to partial and unsatisfactory explanations.

In *The Hungry Earth*, the audience is informed that 'we are about to take you on a heroic voyage of the Bahumutsi Drama Group'.[31] It is a voyage which spans a vast historical space, time and experience. *uNosilimela*, on the other hand, describes itself as 'a story of self-understanding, self-discovery, love of your neighbour and love and respect for the laws and religion of your civilised forefathers'.[32] Both plays present powerful collages which link the current oppression and exploitation of Africans with the processes of colonial conquest. These are presented as constituting an uninterrupted and unchanged process and history.

The story of *uNosilimela* is performed at the Great Place of Magadlemzini, King of the amaQhashi in Natal. In *uNosilimela* Mutwa attempts a detailed depiction of an African society that somehow escapes the direct impact of Christianity and colonial conquest. Mutwa is then able to present to modern audiences his vision of a 'traditional' African society. The first parts of the play are a cultural inventory of the daily life patterns, cultural rituals and practices of the amaQhashi. They are presented, on the whole, as a well-ordered society which peacefully co-exists with other black nations and appreciates the political importance of unity between blacks. The factors that lead to the disintegration of the amaQhashi are internally located and they revolve, mainly, around incidences of cultural mutiny. uNosilimela commits the most serious act of cultural treachery when she strikes her step-mother 'an open-handed blow with the back of her hand'. The severity of her action leads to the appearance of an ancestral spirit with the task of punishing and cleansing both child and society: 'The hand that strikes the mother is cursed throughout the land! Expel that child from your household … The cattle will die, the crops be burnt by the sun'.[33] Initially uNosilimela registers her exile as a release from the 'tribal stuffiness and restriction' but her exile marks, instead, the beginnings of her 'wanderings and pains'.[34] The communities that she passes through and her experiences are the epitome of oppression, corruption, cultural decadence and violence. uNosilimela's degeneration into being 'rubbish upon rubbish' presents a powerful contrast to her stay with the amaQhashi. She is then instructed by the Earth Mother to leave Johannesburg for 'the pure open spaces where the truth' will be revealed to her.[35] Upon her return to the amaQhashi, Johannesburg and South Africa, with the exception of Natal where the amaQhashi are based, are destroyed in an apocalyptic ending.[36]

The Hungry Earth is narrated by mineworkers whose daily descent into the hungry bowels of the mines is symbolic of the historical predicament facing Africans as a nation. We are presented in five scenes with accounts of colonial conquest, the frontier wars, Isandlwana, Umgungundlovu plus imperialist and capitalist exploitation of the continent, child-labour, mineworkers and the government's apartheid policies. Africans are arrested for influx control infringements and deported to the homelands; they are assaulted, interrogated, discriminated against and their families separated by the migrant labour system.

The form of *The Hungry Earth*, its short scenes and eclectic paging through history, works against the clarity of Maponya's propositions. There is a sense that Maponya has a utopian vision of pre-colonial African societies. There are fleeting references to 'those vast tracts of land that are still in their virgin state'. It is only after colonial conquest that social contradictions are supposed to manifest themselves in African social formations.[37] The construction of egalitarian pre-colonial African societies in *uNosilimela* and *The Hungry Earth*, is intended to challenge eurocentric portrayals of pre-colonial African societies as stagnant or characterised by incessant tribal conflicts. Yet the exorcism of social contradictions comes ironically close to being an inverted restatement of eurocentric perceptions of pre-colonial African societies.[38] It can also be easily recast 'into the rhetoric of a classless black modern South Africa'.[39]

The embrace of a utopian vision of the past tends to lead to a moral critique of colonialism. Colonisation is then metaphorically presented as having been precipitated by the ingratitude, deception and greed of African individuals or whites.[40] The struggles of organising resistance become, at times, the source of frustration and lead to a sad judgement on humanity: 'If we could really feel the pain, the pain would be so great that we would stand up and fight to stop all the suffering ... and apartheid would end. Ah, we would all know what love is.'[41] Moralistic critiques are problematic because contained within their judgemental and metaphoric analyses are profound displacements of social contradictions and they also contradict, (by, for instance, blaming colonisation on the gullibility of Africans), the heroic history and struggles that are supposed to be retrieved and celebrated. *uNosilimela* and *The Hungry Earth* make clarion calls for Africans to resist apartheid and to embark upon forms of cultural and political resistance. The names of the three progressive characters in *The Hungry Earth*, Matlhoko, Usiviko and Beshwana, Sufferings, Shield and Loin-cloth respectively, encapsulate the nationalism operative in the play: 'MOTHER AFRICA WAKE UP/AND ARM YOURSELF/WIPE THE TEARS OF YOUR BRAVE/MOTHER AFRICA WAKE UP/LEST UMLUNGU RAPES YOU ... '.[42]

The critique of oppression and exploitation in *The Hungry Earth* and Manaka's *Egoli*, (both plays also attempt to foreground the struggles of black workers), is based on the identification of apartheid as the primary cause of Africans' suffering. The historical but contingent links between apartheid and capitalism are, at best, dramatised as a seamless apartheid conspiracy. The result is a considerable silence on work-place conditions and exploitation and the potential for black workers to make profound critiques of their experiences. Black workers, and especially migrant labourers, are presented as baffled by the politics that regulate their lives and all they manage to do is develop a stoic resilience.[43] Otherwise the presence of workers on stage frequently serves as a source of dramatic comedy because of their inability to cope with city life and, even, to speak English. Stereotypes of the 'country-bumpkin' or 'Jim-comes-to-Jo'burg' abound in black theatre as both theme and character.[44]

Black theatre does not uniformly predicate the resolution of contradictions in South Africa on the exercise of a political and militant nationalism. A significant proportion of black theatre emphasises religion, familial and cultural virtues and communal strengths as the best ways in which to challenge apartheid. Gibson Kente's plays are typical in this regard and they have exercised a considerable influence on township performances. Kente's most important imprints are the popular aesthetics of his plays and their deep-seated and felt moralistic content. A Kente play combines dialogue, dance, music, mime and tableau into an evocative melodramatic spectacle that has sensory appeal because it is profoundly informed by township popular culture, its slangs, fashions, topical issues, music and dance styles. The egalitarian impulse of the Kentesque form is matched by his predisposition to focus on the day to day struggles of his characters, drawn from ordinary people, depicting and celebrating the lives they have wrought out of the hostile and degenerate urban landscapes. Politics is always present in the Kente project but it is nothing more than a surface reality, an aberration that masks the fundamental moral conflicts that challenge individuals and society. *Too Late* was first staged in 1975 and, like *I Believe* and *How Long?*, it privileged politics beyond its customary secondary status. Kente's moral intents are not displaced from their central location. It is rather that the social cohesiveness of the family and the community, the traditional repositories of culture and virtue, are challenged by political processes.

Too Late commences with a family and community that is socially and psychologically fractured. Madinto, a shebeen owner, is a single parent and mother to Ntanana who is 'cripple, touchy ... (and) ... slightly retarded'.[45] The two of them are joined by an orphaned teenage boy Saduva. He establishes a warm relationship with community members and with Ntanana who, because of her physical handicaps, knew 'that it was unlikely she would ever get a boyfriend and so Saduva was a psychological substitute'.[46] People who suffer from some kind of physical disability are one of the key symbols of innocence and virtue within the melodramatic narrative. Children and the deaf, blind and dumb often possess a sense of truth, affection and perception exceeding their age, experience and physical disability.[47]

Madinto resorts to selling liquor because, she tells us in song: 'I have no other way (To make ends meet)'.[48] This sets her on a collision course with the police who are the most visible symbol of an impersonal, petty and corrupt officialdom. Madinto's predicament is presented as metaphorical of the social conflicts which confront township dwellers and how they are frustrated into anti-social acts such as alcoholism and petty thieving. The social outlaw identities that community members embrace do violence to their personal sense of morality and bring them into constant clashes with the police, ending in their imprisonment.

The children left alone represent the family in its most vulnerable state. It is at such moments that Kente's aesthetics and morality come into their own. Physical gestures, singing instead of dialogue, music and tableau all combine to produce excesses of meanings:

Bus rank in Soweto. It is late Friday afternoon. Ntanana is anxiously waiting for Saduva at the rank, with pale hungry lips she screens every bus load for him. It being Friday and people salaried, they pass her chewing something or other — fish and chips, fruits, sweets and so on. Ntanana's eyes cannot resist following their hands as they travel to their mouths. She even swallows saliva.

At one stage someone throws away orange peel. Ntanana just waits for the owner to disappear and goes for it. Her plight is enhanced by swelling voices in the winds, humming a touching hymn, "Ndilahlekile" I am lost (Enter Totozi). Finds her still feasting on an orange peel ... (Totozi) touched — battling to hold her tears back.[49]

The arrest of Madinto and Saduva for illicit liquor selling and for 'failing to produce' a pass provides the narrative with its most powerful signs for denouement. The narrative dismisses their 'crimes' and it focuses us instead on the baseness of a system bent on destroying family life. For instance, Madinto is primarily arrested for refusing another debased role that is forced on her, that of prostituting herself to Pelepele, the local policeman. Her decision to sell liquor is also presented as a defence of the social values of virtue, childhood and motherhood. Kente draws these links in a scene of tender pathos when on her release from prison, unaware of the death of Ntanana and with voices singing 'Ntanana kamama', she picks up a toy next to a dustbin and 'like a baby she hugs it and admires it' as she joins in 'Ntanana kamama'.[50]

In prison Saduva's experiences lead to a radical change in his character. Saduva summarises his character change with a simple rhetorical challenge to society: 'You don't expect me to be dumped in the wilderness with lizards and snakes and still come out the same'.[51] The moral of the play is straightforward: unless the social violence that regulates black life is redressed it will inevitably release its own equally destructive counter violence. The forms of violent responses possible are characterised into two types. The degenerate fall of once-virtuous individuals like Saduva into crime and hate and, secondly, the equally unwelcome possibility that black people could embark on forms of political and economic protest and action. The play's two possible endings conclude with the same warning to the authorities — who are presented as the only ones capable of any meaningful political intervention — to do something 'Before it's too late'.[52]

Spectacle, excess, and hyperbole are the frequent adjectives that are used, often pejoratively to describe melodrama. Such descriptions fail to convey the efficacy of cathartic rituals that melodrama re-creates in performance with its audiences. In *Too Late* the emphasis on experientially based rituals is an extension of its rejection of rationalist solutions, practical resolutions which, in South Africa, would be predicated on some form of political action. Instead Kente gestures towards the capacity in all of us to do good as the most feasible solution. The township community in *Too Late* possesses an indelible strength because of the communal sensibilities of its inhabitants. This worldview is nourished by the church which acts as the final refuge of the community. The interventions of the local priest, Mfundisi, who is critical of the support Christianity has given to apartheid, are the only ones, coming from blacks, that Kente approves of.

Woza Albert!, a collaborative work by Percy Mtwa, Mbongeni Ngema and Barney Simon, bridges, in many ways the different political solutions suggested in black theatre. *Woza Albert!* developed from a concept which Ngema and Mtwa had while they were touring as actors in Kente's *Mama and the Load*. *Woza Albert!* has as its narrative axis the fantastic question: what would happen if Morena, Jesus, in his second coming decides to land in the South Africa of the Eighties? How would the racially polarised communities view his responses to South Africa's political and socio-economic contradictions?

The narrative structure of *Woza Albert!* is divided into two main parts: firstly, a series of vignettes in the form of radio and television interviews with blacks. They are asked how they would respond to Morena's possible visit to South Africa and what they would expect him to do with regard to their welfare and that of blacks in general. The second part ensues when the improbable occurs and Morena arrives in South Africa and sides with the poor and oppressed masses. He is consequently arrested, escapes twice — on a cloud and by walking on the waters from Robben Island — and is killed by a torpedo during the latter escape. He again resurrects — the third coming? — this time together with the symbolic heroes of the liberation struggle, Albert Luthuli, Robert Sobukwe, Lilian Ngoye, Ruth First, Braam Fischer and Steve Biko. They are joined in a victory dance, the play's finale, by Zuluboy who stands as a symbol for the masses.

Apart from exploring the human suffering that confronts Africans as a result of apartheid, *Woza Albert!* also considers the resistance options open to Africans. *Woza Albert!* covertly translates this motif into a conflict between good and evil, Morena and his followers against the evils of apartheid. Equally important in the play's discourse is the consideration of the kind of Christianity that is relevant in South Africa. This is indicated in the play's rhetorical inversion of the prophecy of the second coming and the depiction of Christ as being concerned with the socio-political and spiritual well-being of people.[53] The enunciation of Christianity in *Woza Albert!* is similar to that advanced by the adherents of contextual theology and black theology. Both were influential social currents in the Seventies and especially within the Black Consciousness Movement.

One can see parallels with Kente's *Too Late* here and we can regard the doubting Thomases, Zuluboy and the musician, as variations of Saduva.

But whereas Kente called on the authorities to resolve the social conflicts, *Woza Albert!* offers somewhat ambiguous political solutions. In both plays, however, the doubting Thomases are won over by the power of religion. *Woza Albert's* typification of Morena's resurrection and interventions, which result in liberation, suggests either a complete predisposition towards divine intervention or political activism that is organised around Christianity. This ambivalence is reflected in the ending of the play which is a recreation of Morena's third resurrection. We leap from his death to the political victory of Africans with little account of the development or the link between these two phases. We can conclude that there is no need to specify what has been demonstrated by implication in the preceding scenes and what is after all a well known prophecy fulfilled. On the other hand, this silence can be read as reflecting the uncertain balance of power characterising current political struggles in South Africa. The songs and the victory celebration in *Woza Albert!* suggest, on the other hand, nationalist resistance. The victory dance is also ambiguous because it represents a political and racial unity that currently does not exist. Is it signifying unity as a prerequisite for liberation, or liberation as the prerequisite for unity, or both?

Notes in Conclusion

Black theatre, in its responses to apartheid, attempts to say everything and if a unifying theme can be found it is that of apartheid. An ogre of a theme, forever present, expansive and melodramatic as the plays themselves. At times the plays gesture, thematically, in all directions in a spectacular fashion with little analysis and contextualisation. It is as if the practitioners are confident that their audiences, and history, know and feel the story that is being retold and that they will make the necessary contextualisation. Their task is merely to reveal what is being repressed, to say what is being whispered and to demonstrate what will or must happen. Melodrama, it has been noted:

> comes into being in a world where the traditional imperatives of truth and ethics have been violently thrown into question, yet where the promulgation of truth and ethics, their installation as a way of life, is of immediate, daily, political concern.[54]

The efficacy of the morality operative within black performance cannot be dismissed. It spans a wide range of plays including those which consciously foreground history, politics and resistance in their discourse, such as *The Hungry Earth* and *uNosilimela*, to the dramas of Kente and their concern with the social experiences of urban dwellers. Melodrama speaks eloquently and profoundly elicits and communalises individual experiences of oppression and exploitation. It also confirms that, at the end of the day, righteousness shall triumph over injustice.

It is at such moments, when a moral discourse subsumes critical analysis and representation, that the plays sometimes depreciate the social and political clarity of their narratives. They are then rarely able to identify anything more than apartheid's overt manifestations, its grotesque violence, its destructive impact on human life and its imminent fall. Obviously the achievement of the latter conditions is in itself no mean political feat but frequently it is accompanied by simplifications, romanticism and contradictory formulations on South African history and political struggles. The results of these limitations can be seen in two areas that, in turn, have crucial political consequences.

Black theatre, in its content, has taken very little on board that has explored the specific concerns of the lower classes, workers and women. Recent productions emanating from the trade union movement have been more sensitive and democratic in their content, dealing with worker issues and community-centred ones. In *The Long March* the oppression and exploitation experienced on the factory floor is connected to its articulation with socio-political instances. There is concomitantly an equally marked emphasis on embarking on socialist projects and developing working class initiatives, participation and leadership. Secondly, black theatre has been unable to organise its internal structures differently from those characterising the social formation. African males predominate as performers, whites as 'skilled technicians' who mostly direct, and African women are reduced to the periphery in both numbers and status.[55] Within independent black initiatives this schema takes on a class rather than racially pronounced character. A great deal of exploitation, human, economic and political, is operative as a result, in the practice of black performance. It is imperative, then, that black performance address itself to the development of the politics of its counter narratives and that this process be extended, equally, to the ways in which theatre is socially organised in South Africa.

---

1 For a discussion of workers' theatre see my article 'Performing History of the State: Notes on Working Class Theatre', *Radical History Review*, 46/47 (1989).
2 B. Huss, 'Education Through The Drama', *Native Teacher's Journal*, January 1921, p. 48.

3 For a more detailed, if still tentative, discussion of Huss, and African uses of theatre in the period 1900-1940 see my paper All Work and No Play Makes Civilisation Unattractive to the Masses: The Emergent Formations of Theatre Amongst Africans from Fr. Bernard Huss to the Bantu Dramatic Society, Paper presented to the Division of African Literature Work in Progress Seminar, University of the Witwatersrand, 18 October 1989.

4 M. Cropper, Possibilities of Teaching by Drama, *The South African Outlook*, 1 March 1932, p. 59.

5 B. Huss, Education Through The Drama, p. 49.

6 See T. Couzens and N. Visser (eds), *H.I.E. Dhlomo, Collected Works* (Johannesburg, 1985) and N. Visser (ed.), *Literary Theory and Criticism of H.I.E. Dhlomo,* published as a separate issue of *English in Africa,* 4, 2 (1977).

7 A. Hoernle, The Bantu Dramatic Society at Johannesburg, *Africa,* April 1934, p. 223.

8 See N. Visser (ed.), *Literary Theory and Criticism of H.I.E. Dhlomo,* p. 38.

9 Interview published in *The Rand Daily Mail,* 8 May 1933.

10 J.C.W. Van Rooyen, *Censorship in South Africa* (Johannesburg, 1987), p. 3.

11 The results of the conference included the coordination of cultural practices on a national level through the Department of National Education, cabinet approval of a five-year plan to fund the arts and the setting up, in 1963, of four regional performing arts councils. See the *Report of the Commission of Inquiry into the Promotion of the Creative Arts* (Niemand Commission), August 1977, p. 3.

12 *The Star,* 7 March 1969.

13 *S'ketsh,* Summer 1975, p. 15.

14 *S'ketsh,* Winter 1975, p. 5

15 *The Attorney-General's Report, 1975: Documentary Exhibits, Charge Sheet and Other Materials for the 'Treason Trial',* p. 4.

16 *Rapport,* 13 May 1973.

17 For a presentation of the general harassment of individuals and groups involved in black theatre at about this time see Blackout clamp on Black Theatre in *The Star,* 6 June 1976.

18 See S.T. Greenberg, Ideological struggles within the South African state and D. Posel. The language of domination. 1978-1983. In S. Marks and S. Trapido (eds), *The Politics of Race, Class and Nationalism in Twentieth Century South Africa* (London, 1987).

19 Niemand Commission, 1977, pp. viii, 75.

20 *Report of the Commission of Inquiry into the Promotion of the Creative Arts* (Schutte Commission), March, 1984, pp. 1-4.

21 Van Rooyen, *Censorship in South Africa,* p. 12.

22 Ibid., p. 118.

23 Ibid., p. 11.

24 See The Address by the Minister of National Education, Mr F.W. de Klerk, on the occasion of the establishment of the Foundation for the Creative Arts in *South African Arts Calendar,* 14, 1 (1989), pp. 4-5.

25 See *The Star,* 25 May 1988 and *The Weekly Mail,* 20–26 May 1988 and 3-9 June 988.

26 M. P. Gwala, Towards a National Theatre. In *South African Outlook,* 1973, p. 132.

27 M. Manaka, *Egoli city of gold,* Johannesburg, n.d., pp. 3-4, emphasis added.

28 T. Couzens and N. Visser (eds), *H.I.E. Dhlomo, Collected Works,* p. 93.

29 M. Manaka, *Egoli,* p. 4.

30 See the following for various expositions of these objectives: S. Biko, *I Write What I Like* (London, 1984), pp. 69-72, 92-96; M. P. Gwala, Towards A National Theatre, pp. 131-33 and M. Manaka, The Babalaz People in *Staffrider,* 4, 3 (1981), pp. 32-34.

31 T. Hauptfleisch and I. Steadman, *South African Theatre: Four Plays and an Introduction* (Pretoria, 1984), p. 151.

32 R.M. Kavanagh, *South African People's Plays* (London, 1981), p. 8.
33 Ibid., p. 26.
34 Ibid., p. 26.
35 Ibid., pp. 48.
36 Ibid., pp. 58-61.
37 T. Hauptfleisch and I. Steadman, *South African Theatre*, pp. 153-55.
38 See L. White, Literature and History in Africa, *Journal of African History*, 21 (1980), pp. 539-540.
39 K. Sole, Identities and priorities in recent black literature and performance. Paper presented at the conference on Economic Development and Racial Domination, University of the Western Cape, 8-10 October 1984, p. 13.
40 T. Hauptfleisch and I. Steadman, *South African Theatre*, p. 153.
41 Ibid., p. 151. *Egoli* delivers the same verdict: 'There is no brotherly love, that is what is wrong with this country.' Manaka, *Egoli*, p. 9.
42 Hauptfleisch and Steadman, *South African Plays*, p. 155, emphasis in original.
43 See Manaka, *Egoli*, pp. 15-16.
44 See *Asinamali* in D. Ndlovu (ed.), *Woza Afrika! An Anthology of South African Plays* (New York, 1986), pp. 203-209.
45 R. Kavanagh, *South African People's Plays*, p. 68.
46 Ibid., p. 118.
47 My discussion of melodrama draws upon Peter Brook's excellent discussion of the genre in his *The Melodramatic Imagination*, (New York, 1984).
48 Ibid., p. 102.
49 Ibid., p. 111. See p. 113 for a similar presentation of the death of Ntanana.
50 Ibid., p. 115.
51 Ibid., p. 118.
52 Ibid., p. 123. The titles of Kente's plays tend to gesture towards their content, inter alia, *Can You Take It?*, *Mama and the Load*, *The Taximan* and *The Schoolgirl*.
53 D. Ndlovu, *Woza Afrika!*, p. 43.
54 P. Brook, *The Melodramatic Imagination*, p. 15.
55 The issue of sexism is, silently, contentious in black theatre. For the most recent glorifications of the subordination of women see Ngema's *Asinamali* in D. Ndlovu, *Woza Afrika!*

Trends in Zimbabwean Theatre Since 1980

STEPHEN CHIFUNYISE

At independence in 1980, Zimbabwe's black majority government adopted a policy of reconciliation as a strategy of transforming black-white relations which for over ninety years had been characterised by stark inequality. The effect of the policy of reconciliation was further enhanced by the formation of a government of national unity which included in its cabinet some members of the white minority regime. Theatre in Zimbabwe since 1980 has, in the main, been a response to these policies of reconciliation, non-racial development and socialism. Thus an analysis of Zimbabwean theatre is in many ways an assessment of the successes of and obstacles to the development of a non-racial and socialist culture in Zimbabwe. Since 1980 a number of trends in Zimbabwean theatre have developed. The first trend is that of theatre that had its roots in the liberation struggle in guerrilla camps in Mozambique and Zambia and inside the country's liberated zones. This is the theatre used by combatants to articulate the people's role and aspirations in waging a war of liberation. It was used to effectively tell the story of colonial occupation and the revolutionary history of the people's resistance since 1896. In the liberated zones inside the country, an all-night song-dance-political rally called *Pungwe* became the medium for the dramatisation of the people's struggle (*Chimurenga*) and the inevitable defeat of colonialism in Zimbabwe.

This dynamic use of the diverse and popular forms of indigenous performing arts, for instance traditional dance, ritual dances, poetic recitation, chants, slogans, songs and story-telling, enabled the combatants to mobilise the peasants to articulate their opposition to the settler white minority regime, and to consolidate the peasants' solidarity with the liberation struggle despite the punitive strikes by the forces of the Smith regime. The *Pungwe* enabled the combatants to concretise the ideology of socialism as an instrument of transferring political and economic power to the indigenous people of Zimbabwe.

In some ways, the new artistic experience forged largely in the guerrilla camps was not fully exploited once the war had ended. At independence, theatre artists who had been involved in the use of theatre as a revolutionary tool for articulating both the experience and the ideological dynamics of the liberation struggle returned home from Mozambique, Zambia, Tanzania, Europe, America and many African countries. Those who had been pioneers of this radical and innovative theatre were, upon their return home, either appointed to senior government positions or absorbed into the newly integrated national army. They did not find the time or the structures to use their experience in the development of theatre in independent Zimbabwe. The crucial absence of structures with high social and economic status for cultural workers was the main factor responsible for the disappearance of performing artists who had been very prominent in the war of liberation. Thus a valuable opportunity to make maximum use of a novel form of theatre in the newly liberated society was lost.

However, there was some continuity: many rural schools where the war of liberation had raged viciously continued with this trend of revolutionary theatre. Chindunduma Secondary School's *Takaitora Neropa* (We Took the Country by Bloodshed), performed in 1983, is an example of such theatre. Many other rural schools created plays on the war of liberation, its victims and its heroes. Another example of this theatre is Chaminuka Youth Training Centre's production of *Rivers of Blood* (1985) which dealt with the bombings by Rhodesian forces of children and youths in various refugee camps in Mozambique. The objective of this type of theatre was to conscientise the people of Zimbabwe about the history of the revolution. It aimed also to articulate the resolve of the people of Zimbabwe to defend their independence, especially in view of acts of destabilisation by South Africa and others which had already threatened Mozambique's survival and which for a long period disrupted peace and development in the Matabeleland Provinces of Zimbabwe.

Consolidation of 'white theatre'

In the heady early days of the post-independence era, white cultural institutions responded to the new policies of reconciliation, a non-racial society and non-racial cultural development with extreme caution. One such institution was the National Theatre Organisation (NTO) which had grouped together 'whites-only' clubs operating from what had been 'whites-only' playhouses and little theatres in Harare (Salisbury), Bulawayo, Gweru (Gwelo), Mutare (Umtali), Masvingo (Fort Victoria),

Kwekwe (Que Que), Kadoma (Gatooma), and other urban centres and mining towns. During the Rhodesian era, these theatre clubs had focused all their energies on policies that encouraged a separate cultural life and stressed a common 'European' heritage. The long-standing practice of bringing adjudicators from Britain for the annual theatre festival was intended to ensure that the kind of theatre which developed in the colony was consistent with that of Britain. And so the sense, or perhaps the illusion, of intimate links with the distant yet close mother-culture was carefully fostered.

However cautious, there were nevertheless significant shifts in the policy of the National Theatre Organisation after independence. The central trend became that of trying to draw to itself black theatre artists who would authenticate it as 'national', thereby enabling it to continue obtaining financial support from the new black government and the private sector. While there were no significant changes in its European theatre orientation, these accommodative gestures were interpreted as extending theatre skills to blacks who were said to have been denied such assistance during the colonial era. Although black theatre artists became members, there were no significant changes in the association's objectives, choice of plays by its clubs, the target audience, the ownership and use of theatre facilities. As the policy of reconciliation had ruled out nationalisation of economic institutions, there was no danger of cultural facilities such as the well-equipped and white owned theatre facilities being nationalised. Neither did the policy cause any change in the attitudes of city councils and multi-national companies which continued to give the white theatre establishment preferential financial support, in spite of the mass cultural demands of the new social order.

Thus in many ways there was nothing that challenged the 'white theatre' to transform or to accommodate to the new idea of a non-racial culture. The black theatre artists who joined the National Theatre Organisation at independence were determined to introduce into the white theatre establishment the kind of theatre that was consistent with the expectations of the new social order. Yet their impact, though initially significant, did not have any substantial effect on the nature of the white theatre establishment. One theatre club, which at first seemed to be moving in a new direction, was the Sundown Theatre directed by John Haigh. The club featured some of the country's leading black actors such as Walter Mparutsa, Dominic Kanaventi and John Indi. Its choice of Athol Fugard plays such as *The Island* and *Master Harold ... and the Boys* challenged the orientation of the white theatre establishment by discussing life in apartheid South Africa. However, this group did not go beyond this; they did not produce plays which dealt with life in Rhodesia which challenged the racist attitudes of white Zimbabweans. This suggests, possibly, that a kind of self-censorship was operating, because of the group's respect for the sensitivity of white Zimbabweans to such themes. The fact that the group produced these plays in the expected western theatre tradition and that it did not feature traditional performing arts, made its success insignificant in the broader development of Zimbabwean theatre.

Another pioneer theatre club to join the white theatre establishment was the People's Theatre Company whose production of Ben Sibenke's *My Uncle Grey Bonzo* made a tremendous impact in the 1982 National Theatre Organisation's annual theatre festival. The Company's other productions such as *Murume Murume* (1983) *Chidembo Chanhuwa* (1984) and *Dr Mazuma and the Vipers* (1987) showed quite clearly a new emphasis in Zimbabwean theatre, namely seizing the responsibility to discuss local issues. Other black theatre clubs have subsequently strengthened the concept of presenting in the National Theatre Organisation festival locally written plays which tackle local issues. A good example of this is Amakhosi Theatre with its production of Cont Mhlanga's *Nansi Lendoda* (Here's this Man) which won the best play of the year award in the National Theatre Festival in 1987. *Nansi Lendoda* discussed such problems and negative tendencies as corruption, nepotism, bribery, and sexual harassment at places of work and regionalism in independent Zimbabwe. Amakhosi's most successful play, *Workshop Negative,* dramatised the contentious and sensitive issue of corruption in high places and the fact that some of those leaders guilty of corrupt practices were championing socialism. Another key group was the Zimbabwe Arts Production which featured Dominic Kanaventi and Walter Mparutsa in collaboration with Andrew Whaley in the production *Platform Five* — the winner of 1988 National Theatre Festival's best play award.

In contrast to the energetic engagement with local issues shown by the black theatre groups affiliated to the National Theatre Organisation, white theatre clubs have totally ignored locally written and African plays. This has made their contribution to the development of Zimbabwean theatre negligible. Most of the movement's outstanding directors have remained as isolated from the theatre of the majority as they were in the pre-independence era. Neither have they been exposed to many exciting experiments in other theatre movements of independent Zimbabwe. Government sponsored theatre workshops which have aimed at democratising the acquisition of theatre skills have not been patronised by these directors, either because of their restrictive production schedules or because they have been seen as being irrelevant to the development of Zimbabwean theatre.

The National Theatre Organisation has to a large extent organised its year around its annual theatre festival and it is this festival that has been the chief attraction for many of the black theatre groups which became members of the Organisation. Yet here too problems have emerged — in this case around the issue of language. Certainly the theatre festival underwent some changes after 1980, the main change being the introduction by black theatre groups of plays in Shona and Ndebele. Unfortunately, when the organisation realised that foreign theatre artists were unable to adjudicate plays in these languages, it decided that local black theatre artists should be attached to foreign adjudicators. Some clubs then argued that the arrangement disadvantaged plays in indigenous languages. This led to the idea of co-adjudicators, a foreign adjudicator for plays in English and a local adjudicator mainly for plays in indigenous languages. It soon became evident that the inclusion of local theatre artists as adjudicators encouraged many black theatre groups to enter plays featuring a wide variety of indigenous performing arts in the country's indigenous languages. This infusion of new theatrical groups provoked a sharp and largely negative reaction.

Thus in 1988, the non-participation in the annual festival by the most well-known and well-established white theatre clubs was a sign that these clubs resented the success of black theatre groups which entered predominantly locally-written plays featuring indigenous languages and discussing local issues. White theatre clubs believed that such plays were awarded top prizes mainly because of their content and that the aspect of relevance of the content of plays overshadowed the artistic criteria for determining the best theatre productions. The festival has, therefore, begun to raise crucial questions on the role of competitive theatre in the development of Zimbabwean culture. The question of co-adjudicators has highlighted the fact that a trend has developed since 1980 which shows that white Zimbabweans are not prepared to produce African plays and plays which deal with the concerns of Zimbabwe. It is a trend that limits the contribution of white theatre to the development of non-racial culture in Zimbabwe. It also threatens to undermine the significance of the excellent work of the black theatre artists in the development of Zimbabwean theatre, as these artists become preoccupied with theatre for competitive festivals which are completely cut away from their own communities and the working class.

University Theatre

Another trend in Zimbabwean theatre is that illustrated by the University of Zimbabwe's Faculty of Arts Drama which began in 1984 with the appointment of Robert McLaren as drama lecturer. The most influential aspect of the Faculty of Arts Drama has been its annual major productions projects which have featured the participation of University students and lecturers, workers in the university and outside the university, secondary school teachers and pupils and non-university performing artists. This wide cross-section of participants has encouraged the use in these productions of an equally wide selection of indigenous performing arts, indigenous languages, a variety of theatre techniques and a wide diversity of themes. The Faculty of Arts Drama's major productions have included *Mavambo* (First Steps) — an adaptation of Wilson Katiyo's Novel *Son of the Soil* (1984), *I will Marry When I Want* (1985) by Ngugi wa Thiong'o and Ngugi wa Mirii, *Kremlin Chimes* (1987) by Nikolai Pogodin and *The Contest* (1988) by M. Rugyendo.

The major productions have turned the University of Zimbabwe into a cultural workshop where the talents and experiences of academics are married with those of artists and workers outside the university to produce illustrative theatre which appeals both to university and out-of university audiences. They have also successfully fulfilled the Faculty of Arts Drama's objective of using drama 'to develop an ideological direction in key with the most progressive elements in Zimbabwean society as represented by the liberation struggle, the struggle for majority rule, the struggle against racism, colonialism and the struggle for a socialist Zimbabwe'.[1] During the creation of major productions, drama students have acquired traditional performing arts skills not normally included in the University's drama courses.

These theatre productions have helped to demystify the idea of the university as an ivory tower by showing how students can learn from the working class skills necessary in the production of Zimbabwean performing arts. The working class has therefore come to the university campus not merely to consume but also to create, together with the university students, unique Zimbabwean theatre. In the production of *The Contest* and *Kremlin Chimes*, for example, major roles were taken by workers from outside the university.

Faculty of Arts Drama's major productions have also demonstrated that African Universities can become experimental workshops in the promotion of the performing arts of the African Continent. In *I Will Marry When I Want*, for example, most of the music and dance materials were drawn from Kenya and were taught by Ngugi wa Mirii who was a co-producer. Therefore the performance of the play became a pan-African cultural festival where students became cultural animators of performing arts of other African countries. This is consistent with the Faculty of Arts Drama's objective of contributing to the development of Zimbabwean theatre by basing 'its work on the lives, experiences, thoughts and culture of the Zimbabwean people and their brothers and sisters in other parts of Africa'.[2]

An important development brought about by this trend of theatre is the drawing into the university campus of audiences from different parts of Harare. Such non-racial audiences have been attracted by the wide diversity of performing arts featured in the productions: these have included, the varied choice of material for dramatisation, the unique use of English and the wide use of Shona and Ndebele in the plays, the adventurous use of a variety of theatre techniques and, most importantly, the fact that each production has introduced some aspects which have helped to illustrate what should constitute Zimbabwean theatre. In a newly independent African state that is determined to undermine the effects of almost a century of cultural domination, such theatre productions become effective tools in the struggle for cultural independence.

Another significant trend has been the pioneer work that has been produced as part of practical drama courses by students of English, African Languages, and Modern Languages. Productions such as *The Adamant Eve* (1985), *Seri Kwesasa/Okumsemsamo* (1985), *Zino Irema/Izinyo Lomthakathi* (1986), *Upenyu Here?* (Is This Life?) (1987), *Watch Me Fly* (1988) and *Chokwadi Ndechipi?* (What is the Truth?) (1988) have all illustrated the role of drama in national development, the advantage of collective-playmaking, and the dominant place of indigenous languages and performing arts in Zimbabwean theatre. This drama has enabled the University community to articulate its ideological orientation, express its understanding of the socio-economic and political realities of Zimbabwe and Southern Africa as well as critically examine itself and its relationship with the wider Zimbabwean society.

University as a Workshop for Political Theatre

Since 1980, most of the plays written by Zimbabwean playwrights fit well into the category of political theatre. The University of Zimbabwe's Drama Club has also played a role in this trend of theatre development. In 1984 the University Drama Club's production of Habakuk

Musengezi's *The Honourable MP* was the beginning of a trend in critical political theatre. *The Honourable MP* examines the contradictions which dominate the lives of politicians in independent Zimbabwe who advocate socialism while depending for their survival on the capitalist economic infrastructure. The establishment in 1985 of Zambuko/Izibuko Theatre as a university-based theatre with lecturers, students, workers, non-university students and unemployed youths as members effectively turned the university into a workshop for political theatre. Zambuko/Izibuko Theatre's most popular example of 'collectively-created' political theatre is *Katshaa!* (1985) — an anti-apartheid play that 'talked to Zimbabweans about the South African political struggle'[3] *Katshaa!* was created with an aim of winning the support of the people of Zimbabwe in the elimination of apartheid. Another example of Zambuko/Izibuko political theatre is *Samora Continua* (1988) which dealt mainly with the history of the Mozambican revolution and the place of the late Samora Machel in that history. These collectively-created plays have a political thrust which has made them suitable for commemorative and solidarity events and conferences. They have also effectively demonstrated how theatre artists, political and social scientists can use the performing arts to articulate effectively and collectively the people's ideological consciousness as well as the various facets of the revolutionary struggle in Southern Africa.

Challenging Male Chauvinism

Plays dealing with issues relating to women have also been a significant trend in the development of drama in Zimbabwe since 1980. Vashandi (Workers) Theatre's first major play soon after its formation in 1985, *Madzimai Pabasa* (Women at Work) presented the workers' view of sexual harassment at work places especially in factories and industries. This play successfully showed the vulnerability of uneducated women and tried to argue that women were involved in sex-for-job activities in order to guarantee their survival and that of their children. *Madzimai Pabasa* also attempted to articulate the need for laws to protect women against sexual harassment at work-places. But probably the most important point made by the play was that the re-orientation of men was as important in the eradication of male chauvinist tendencies as the education of women on how to fight such tendencies together.

The University of Zimbabwe Faculty of Arts Drama's *The Adamant Eve* (1985) whose production coincided with the last year of the Decade of Women, was based on research findings and media reports on the rights of women in Zimbabwe. *The Adamant Eve* which was described as 'an echoing chamber of women's voices'[4] questioned some of the male chauvinist customs and attitudes dominant in Shona and Ndebele cultures and in contemporary Zimbabwe. It exposed various types of sexual harassment of women at work places and articulated the role of women's organisations in the conscientisation of women in their struggle for equal rights.

In 1986, Vashandi (Workers) Theatre produced a topical dance-drama, *New Age*, the main aim of which was to explain the significance of the progressive Age of Majority Act. The Act brought down the age of adult suffrage to eighteen and abolished the colonial laws where 'African Women' were never considered adults throughout their lives. Before marriage, the 'African Woman' in colonial Rhodesia was under the custody of her father. Once married, that custody was transferred to her husband. The dance-drama dealt with the seduction of a girl who was an adult under the new law; and the demands made by her father for seduction charges to be paid instead of the girl receiving such payment as is provided for in the new Act. It highlighted the traditional customs of the people of Zimbabwe and expressed concern at the fact that the promotion of some aspects of custom and tradition gravely undermined the implementation of this progressive piece of legislation.

Just for Women Theatre, formed in 1987, has consistently occupied itself with women's issues. Its major production, *Waringa* — a dramatisation of an excerpt from Ngugi wa Thiong'o's Novel *Devil on the Cross* is a very eloquent portrayal of sexual harassment of women at work places and the predicament of educated young women. Although set in Kenya, *Waringa* articulates issues of major concern to working women in Zimbabwe. The play has been presented mainly at women's conferences and seminars. Other theatre groups have also focused on the contentious issue of women's status in the new Zimbabwe. One of the most travelled school leavers' full-time theatre groups, Theatrical Manoeuvres on the Stage, has since 1985 regularly featured my play *Not For Sale* which is a social comedy on the issue of *lobola*. The play examines the predicament of a young educated woman who refuses 'to be sold like a chicken' by her parents to her equally educated husband who insists that he must pay everything demanded by her parents!

Another play that deals with women's issues and has been popular in school performances throughout the country is Bertha Msora's *I Will Want* which raises various questions on the rights of girls in marital issues in Shona culture, and shows how complex the Shona traditional customs are. Tsitsi Dangaremgba, in her recent play *She no Longer Weeps* (1988), examines the attitudes of parents and the society to unmarried young women who have children. This play examines the traditional attitudes to marriage and why such women are considered as outcasts and 'prostitutes'. Another Zimbabwean playwright, Cont Mhlanga, has dealt with sexual harassment of underprivileged women at work places in urban areas of Zimbabwe in his play *Cry Isililo* (Cry Mourning, 1984) .

What has been a dominant trend in all these plays, which attempt to challenge patriarchal attitudes, is the use of socialism as a means to end negative male chauvinist traditions and to promote the idea of equality of women in independent Zimbabwe. The role played by women in the war of liberation has been used in some of these plays to condemn tendencies which have been responsible for relegating women to second class citizens and for their subsequent poor social and economic status. Unfortunately the influence of this type of drama has been undermined by a trend in the locally-produced radio and television drama where women have continued to be presented as sex objects and men's property and where the exploitation and domination of women — especially wife-beating! — have been presented as part of a unique cultural heritage. The best known example of such radio and television drama series is Safiriyo Madzikatire's *Mukadota Family* which is based on the most dominant male chauvinist aspects of Shona culture, although most of the episodes of this drama series are set in an urban environment. Other drama series which have consolidated this unfortunate trend are dramatisations of Shona novels. Women are presented in these plays in a way that challenges the provisions of legislation, which has given women new rights since independence. There is thus a tension between the conservatism put out through the medium of radio, and the more radical, modern vision of the live plays.

Expressing Workers' Aspirations

One of the most important actions taken by Zimbabwe's black majority government at independence was the establishment of minimum wage levels applicable to all workers. The class of workers that benefited most from this action was that of domestic and farm workers who had received the lowest and most exploitative wages during the colonial era.

It is therefore not surprising that it is the domestic and farm workers who were the first class of workers to use drama in independent Zimbabwe to express their plight and aspirations. The first drama group of workers to receive prominent press coverage was the Shingayi Domestic Workers Drama Group formed in 1984. The group's play *Shingayi Mumatambudziko* (Be Courageous) (1985) eloquently discussed the exploitation of domestic workers during the colonial era and how that exploitation had persisted in the independence era. Fambidzanai Agricultural Cooperative Theatre Group's production of *Tikiti Wanga Bwana* (My Job-Card Boss) (1986) is an example of theatre that dealt with the plight of farm workers. In this play, a white farmer sells his farm to a black businessman and emigrates to South Africa. The new farm owner, whom the farm workers expect to be sympathetic to their plight, unfortunately turns out to be worse than the former white owner. Eventually, with state support, the workers instigate action that forces the new owner to lose the farm to the workers who form a cooperative.

Bulawayo-based domestic workers' theatre group, Kuwirirana Theatre Production's *Akusimlanda Wami* (It is not my Fault) (1987) was regarded by the *Sunday Mail* theatre critic, T. Nyakunu as 'the most convincing analysis of problems being faced by domestic workers in Zimbabwe. It is a play with a message to employers of domestic workers as well as to all workers in Zimbabwe'. Another workers' theatre group that articulated workers' aspirations was the Vashandi (Workers) Theatre which produced a successful play, *The Movement* (1986), dealing with the problems in the Zimbabwe Congress of Trade Unions (ZCTU) which the group felt made the workers' movement ineffective. The play discussed the need for stronger worker solidarity and advocated trade union education.

In 1987, Manyame Theatre, comprising workers from different sectors of the economy, also examined the problems of workers in its play *Chimbadzo* which showed how they were exploited by their fellow workers when they borrowed money, for emergency cases, and returned it with more than 100% interest. The play showed that exploitative tendencies were also prevalent among the working class itself. One of the most eloquent analyses of the exploitation of workers during the colonial era was *Upfumi ne VaShandi* (Wealth and Workers) (1987) by Zimbabwe Theatre Workers Cooperative. In this play, the exploitation of workers in various sectors of the economy was presented mainly in song and dance. The play articulated the workers' determination to own the means of production and to contribute to the establishment of a socialist Zimbabwe. Andrew Whaley's *Nyoka Tree* (1988), produced by Meridian Theatre, examined the racial dimension of employer and employee relationship in Zimbabwe. This is a topic that has not been a feature of Zimbabwean theatre. One reason for this may be the fact that art that examines white and black relationship in independent Zimbabwe might have been seen as pre-empting the results of the policy of reconciliation and the idea of creating a non-racial Zimbabwe.

Moses Bhowa's *Ndizvo Here?* (Is This Right?) (1987), performed by the Nyanyadzi Theatre Productions explored the relationship between peasants and the white-collar workers, such as teachers and nurses, who work in rural areas. This play expressed the negative attitude of the white and blue collar workers towards peasants. This was indeed a new dimension as it was theatre that articulated the class positions of workers in independent Zimbabwe and showed the absence of solidarity among members of the working class caused by weak class consciousness.

Grassroots Theatre

In 1982 the Zimbabwean government employed two Kenyan theatre artists, Ngugi wa Mirii and Kimani Gecau of Kamiriithu Theatre Community to help in the establishment of community-based theatre in Zimbabwe. The two theatre artists were attached to the Zimbabwe Foundation for Education with Production (ZIMFEP) which created a community theatre project as part of its programmes. In order to demonstrate various concepts of community-based theatre, the two theatre artists worked with Chindunduma Secondary School, one of ZIMFEP's first schools for ex-combatants and orphans of the war of liberation, to produce *The Trials of Dedan Kimathi* by Ngugi wa Thiong'o and Micere Mugo. In producing this play, the dramatists used the student's own experiences in the war of liberation and the community's performing arts. The success of the tour of *The Trials of Dedan Kimathi* to various parts of the country showed that many communities were starved of theatre and demonstrated the need for community-based theatre throughout the country. The tour also demonstrated the type of theatre that appealed to the grassroots and underlined why the success of community-based theatre depended very much on the use of performing arts common in the community and dealing with the community's concerns

The promoters of the idea of community-based theatre received a tremendous boost from the African Workshop on Theatre for Development which was held in Zimbabwe in 1983. Popular theatre artists and other pioneers of theatre for development from 22 African countries used the workshop to experiment with the theatre for development processes which showed how the community can use theatre to identify development problems, seek their solutions and agree on programmes of collectively implementing the problem-solving strategies.

Since 1983, the Zimbabwe Foundation for Education with Production has joined hands with the Department of Culture in promoting the establishment of theatre on the community level and the idea of theatre development. This has been done through theatre skills workshops at district, provincial and national level where techniques in collective-play making and theatre for development processes were demonstrated. It is these workshops which have led to the establishment of theatre groups at the grassroots level through out the country.

By 1986, when the community-based theatre groups formed the Zimbabwe Association of Community Theatre (ZACT), a unique community theatre trend had been established. Non-competitive solidarity theatre festivals became the dominant feature of ZACT. This was demonstrated by its 1986 Solidarity Theatre Festival in recognition of the Non-Aligned Movement's anti-imperialist stand and solidarity with the struggling people of South Africa and Namibia. The festival was held during the 8th NAM Summit in Harare. Collectively-written plays performed in the one-week solidarity festival included *The South African Prisoner* by Manyame Theatre, *Goodbye Apartheid* by Tafara Theatre Productions, *The Boy Who Went To Jail* by Shingai Domestic Workers' Theatre, *We Shall Strike Harder* by Vashandi Workers Theatre, *Revolution* by Chidhembo Theatre, *Liberation Struggle* by St Michael's Church Theatre and *Katshaa!* by Zambuko/Izibuko theatre. These plays were performed in various communities and workers' townships.

Another significant trend established by the Zimbabwe Association of Community Theatre was its adoption and publication of a political calendar in 1987 in which community-based theatre groups participated in the commemoration of national and international days. These included Independence Day, Workers' Day, United Nations Day, World Health Day, World Literacy Day, South African Youth Day (Soweto Day), Heroes Day and World Theatre Day. This encouraged community-based theatre groups to create plays for these commemorative days and these performances became regular community-based theatre festivals. The strategy of collective-play creation has enabled these theatre groups to present performances that deal with issues of concern to the community and are consistent with the themes of these national and international days.

The obvious power of grassroots theatre has led to further initiatives. Local and international non-governmental development agencies who have become familiar with the work of community-based theatre groups and the effectiveness of community theatre festivals as vital media for development, have established links which have led to the promotion of campaign plays. These are plays created to support country-wide campaigns in such areas as primary health care, literacy, cooperatives and environment education. Using theatre for development techniques, community-based theatre groups have used scientific data and technical information provided by development agencies and government departments to create campaign plays which have been sponsored for performances outside the groups' own communities.

One of the most significant trends brought about by the grassroots theatre movement has been the establishment of full-time theatre groups mainly comprising school leavers. By the end of 1988 there were nine full-time groups in the Zimbabwe Association of Community Theatre. A unique feature of this full-time theatre is that it is mainly a form of travelling theatre to schools and colleges. For many years, the established theatre and the white-dominated National Theatre Organisation claimed that professional theatre was not possible in Zimbabwe. It is this travelling theatre trend that has made the most significant impact in the promotion of Zimbabwean theatre in the remotest parts of Zimbabwe. A major feature of these travelling theatres are the workshops which are held for drama clubs in schools and for newly formed community-based theatre groups. These workshops have dealt mainly with collective play making, theatre for development techniques and the use of indigenous performing arts in the production of theatre. The workshops have not only helped in the promotion of theatre skills in rural areas but have helped in the identification of community-based performing artists who have acted as resource persons in the use of indigenous performing arts in theatre.

Zimbabwe Association of Community Theatre's political orientation and its policy of solidarity festivals has established very strong links with liberation movements of South Africa and Namibia as well as with community-based and popular theatre movements in Botswana and Zambia. Contact with theatre artists in the liberation movements has helped community-based groups to create useful and relevant political theatre on Southern Africa. Other contacts have been established through a performance tour of Botswana by such groups as Zimbabwe Theatre Works, Iluba Elimnyama Theatre Productions, Amakhosi Theatre Productions and Taako Theatre. Successful performance tours of Zimbabwe have been undertaken by Zambia's leading 'theatre for development' group, the Kanyama Theatre Productions. These contacts have become the most dominant cultural exchange programmes initiated and implemented at the grassroots level with neither state financial support nor the use of government administrative structures. This trend has the potential to develop into a movement of cultural exchange between the various grassroots cultural organisations in Southern Africa. It could also lead to the establishment of sub-regional, non-competitive and solidarity theatre festivals at grassroots levels.

Cultural Gala Drama

Since 1985 a trend has also developed where drama features prominently in the Independence Anniversary Cultural Gala which is attended by the nation's political and civic leaders and representatives of various mass organisations. Most of the people who attend this state occasion are not regular theatre goers. Therefore, the Independence Anniversary Cultural Gala has introduced drama to many people who would normally have no time for it or who live in communities which have no access to drama.

The drama that has been presented in all cultural galas has tended to use a variety of agit-prop theatre techniques and a wide diversity of performing arts such as traditional dance, poetic recital, revolutionary (*chimurenga*) songs, story-telling, chants, slogans, choral music, mime and dance-drama. The use of these predominantly traditional performing arts and the use of Shona and Ndebele has made it possible to present a drama that appeals to a wide cross-section of the Zimbabwean society as well as one that is easily adaptable to the theatre-in-the-round formation dictated by the structure of the Harare International Conference Centre where the gala is presented annually. Another very significant feature of the 'cultural gala drama' is the consistent trend of dealing with very current national concerns and problems as its content. In 1985 the drama consisted of an excerpt from Zambuko/Izibuko Theatre's *Katshaa!* The following year Chidembo Theatre presented Aaron C. Moyo's *Kuridza Ngoma Nedemo* which examined the issue of land resettlement and the type of land reforms Zimbabwean peasants expected at independence. In 1987 the drama took a panoramic view of the major political events of that year and their implications for socialist development in Zimbabwe. The 1988 drama traced Zimbabwe's political history from the first anti-colonial resistance of the 1890s to the signing of the unity accord between ZANU (PF) and PF-ZAPU in 1987. Those who attend the Independence Anniversary Cultural Gala therefore expect the drama item to make very important political statements. They expect the drama to be an example of critical but constructive art, one which shows how theatre artists can play a role in the promotion of the ideological consciousness consistent with the aspirations of the majority of the people of Zimbabwe.

So far, the fear that such drama, supported by the state and featured in state-sponsored programmes would be used as a tool for 'domesticating' the people and appeasing the political leadership has not been justified. In both the 1987 and 1988 dramas there were vivid portrayals of political leaders who were preoccupied with activities which President Robert Mugabe had condemned. Therefore the 'cultural gala drama' has

demonstrated that political theatre does not have to be confrontational
and disrespectful to be critical and revolutionary.

Although many skills training workshops on 'community based theatre'
and 'theatre for development' have been held since 1983, they have not
offered as comprehensive a training in a 'collective-drama-making
process' as the preparations of these cultural gala dramas. Once the
gala's implementing team has decided on the overall theme of the gala, a
team comprising representatives of Zimbabwe Writers Union, University
of Zimbabwe's Faculty of Arts Drama, The Zimbabwe Foundation for
Education with Production, the Zimbabwe Association of Community
Theatre, Zimbabwe Integration Through the Arts and the National
Theatre Organisation meet to produce the drama's story line. The
'cultural gala drama' is then collectively created by members of a number
of community-based theatre groups over a period of four to six weeks.
The end-product has often taken care of various political views of the
cast and those of the cultural gala implementing committee. The
rehearsals of the drama have also become theatre training sessions in
order for all the members of the cast to reach high levels of competence
in traditional dancing, playing of traditional musical instruments and
acting. The most revolutionary aspect of the 'cultural gala drama' has
been the idea of collective-directing. In some cases the entire cultural
gala implementing committee consisting of dancers, musicians,
dramatists, writers and visual artists has taken part in collective-directing
of the drama. Another very important aspect of this 'cultural gala drama'
is that it has been presented by school leavers who have taken theatre as
a full-time profession. The occasion has therefore enabled parents to
have a taste of professional theatre and to appreciate that full-time
theatre is a worthwhile occupation.

Conclusion

In this discussion, I have tried to show that since 1980, Zimbabwe has
witnessed a most dynamic development in the field of theatre. The
various trends discussed above have been caused by a rapidly
transforming socio-economic, political and cultural environment on the
one hand, and attempts by sections of Zimbabwean society to resolve
contradictions created by the long history of cultural and political
domination, on the other. This diversity of theatre development is without
doubt an indication of the level of freedom of expression and association,
although some plays in their forthright criticism of topics like corruption
have met with a measure of resistance. Also important has been the result

of the influence of the political situation in South Africa on the production of culture in Zimbabwe.

Unfortunately the mass media in Zimbabwe have not been adequately equipped to assess the different and innovative trends of theatre in the country. This weakness has been caused, to a great extent, by the continued dominance of the mass media by those associated with the movement for the consolidation of 'white theatre'. The absence of grassroots publications and the inability of grassroots mass cultural organisations to use formal mass media has also led to the inadequate exposure of the success and the popularity of grassroots theatre trends in Zimbabwe. The tension therefore between a vital theatre movement reflecting people's aspirations and mass media which are unresponsive, even hostile, to this new theatre has yet to be resolved.

In the event the youth theatre collapsed as the membership melted away, some sent to their rural homes, others managing to find employment, yet others simply demoralised by the absence of their friends. But work on the women's play continued into a further year after another performance discussion with the authorities. It was realised that for the women, who had in the meantime formed themselves into a catering co-operative called *Budiriro* (Success in Shona) the crucial concern was an improvement in their earning capacity. They came to doubt that the ongoing dialogue with the authorities was sufficient reason for continuing to work on the play. It was decided that to demonstrate the students' sensitivity to the issue of the need for material assistance, two of the students would stage a performance of the play, *Egoli* by South African playwright, Matsemela Manaka, in order to raise funds for them.

The origins of this performance are interesting in themselves. The students had performed an extract from the play as a practical assignment in their first year. This had been so successful that they went on to stage the entire play, both at the Univerisity and at other venues in Harare, Bulawayo and so-called Matabeleland. Posters were put up in Mbare and the women were provided with invitations to distribute among their friends in the hostels. Very few turned up. This was also true of the 'performance' for the local authorities later on. While most of those invited by the students attended, those who it was expected would be mobilised by the women, namely the community, did not. It became clear that the women were either not able or not willing to mobilize community support for what they were trying to do.

Another aspect of this round of the work was that the efforts to develop in-character discussion within and during the performance, were becoming more successful. Thus the discussion between the women of the Budiriro Co-operative and the authorities was ultimately relatively effective and produced tangible results. Yet these gains were in themselves problematical. For instance, a foreign-based organisation offered to provide fridges. The offer ran into problems when the women realised that it was also being extended to the other women's co-operatives with whom they shared the dining room.

A number of conclusions suggested themselves after this, the final round of the University's work with the women of Matapi. Firstly, it became clear that the University is a very viable pad from which to launch pilot projects but it is not by itself able to sustain and carry through theatre for development work with the consistency, commitment and tenacity that would be required to transform a pilot scheme into an effective campaign. It is therefore essential that theatre for development work be based in specialist structures either outside or relatively autonomous of educational institutions.

The inability of the women to mobilise their own community to participate in the process — or even to attend fund-raising performances — indicated the need to be highly flexible in the planning of theatre for development projects. The only way to have enlisted the participation in any numbers of the Matapi residents would have been by demonstrating that the drama the women were doing could be entertaining enough to sacrifice, for an hour or two, either relaxation in the beerhall or the struggle for survival. Theatre as a process of analysis and discussion is not likely to do that. It became clear that work needed to be done with the women to produce a more formal play, hard-hitting, topical and artistically entertaining and effective.

Finally, the students' own play, *Chero Tiri MuHarare,* proved to have exactly those qualities. It was in itself an example of community theatre in so far as the roles of the children were played by volunteers from a nearby primary school. The Matapi women were invited to a performance after which a discussion was held commenting on the development from the material as part of the theatre for development process to that of a fully-fledged polished theatre performance.

Thus a strategy with which to continue the work begun in Matapi — had there been a structure with the autonomy and organizational capacity to carry it through — would have been to mobilise the Matapi community into the debate through performances of *Chero Tiri MuHarare* or a more entertaining formal play by the women and then to perform either one or both plays widely to a wider audience, attracting in the process as much publicity as possible to the plight of the people of Matapi. The combined pressure of a mobilized Matapi community and a nation made aware of their situation might, in the long run, have sparked off significant moves to bring about changes.

However, *Chero Tiri MuHarare* stressed that the underlying causes of phenomena like Matapi are to be found in a system in which people are either unemployed or employed but not paid enough to ensure a decent livelihood — which brings us back to the question raised at the outset concerning the long-term validity of theatre for development. Such a system has to be revolutionised and for a theatre that promotes such exigency the only genuine basis for development is revolution. The theatre worker must ultimately make a choice — theatre for development as a reformist attempt to make a bad system easier to put up with or theatre for development as a revolutionary bid to transform that system in the interests of those who suffer at its hands.

1 Notes on programme of the Faculty of Arts Drama's production of *Chokwadi Ndechipi?/Iqiniso yiliphi?* (Which is the Truth?).

2 Notes on programme of the Faculty of Arts Drama's production of *Zino Iremal/Izinyo Lomthakathi* (The Wizard's Tooth) (1986).

3 Notes on programme of Zambuko/Izbuko Theatre's production of *Katshaa!* (1985). The text has now been published.

4 Notes on programme of the Faculty of Arts Drama's production of *The Adamant Eve* (1985).

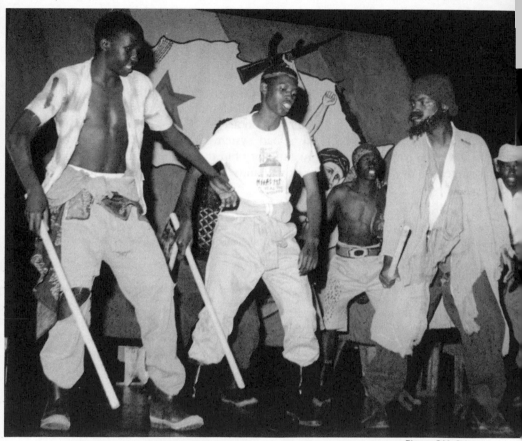

Actors from the Mufakose-based theatre group, Chevhu NdeChevhu, and others in a scene from Zmbuko/Izibuko's *Mandela, The Spirit of No Surrender* (See Theatre for Development in Zimbabwe).

Backstage on the Frontline: Iluba Elimnyama — a Bulawayo Theatre Collective

EVIE GLOBERMAN

Community-based theatre has become an increasingly popular mode of cultural expression in Zimbabwe since Independence in 1980. In Bulawayo, the capital of Matabeleland North Province, there are now thirty-four theatre groups operating in the high-density suburbs or townships, more than double the number that existed in 1986. Comprising mainly unemployed school-leavers, township theatre groups produce plays that reflect the socio-political concerns of students, workers and peasants. In this short piece I want to concentrate on a play by one such group which focuses on women's issues in the country. Besides tackling this necessary but still neglected area, the group has addressed itself to other political issues such as the need for unity in the country, in *Bloodbrothers*, and the South African question, in *Manqoba* and *Blackfist — Lingesabi*.

Iluba Elimnyama (Black Flower) Experimental Theatre Workshop is typical of the many township drama groups currently producing shows in Bulawayo. Based in a ramshackle, concrete-slab clubhouse in Njube township, Iluba operates as Bulawayo's first theatre collective. The group has six members, two women and three men, a balanced gender mix that is rare for theatre groups in the city. Many parents still disapprove of theatre as an occupation for their daughters, preferring unemployed young women to help out in the family home rather than become too intimately involved in working with the single men who dominate the community-based theatre movement. The women in Iluba have had to overcome family resistance to their chosen work, as well as learn to assert themselves within the group. Like most township companies, Iluba writes, directs and produces original plays. Themes are chosen during 'brain-storming' sessions, where a wide variety of possible subjects are considered. The group comes to a consensus over artistic matters after democratic debate, a process that Iluba has perfected in recent years.[1] Plays are built through a process of improvisation and discussions, with the final product roughly scripted in the end. Because of the improvisational nature of the work, it is common for sections of the play to remain flexible. Thus scripts are not available in final or published versions, and often consist of individual parts hand-written on sheets of paper in the possession of the actors. Actors also frequently improvise during performance and incorporate topical news items or jokes into a scene. The language of production is mainly Ndebele, although the group switches to English and Shona with ease when they wish to.

The members of the Iluba collective adopted drama as a profession in 1986. A few of the actors left other occupations, such as piece-work embroidery and Red Cross work, but the majority of township theatre workers have spent their post-school years searching unsuccessfully for employment. Like other township actors, Iluba are directly involved in the social and economic hardships faced by Zimbabweans and their plays translate these experiences into performative texts that have become a popular form of community entertainment. Their performances usually take place in community halls which have very few production facilities. Plays are performed with a minimum of sets, costumes and props, and lighting is provided by low watt electric bulbs hanging bare from the ceiling. The frugality of the shows reflects the financial constraints under which they and other township groups operate, but the simplicity of the productions does not undermine the dynamic energy of the plays.

Like most groups, Iluba opens a production with a curtain raiser of 'traditional' songs and dances. Audiences have come to expect this musical prelude which gives the spectators a chance to gather and settle into their seats, and also functions as a kind of 'bonus', hearkening back to the custom of giving the first customer in the market some extra tomatoes as a gesture of goodwill. Certainly music and dance are integral to Iluba's plays, and are used to comment upon the action, link scenes together and encourage audience participation. The principle of directly involving the audience is central to the group's artistic practice. Members of the community are invited to give comments about a production after a performance, and local people who happen to come into the rehearsal hall are encouraged to offer opinions about the work in progress.

Impilo-le (Oh, this life) was Iluba Elimnyama's first full-length production and directly confronts the question of gender and equality in a post-liberation era that still has to wrestle with patriarchal attitudes which permeate many aspects of society. The Khoza family in *Impilo-le* make up a typical township household. The father works as a City Council gardener, earning barely enough to support his wife and two children. Mrs Khoza, an employed housewife, operates a shebeen from the home in an effort to contribute to the family's income. The action of the play chiefly concerns the Khozas' son, Vuma, and his younger sister, Senzeni.

Like thousands of school-leavers in Zimbabwe, including most township actors, Vuma has passed his 'O' Levels but is unable to find a job. Frustrated by his situation, Vuma teams up with a gang of *tsotsis* (thugs), who tempt him with the potential profits of a planned shop-lifting caper. He soon becomes disillusioned with this and returns to his family a repentant man.

Senzeni's story highlights the situation faced by many girls in the country. She becomes infatuated with Max, a married man who frequents Mrs Khoza's shebeen. Believing that Max is in love with her and knowing nothing of his wife, she neglects her schooling to spend time with her new 'sugar-daddy'. She falls pregnant, suddenly she is desperate and terribly alone.

Iluba's intention in the clinic scene, where Senzeni discovers her pregnancy, was to show how young women are abandoned by the community at a time when they most need support. Dr Sibindi, the insensitive clinic doctor, informs Senzeni of her condition, and in spite of the young woman's obvious shock and impending panic, congratulates her as he rushes off to conduct his hospital rounds. The clinic nurse rather officiously instructs Senzeni to eat eggs and drink milk, answering questions about abortion with a resounding negative. In Zimbabwe abortion is not a legal option for healthy young women like Senzeni. The alternative that first springs to Senzeni's mind is to 'dump' the child immediately after it is born, a horrible option that in 1986 was receiving frequent national press coverage. Many young mothers without any means to support their illegitimate offspring were abandoning babies in drainpipes, rubbish bins and public toilets. Iluba discovered in researching this play that township clinics often humiliate unmarried women who request family planning devices, accusing them of being prostitutes. To avoid such embarrassment, young women often remain unprotected against conception. The irony is that when these women do become pregnant, their boyfriends frequently deny paternity and accuse the women of being whores; the infuriating argument of such men is that if their girlfriends have slept with one man, they must have slept with others!

Senzeni's plight is indeed a representative one. Her family and lover reject her; Max refuses to accept any responsibility for the child, and his wife from the rural areas makes it very clear that she will not accept a polygamous marriage, a possible method of resolving this kind of situation. Increasingly depressed, Senzeni returns to her father's house, only to be driven away once she has confided her condition. The Iluba actors wanted *Impilo-le* to do more than just present a case history of 'sugar-daddies' and 'baby-dumpers'. They felt the play should provide a critical commentary on a very important social problem. When they were struggling to write the ending of the play, the first obstacle that the group had to overcome was their automatic tendency to condemn the woman and excuse the man. Many actors, including some women in the group, felt at first that Senzeni alone should be held responsible for her condition. Max was exempt from blame because he is a man, and real men should not be expected to control their sexual urges! Iluba's initial bias against Senzeni reflected the chauvinistic views of the community, and it was a brave step for the group when they chose, after much debate, to offer a conclusion to the play that challenged the attitudes of their elders.

In the last scene of *Impilo-le* the entire family gathers at the Khozas' house for the final resolution. Before Senzeni's entrance, there is a short scene in which the young woman returns to Max's house and threatens to take him to court for paternity and maintenance. This action, modest as it might seem by western standards, was greeted with thunderous applause by female members of the audience, leaving the actors little doubt of how many women have not had the confidence to demand even basic rights for themselves and their children. Fearing negative publicity, Max finally agrees to follow Senzeni to her parent's house in the company of a relative who will act as his spokesperson. According to Ndebele custom, Max cannot speak directly to Mr Khoza, who is considered to be the injured party.

Having Max accompany Senzeni to her parent's home was considered a bold and revolutionary step. Audience members were amazed at Senzeni's courage, and waited with eager, vocal anticipation to see a 'sugar-daddy' being forced to apologise to a father for 'damaging' his 'property'. Mr. Khoza has paid *lobola* (brideprice) for his wife, and thus the children of the marriage belong to him. Women are traditionally, although not legally, considered to be minors regardless of age, which is why Khoza not Senzeni, negotiates with Max's relative.

The scene tries to combine traditional and modern ideas to suggest that women like Senzeni, should be re-integrated into their families, thereby averting the 'baby-dumping' scenario. In the end, Max agrees to pay maintenance for the child once it is born, a promise that was greeted with female ululations and cheers.

The play highlights the difference in the treatment of the son and daughter in the Khoza family, thus bringing gender discrimination into the play's ambit. When Vuma confesses his role in the theft of a radio, his parents are disappointed, but they do not at any time give the impression that he will be rejected by the family. Senzeni, on the other hand, is driven from the house with only a blanket and a few scraps of clothing when she admits her pregnancy. The boy's punishment is to be sent to his grandmother's village to plough for a season, during which time he is expected to reflect upon his past mistakes. Senzeni is not treated with the same degree of tolerance, and is not automatically given a chance to make amends to the family. The inequitable treatment of sons and daughters was not adequately addressed in the play, although audience members were invited to engage in critical thinking about their own prejudices against women.

In 1988 the government announced progressive legislation governing the maintenance of children belonging to legal, traditional and common-law marriages. *Impilo-le* was toured throughout Bulawayo in 1987, while in other parts of Zimbabwe theatre groups produced their own versions of 'baby-dumping' plays. Products like *Impilo-le* helped to focus government and public attention on the need for strict legislation to protect unemployed mothers from being left economically stranded by the fathers of their children.

---

1 Iluba Elimnyama trained for two years under Theatre Project, a Bulawayo City Council school-leaver drama programme set up by the author in August 1986, and funded by CUSO, a Canadian aid agency that works closely with the co-operative movement in Zimbabwe. I worked with the group from August 1986–August 1988. The training involved daily classes in improvisation, movement, mime, mask, voice and play-making, as well as seminars on theatre administration and group work.

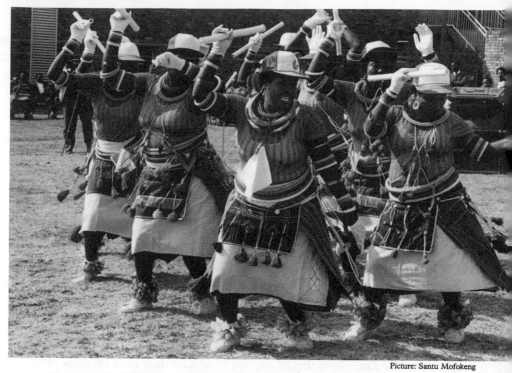

Women's *kiba*: Ditšhweu tša Malebogo performing at Funda Centre, Soweto.

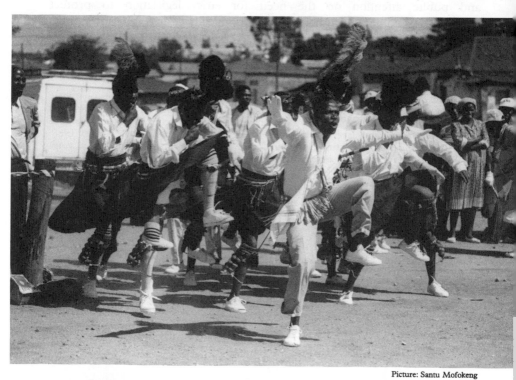

A group performing men's *kiba:* the regimental song *monti* in Alexandra Township, Johannesburg.

Basadi ba baeng/*Visiting Women: Female Migrant Performance from the Northern Transvaal*[1]

DEBORAH JAMES

A concern with female migrant performance and its relationship to that of migrant men reveals two major, and linked, areas of neglect in the literature about the Southern African region. The first is a gap in the literature on migrancy and on the accompanying processes of land deprivation, rural deprivation, and the like. Approaches in the 'political economy' vein to understanding migration tended to overlook the cultural processes through which people came to terms with, and reconstructed for themselves, the migrant experience. This emphasis has been counterbalanced by recent writings, some of which have been specifically concerned with poetry, song lyrics, and performance.[2] But, with the exception of Coplan's work on *lifela* aurature from Lesotho, none of this work has taken account of the emergence or development of women's genres alongside those of men.[3]

A look at the literature specifically devoted to gender issues in Southern Africa indicates little attempt to redress this imbalance. Recent studies of changing gender roles have left us with an awareness of the economic and political underpinnings of these roles, but with little understanding of the way they are culturally constructed or enunciated.[4] Specifically, writers have neglected to investigate the transformations of female performance and practice of such things as music and oral literature. Again, there are exceptions, but these deal primarily with rural-based genres rather than with those emerging in the context of migrancy.[5]

This paper, attempting to address some of these unanswered questions, will examine a migrant performance genre of men and women from the northern Transvaal. The male form of the genre, based on rural performance, has evolved during nearly a century of rural-urban migration. Migrant women's song and dance, although similarly linked to pre-existing rural performance, has only recently claimed an identity equivalent to that of men. The fact that men's and women's music have been defined as versions of the same genre obscures a number of discontinuities, both social and stylistic.

Socially, male migrant musicians have their origins in areas and socio-economic circumstances very different from those of the members of their female partner-groups. Where the men have played the same music since childhood, most of the women began to play in the 'traditional' style, borrowed from rural women, only after coming to town to find work. Stylistically, the strong continuities in men's music and dance give it the quality of a heroic discourse, rooted in an idiom which celebrates the glorious past of independent chiefs. Women, claiming definition within this genre which was previously the proper domain of men, have used its grandiose and heroic idiom, but at the same time subverted it. They have created an identity which both partakes of and distinguishes itself from that of men.

The annual party of SK Alex

At the piece of open ground next to the No 1 Men's Hostel in Alexandra, the dance group *SK Alex*[6] held its annual party one Sunday late in 1990. They spent their accumulated savings from the year's performances on a variety of drink and food, of which the most important item was a sheep which was slaughtered at midnight on Saturday and by Sunday morning was cooking in a series of black pots on an open fire. The honoured guests, who arrived at midday, were *Bapedi Champions*, a group representing the same home area in the northern Transvaal, but based in the Benoni township of Daveyton. Immediately after their arrival in a hired bus, the visitors alighted and prepared to dance. While the women, already dressed in *diaparo tša setšo* (traditional dress) stood to one side, the men, still wearing their best Sunday suits, did a performance of the regimental song *monti* to greet their hosts. Grouping themselves on one side of the drummers who began to play a set of hide-covered drums, the men created a polyphonic texture of sound, each blowing a recurrent note on a single aluminium pipe hanging around his neck on a piece of thong, and then commenced the dance itself. It was accompanied by such invocations as:

'we want to please those who have invited us: whatever food has been prepared here is for us, so we must please these people'.

The hosts, *SK Alex*, also dressed in suits, responded with a similar greeting.

The women partners of both groups, already in dance uniform, then performed in their turn. Their dress was layers of different coloured cloths tied around the waist, embroidered cotton smocks, headcloths of netting or velveteen, numerous beaded necklaces and anklets, and leg-rattles made of plastic from milk-bottle containers. The women sang rather than playing pipes, and their dances were more sedate than those of their male counterparts.

It was only later, after both men's groups had retreated into the hostel to change into full dance regalia — including authentic Scottish kilts, white boxer shorts, white tennis shoes, white shirts with collar, seedpod leg-rattles and headdresses with ostrich feathers and goats' horns — that the fierceness of the competition between them started to be expressed in performance. The groups vied with each other in producing a range of special aesthetic effects never seen at regular practices. During a kicking dance step one man created great hilarity by 'losing' a shoe which soared high above the heads of the spectators; another man 'borrowed' a hat from a member of the audience as a dance prop, only to be outdone by a member of the competing group who 'borrowed' a small child from its mother for the same purpose. The man eventually judged best dancer by the crowd, as measured by the amount of money thrown to him, engaged in an acrobatic display which involved equal measures of simulated aggression and comical self-mockery, and which ended with him turning somersaults and falling with mock surprise in the dust.

In similar vein, the women's groups had kept some of their most striking *papadi* (dramatic tableaux; lit games) for this stage of the competition. The host group put on an act in which a sick person, after first consulting a *ngaka* (traditional healer) for a cure, was then taken to a medical doctor in a white coat who examined her with a stethoscope and prescribed some bright pink medicine. The visitors, to the crowd's delight, produced a 'monkey' — a woman clothed in overalls and a gorilla mask — who swaggered among the dancers and made as if to frighten the children in the audience.

The dancing and acting in this second phase of the event was no longer designed to please the hosts, but to outdo them. 'We are two groups, and we must compete, just like Pirates and Chiefs'.*

*Two of the most popular South African football teams.

The musical style or genre which was danced and sung at this event is known as *kiba*.[7] Based on a series of rural styles used by Sotho-speakers from the northern Transvaal, it is played widely on the Reef and in surrounding areas of industrial and domestic employment. In the compounds of mines, power stations and factories, where it acquired many of its present features, and where it was encouraged by management as a form of competitive recreation, it developed as an exclusively male genre. Since the onset of female migration from a number of areas in the northern Transvaal during the 1970s, and in the less restrictive environment of the townships, *kiba* has acquired a female version.

Migrant women's musical performance, by seeking definition as *kiba* alongside men's, has sought to share a physical and conceptual performance space with the musical performance of migrant men. Emergent or recently emerged from a series of rural styles, its capacity to reconstitute itself in new contexts, and to infiltrate pre-existing styles, has facilitated its incorporation as part of *kiba*. But within this overarching genre, two rather different gender-specific sub-styles can be distinguished.

Men's *kiba*, danced while playing on aluminium pipes, takes its name — *dinaka* — from these instruments, while women's *kiba*, danced while singing, is called *koša* (song). In each case, the terms are descriptive of the specific techniques used to produce musical sound: pipe-blowing and singing respectively. As will be seen, these differences in musical technique are linked to other important differences between men's and women's *kiba*.

The distinctions are de-emphasised, however, by the clustering of the two sub-styles within a single genre. *Koša*, or women's *kiba*, has an ambiguous status. While it actively engages in the projects of men's *kiba*, it also retains a separation from the world of male migrant performance. This paper seeks to explore both the commonalities between men's and women's performance, and the new flexibilities and unorthodoxies which women have introduced into this originally male genre.

Borrowed instruments, old songs

Two assumptions underlie much of the ethnomusicological study of Southern African societies. The first is that music was integrated into the structures and activities of rural life in a very profound way. The second is that this music obeyed relatively fixed stylistic canons. These combined assumptions focused attention away from the phenomenon of stylistic change, and away from the existence of styles which might be less central to a community's life.[8]

Assumptions of this kind have been shown to be flawed. Our attention has recently been drawn to the existence of marginal or peripheral arts which exist alongside mainstream ones in rural society: to the existence, for example, of personalised commoner praises alongside those with which chiefs and rulers celebrate their power. It is often these unofficial genres which become the basis for transformed cultural forms in an urban or migrant context. *Lifela*, through which miners from Lesotho announce and elaborate their identity as workers, originated in boys' initiation songs rather than in chiefly praises. Zulu men's migrant guitar styles transform an individualised tradition of women's songs of love and courtship, rather than drawing from songs of communal or political import.[9]

In similar vein, the northern Transvaal-based genre of *kiba*, in both its male and female versions, grew out of rural performance styles which were neither under chiefly control nor tied to events of general ritual significance. Both were thought of as *dipapadi* (games), and were performed, by groups or teams of youths, at occasions such as weddings, or at competitions held at neighbouring villages at which a rich patron might supply beer or present a goat as a prize for the winning group.[10]

Kiba, in its male form as a pipe dance, is said to have been imported. Its place of origin varies with different accounts: some say it comes from Venda (where a similar dance has long been linked to national political occasions), some from Zimbabwe, and some simply from 'the north'. Although the details of its origins need not concern us here, the fact that players are so insistent on its provenance outside their own area seems to endorse its status as a peripheral form of cultural expression, free to be defined as 'play' and later to become the major vehicle of a new migrant identity since, unlike its Venda counterpart, it has remained beyond the ambit of rulers' jurisdiction.[11]

This stress on importation is even more pronounced in the case of migrant women's *kiba*, the sung form of the genre, which developed out of a succession of female rural styles. Informants describe these as having been acquired by local populations from some other area — 'we got it from GaMphahlele', 'one of us saw this being danced at GaMasha, and the others learned it from her'. Newer women's songs, imported into villages and replacing older ones in this way, were thought of as 'fashions'. They swept through the countryside, and often contained lyrics of great national topicality alongside those referring to more domestic and area-specific concerns.

In the Pedi heartland *Sekhukhune*[12] during the 1940s, great-grandmothers now in their seventies spent most of their leisure time between initiation and marriage singing *mararankodi*, with lyrics commenting not only on the trials of coping with in-laws, and lamenting the absence of migrant brothers, but also singing of the dangers of the Germans whom many of their men had gone to fight.[13] Women of a slightly younger generation sang *tshutshumakgala* (train), which referred to the struggle of Pedi cultivators and migrants against attempts by the South African state to govern them through the Bantu Authorities system. Subsequent fashions, sung by a succession of younger women, were *makonkwane, eya eya, mankgodi, marashiya,* and *makgakgasa.*[14]

Local accounts, in describing the origins and development of both men's *kiba* and of women's rural styles, thus emphasise their exotic origins. Such an emphasis might seem to contradict informants' insistence on the music's long-standing association with *sotho* tradition.[15] But the borrowed or imported elements have not intrinsically altered musical content. Rather, they have provided novel ways of rendering old songs.

When *dinaka* (pipes) were adapted from Venda or from 'up north', they were used to play songs phrased in the six-note scale of northern Sotho/Pedi music, rather than the eight-note scale of the Venda pipe dance. The borrowing of the instruments did not change the songs, except by 'submerging' their original lyrics as will be shown further on.[16]

A similar adoption of a new instrument to play old melodies occurred with the later introduction of the *harepa* (German autoharp or zither). Kirby, surveying Southern African music in the 1920s, found that 'whenever possible the native owner of an autoharp has his instrument tuned by a European'.[17] But by the time of the first Gallotone recordings in the 1940s, northern Sotho musicians were tuning the instrument with the northern Sotho/Pedi six-note scale. The *harepa*, although western in origin, became assimilated as part of pagan or traditionalist culture, and was shunned by members of the mission elites: a process which was repeated with tradestore instruments in other areas of the country as well.[18] Rather than imposing or suggesting a switch-over to European melodic or harmonic forms, this instrument in Sotho hands allowed for a more effective realisation of indigenous musical principles than did the original instrument — in this case the plucked reed *dipela* — which it replaced.[19]

The adoption of new forms, or the reliance on new fashions, does not then represent a rejection of older songs but rather a revitalisation of them. The development of women's rural genres which resulted eventually in the emergence of women's *kiba* illustrates this point. Through a complex series of reciprocal interactions between town and country, women in both rural and urban areas began to perform in a style previously recognised as the preserve of men. This has been the most recent and certainly the most radically different of the 'fashions' which women's music has taken unto itself. Once again involving borrowed instrumentation, this change has led to women's use of the full set of four drums (*meropa*) instead of the single long drum which previously accompanied their song/dance. But despite being named *kiba*, the genre has not borrowed the *dinaka* (pipes) of men's music. Its notes are sung ones.[20]

The naming of the new fashion or style shows something of its gender ambiguity. Sometimes termed *koša* but mostly *kiba* when performed by migrant women, it claims an equivalence with its male counterpart. Played by village women, it is often referred to as *lebowa*, indicating the frequent use made of it by new political elites in the homeland. A village women's group is called upon to represent its village at the Lebowa agricultural show, to make memorable the opening of a new school or tribal office, or to accompany its chief to the opening of parliament. It is in its rural women's version that the genre has come closest to becoming subordinate to the demands of local chiefs, largely because of the quasi-clientelist dependence of rural women on these chiefs.[21]

The eventual merging of women's with men's music under the rubric of *kiba* was thus the most recent stage in the sequential development of women's rural styles. For decades before this, men's *kiba* had undergone its own development, in the context of the industrial compounds and hostels where most male migrants from the northern Transvaal were living.[22]

Kiba in an urban context

It was on the Reef, and particularly on the mines, where men were often 'hired because of their art' in performing *kiba*,[23] that the genre acquired many of its present features. Here, performers began to be provided with parts of their gradually-evolving uniform by employers: durable plastic shakers to replace the indigenous ones made out of cocoons, headdresses with ostrich feathers and horns, white tennis shoes, and the like. It was on the Reef in the late 1940s and early 1950s that *dinaka* players, originally wearing the black trousers of the *Malaita* gangs,[24] or *thetwana* — a rather restrictive skirt-like garment made of appliqued and beaded cloth — first saw Scottish kilts, and adopted them as part of the uniform for their performances: 'We saw white soldiers wearing Scotch. *Kiba* is like soldiers organised against something, so we too wanted to wear one thing which was similar'.[25]

In the early 1950s, a kilt cost £3, a considerable investment for a miner earning two shillings and sixpence a month. The adoption of kilts was to have a marked effect on the aesthetic of the dance because of the freedom of movement it allowed and encouraged. One of the most applauded effects in current usage is a tossing of the kilt from side to side over the buttocks 'like a peacock', ending with a flourish in which the kilt remains up to reveal (unlike the famed Scottish practice) a pair of white boxer shorts. Such a gesture would have been impossible in the restrictive *thetwana*, and would probably never have been thought of without the impetus provided by the swing of the kilt.

Not only the uniformity of soldiers' dress, but also something of the ethos of regimented soldierly behaviour, found its way into *kiba*. Rank-and-file members were called *masole* (soldiers), and the idiom used to describe membership of a *kiba* group — *go joina* (from the English, to join) — is the same as that used to describe enlisting in a military regiment, or 'joining up'. Although none of my informants fought with the Allied forces in World War II, many older *kiba* players did so. It is probable that much of the imagery of soldiery to be found in present-day *kiba* performance derives from this experience.

In men's *kiba*, these trappings and ideas drawn from the experience of modern soldiery have been combined with the military idiom of an epic precolonial past. Although men's songs have had no words since singing was replaced by the introduction of *dinaka* (pipes) from 'the north', the original words are still known to some participants. These submerged lyrics form the basis of elaborate reflections on the significance of individual tunes, as in this interpretation of the song *madikoti*:

> On arrival home at the *mošate* (chief's kraal) the warrior will have to dance *kati* and say a *sereto* (praise) about himself. The chief ... will say 'a brave man amongst brave men, when I say I am a chief, I am a chief because of you'. He will go to one of his houses, and take one of his daughters who will then be given to the man who made them win the battle ... The chief will praise his daughter, saying 'there you are, my child, there you are with the buttocks of a light-skinned girl who has never walked in bad ways'.[26]

It is not only the lyrics which celebrate the heroic era of chiefly dominance, but the actions of the dance as well. In *segoata-goatana* (the one who sneaks away) and *magana go bušwa* (they refuse to be ruled) the secession by a splinter group from a chief's dominion is described in the lyrics as well as enacted by the performers, who dance backwards in a stealthy way out of the main performance area.

One of the most important songs in the *kiba* repertoire is *monti*:[27]

> *Monti* was a *mogobo*, a situation where warriors from the war will enter the *mošate* (chief's kraal) singing and dancing. When people enter from the war

singing it, it will have a double meaning. You will feel unhappy because some have died in the war, but you will also feel happy and satisfied because you have won the war. With us, as we use *dinaka*, we no longer do this *mogobo*, but instead sing *monti*. It is a regimental song, it is for attacking.[28]

It can be seen from this account that *monti* is conceived of, on one level, as a reenactment of, and perhaps a replacement for, the scenario of warriors returning from a battle. In contemporary use, however, it is a song of greeting in which the ideas of respectful praise and pleasing one's hosts/audience are foremost. The expression of this visiting ethic is tied up with the song's role as introduction and finale to the whole sequence of dances of which the performance consists.

In greeting/introduction, the dancers group together at some distance from the central performance area (defined by the presence of the drums) and dance slowly onto centre stage, where they form a circle and move around the drums; or, in situations with a more clearly defined inside space such as the rural homestead of someone who has invited an urban-based group to play at a party, the performers will assemble in the road or public space outside and dance through the gateway into the yard. At the end of the performance the dancers, having formally greeted and taken leave of their host or audience, will use *monti* again to take them back through the gateway to the public space beyond.[29]

Contemporary women *kiba* singers, performing their own version of *monti*, contribute to its transformation from a song of triumphal regimental return to one of migrant visitation. Women dance with a torch brandished in the right hand and a glove worn on the left; a practice explicitly thought of as substituting for the weapon and shield which members of a regiment once carried in the right and the left hand respectively.[30] But the right hand may also be used to brandish other objects, such as the bottles of soft drink provided by the host. In this context, the action connotes praise and respect rather than aggression.

Much creative effort goes into harnessing the potentially disruptive effects of unbridled competitiveness. The men's song *ke rena baeng* (we are visitors) with its women's version *basadi ba baeng* (visiting women) stresses that the host dancers — equivalent to a football 'home team' — should not feel threatened by the arrival of the visiting dance-group since the latter have come not in a spirit of rivalry but of co-operation, not to set themselves apart but to be included in a broader unity.

In a *kiba* performance such as that which took place at the annual party of *SK Alex*, migrant men combine a number of discourses. By assuming some of the costume and ethos of the Scottish military, they state their membership of a disciplined and purposeful group of urban-based musicians. By referring to the past in which their forebears were ruled over by independent chiefs, they state their identity as inhabitants of particular home areas of the northern Transvaal. And by retaining some of the challenge of battle as a residue of meaning behind the actions of greeting and visitation, they use *kiba* as an idiom of competition with other urban-based groups.

Women's performance emphasises many of the same themes — the idiom of soldiery and 'joining', of fierce competition ambiguously co-existing with regard, and of pride in rural-based identity. In some respects, then, women co-operate with men in the construction through performance of a unitary migrant identity. But in other ways, women's *kiba* performance distinguishes itself sharply from that of men.

There are differences in social constituency and differences in style between men's and women's *kiba*. First, the men and women migrants in a group such as *SK Alex*, although claiming to represent the same home area, came to Johannesburg from two distinct parts of the northern Sotho homeland of Lebowa, where they experienced widely divergent socio-economic and cultural conditions as youths and young adults. The men of *SK Alex* were raised in the villages of the Pedi heartland *Sekhukhune*. All began to play *kiba* as children, and all have followed a well-established migrant trajectory — from compounded employment through to less restrictive forms of labour, in which *kiba* performance played a central role.

Their female co-performers, on the other hand, grew up on freehold land, on white farms or in reserve areas further north, where the influence of mission Christianity lent itself to a musical culture of adolescence which favoured choir, concert and church songs. Some had not sung *sotho* music since early childhood. Many others learned to sing such music, and took to dressing in 'traditional' *sotho* dress, only after arriving on the Reef. The style of music learned by these women from a diversity of rural homes, did not signify, as it did for their male counterparts, a geographical and cultural continuity with a common home area. Rather, it represented an identity which, although constructed on the basis of a female performance culture 'borrowed' from rural women, acquired its meaning in the context of a set of shared urban experiences.

The other differences between men's and women's music are stylistic and will be explored in some detail here. Women's *kiba* has retained its quality as sung music, in contrast to the men's version which is instrumental and blown on pipes. This gives women a greater freedom to improvise, by changing the words of existing songs to suit new contexts, where men's music, although allowing some change of style and of interpretation as described in the case of *monti*, does so more slowly and with less flexibility.

The greater ease of improvisation in turn allows women a greater freedom to comment on issues and scenarios in the present, where men's music tends to be thought of primarily in terms of its epic connotations and its past referents. Women's *kiba* lyrics straddle the epic and the topical. Like other Southern African oral poems such as those discussed in the recent book by Vail and White, commentaries in these poems concern the immediacies of contemporary experience within a structure whose links with previous performance renders them durable and permanent.[31]

Before going on to look at the particular features which demarcate women's *kiba* as a sub-style, we should examine again the way in which migrant performance genres have built themselves on the basis of unofficial rural ones. Although it is true that *kiba* in its rural form was less hidebound and static than many descriptions of traditional music would have us believe, in its urban form it never became as eclectically incorporative of new elements as other more rapidly changing musical forms. Regarded as belonging within the broader family of *mmino wa sesotho* (sotho music), which has tended to be reconceptualised more recently as *mmino wa setšo* (traditional music, or music of origin),[32] it is regarded by practitioners and audience as distinct from these more eclectic forms — *mmino wa kereke, wa sekolo*, and *wa sebjalobjalo* (church, school, and modern music). Unlike these and other more obviously urbanising South African genres, *kiba* has not taken on the ubiquitous three chords of the Wesleyan hymn, the finite song-form of tin-pan alley or the four-square rhythmic patterns of radio jive music.[33]

Although *kiba*'s origin in unofficial genres has thus facilitated its development as a transforming and flexible migrant style which has readily incorporated new meanings, it has, especially in its men's version, been characterised by formal continuities and conventions. Its complex rhythmic patterns, and the descending melodic sequence with the distinctive northern Sotho six-note scale, are much the same today as in the Gallotone recordings of the 1940s, and probably much the same as when, decades earlier, the borrowed end-blown pipes replaced singing as a favoured form of men's entertainment in the Sotho-speaking areas of the northern Transvaal.[34]

Rural men's *kiba* did, then, form the basis for a vibrant migrant style, but it was a style which remained firmly within the bounds of the traditional, as defined both by participants and by outside analysts. Women's *kiba*, while bound by the same scalar and rhythmic canons as men's, gained its greater flexibility from the possibilities of improvising new lyrics.

Women's lyrics: composition and interpretation

Dinaka *is not supposed to be sung by women ... Now men have left it and women are trying to bring it back; that is why we say* 'lebowa'.[35]

In the old days of marashiya [a rural, pre*kiba* style], *there was no* monti [for women]. *We sing it today with our mouths while men blow pipes.*[36]

These two statements capture some of the transformations which have brought female performance into the *kiba* fold. The first was made by Lucas Kgole, a musical entrepreneur who has made several records with a female backing group and who currently makes a living from herbalism in the village of Sephaku, in a district adjoining *Sekhukhune*. *Dinaka*, or men's *kiba*, is more or less defunct in village life. Women, previously excluded from the genre, are seen as having revived it by starting to engage in its performance (albeit, in his case, under the patronage of a male group leader).

The second observation was made by a rural female singer in the *Sekhukhune* village group *Dithabaneng*. It indicates that, while women's songs like *marashiya* were previously named separately, they now have the status of female parallels to standard items in the male repertoire, distinguished from these by being sung rather than rendered instrumentally, and by the much more sedate style of dancing. Women's *monti* shares stylistically with men's a distinctive pattern played on a set of four drums (*meropa*). Similarly parallelled by women's equivalents, and similarly sharing with them easily-recognised drumming patterns, are the other core songs in the men's repertoire: *lerago*, *kiba* (from which the style takes its name), *fesi*, and others (see Tables 1-3).

Table 1: Core songs documented by Huskisson in the 1950s, and still played today

Monti	A regimental song
Lerago	Buttock
Kiba	Stamp, or beat time
Fesi	

Table 2: Additional songs, played by some of the groups met by Huskisson, and still played today

Madikoti	The girl with dimples
Lekwapa	Shangaan (also applied to other non-Sotho speakers)
O le metse	You used to steal
Segoata-goatana	The one who sneaks away
Magana go bušwa	They refuse to be ruled

Table 3: Additional songs played today, not listed by Huskisson

Mahlwa le mpona	You have always seen me
Mojeremane/ke epa thaba	German/I dig the mountain

The standard and easily-recognised rhythm for each song in the male repertoire provides a kind of hook onto which have been hung a range of women's songs adapted from previously-existing rural genres. In some cases, a man's song may have only one female equivalent, but in others it has several, each with its own lyrics, melody and dance-pattern (see Table 4). The resulting multiplicity of women's songs in a group of migrant singers reflects two things: the greater diversity and scatter of home areas, and thus of female rural styles represented in a migrant women's group, and the greater improvisational challenge posed — and freedom allowed — by songs with lyrics than by those without.

If lyrics can be heard and appreciated, they can also be adjusted to enable the precise expression of particular sentiments. It is in the creation of new lyrics, the re-creation of old lyrics, and the constant process of reinterpreting both, that one can see women's music, having sought definition and legitimation within the recognised migrant genre of *kiba*, moving beyond the constraints imposed by this definition to seek acknowledgement as a style of its own.

Table 4: Some men's tunes with women's equivalents

Men	Women		
Lekwapa	Lekwapa		
Lerago	Setimela		
Monti	Legalane	Ke na le ngwana wa mošemane	
Kiba	Lebowa	Sekopa sa maisane	Mpepetloane

If the features of women's *kiba* suggest its recognition as a separate stylistic entity, this distinctiveness is most apparent in its links to older, rural-based female styles. It must be remembered that, for women who did grow up singing *sotho* music, in *Sekhukhune* as well as in places further north, *kiba*'s recent popularity is merely the latest in a succession of fashions. Although the new style of *kiba* has become popular and has replaced older ones in both urban and rural areas, there is a continuity of musical features and of subject-matter. Fragments of older songs are placed into the context of newer ones, which are then reinterpreted by their performers: new lyrics are added which give older ones a different slant and which then provide the basis for an entirely new significance to an older song.

In its continuity with older styles, and in the opportunities it provides for constant re-evaluation and reinterpretation of older lyrics, Sotho women's *kiba* has much in common with the Yoruba women's form of oratory known as *oriki*. One of Barber's claims about this form is that reflections and comments on past practice in the texts should not be seen as part of an 'incomplete historical account', but rather as an indication of the relevance of 'the past in the present' and of the present in the past.[37] Writers who see song texts as repositories of facts about history ignore the formal, textual nature of *oriki* and other, similar forms.[38] In the case of *kiba*, lyrics do contain extensive reference to the past experience of rural women as cultivators and as the stay-at-home wives and sisters of migrant men. But the importance of the past to *kiba*'s constituents is not unmediated, it becomes evident in its refraction through the lens of contemporary performance, and in its reinterpretation by composers, performers and audience.

This observation provides a key to understanding the contrast between the unheard lyrics of *dinaka* (men's *kiba*) and the audible ones of *dikoša* (songs: women's *kiba*). At first glance, this appears as a contrast between a nostalgia expressed in heroic and metaphoric terms for grand public occasions in bygone days, and a concern for domestic situations in the more recent past expressed with critical and often comical directness. *Dinaka* tell of beautiful virgins given to brave warriors in far-off times, while *dikoša*, like other women's genres with similarly domestic preoccupations, comment wryly on the need to conceal an illicit love-affair from one's husband.[39]

This apparent preoccupation with the domestic and mostly rural setting of women's experience conceals the capacity of these songs to undergo a continual process of recomposition and reinterpretation. They are thus not fixed in structure or in meaning, but are characterised by what Barber and others have called an 'emergent' quality. Lyrics which derive from older songs and which on one level might be seen as reflecting on rural women's domestic involvements in the past, on another level express a set of very contemporary and sometimes urban-based concerns, and provide commentary on extra-domestic as well as domestic issues.

The lyrics of these songs, like the West African *oriki* documented by Barber, consist of different parts composed by different people at different times, the most recent contributions being those of the contemporary performer/composer herself.[40] The solo singer adds her own new words to those of an existing song, and sings the resulting combination interspersed with a chorus (usually also the song's title) in which the other singers *dumela* (sing a repeated refrain, lit 'agree'). Not only do solo singers create new lyrics or variations on old ones, audiences and performers construct the song anew at different performances through differing interpretations.[41]

The juxtaposition of old and new elements may at first glance appear confusing: some chorus singers, questioned about the significance of lyrical remnants composed by unknown singers in the past, claim ignorance because they are from 'an old song'. This suggests a throwing together of newer and older elements in a spontaneous and perhaps unconsidered way. But the use of these elements in the hands of accomplished composers, and their interpretation by seasoned performers and audiences, reveals a logical structuring which underlies this apparent lack of design. Themes of the lyrical fragments retained from past performance are often echoed, inverted, or transformed in those of the newly-composed sections.[42]

Through this structuring the relevance of 'the past in the present' is made explicit, and statements of singers' contemporary preoccupations, problems and aspirations are given a transcendent quality which links them to the concerns of previous generations, and to 'tradition'.[43]

The linking of fragments within a broader structure which gives them meaning can be seen in songs which use 'poetic licence' to utter veiled criticism.[44] Negative comments about the present misconduct of an individual chief within the homeland government are placed against a backdrop in which the abstract and transcendent qualities of chiefship are celebrated. Critical comment of this kind relies not only on interpretation by performers but also on informed and receptive audience response. *Dipalela Tlala*, a women's group from the village of Sephaku in a district adjoining *Sekhukhune*, sings a song of praise to the area and to its chief Jack Mahlangu which announces the women's clientelist dependence on him and simultaneously criticises him in a veiled manner.

Dipalela tlala, ko re yeng gae	Defeaters of hunger, let us return home
Bana ba Mahlangu	Children of Mahlangu
Bana ba Jack, ko re yeng gae	Children of Jack, let us return home
Dipalela tlala	Defeaters of hunger
Gopolang Sephaku naga matebele	Remember Sephaku the place of Ndebele
Sephaku, ntsiru ge le ke bone musi	Sephaku, give way, let me see the mist
Ke bone magoši diapara nkwe	Let me see the chiefs who wear the royal leopard skin
A ke bona magoši, ke bona mong arena	When I see the chiefs, I see our own lord
Mong a rena, le ga le ka molatola	Our own lord, even if you say bad things about him
Mong a rena, le koloni ba mo dumela	Our own lord, even in the Cape they greet him
Mong a rena, le Pretoria ba mo dumela	Our own lord, even in Pretoria they greet him.

Although this song appears to be concerned primarily with praise of the area and of the chief, its composer insisted in private discussion that it was critical of him, and that, on hearing the song, village and area audiences would be aware of this. The phrase *dipalela tlala* (defeaters of hunger) is a veiled reference to the chief's support of the introduction into the area of a much-disliked agricultural co-operative, which landed most cultivators deeply in debt and forced them to face, and defeat, hunger and deprivation. The phrase 'even if you say bad things about him', while appearing to invalidate criticism, in fact substantiates it, and the reference to his acceptance in Pretoria disparages him for his role in the state-controlled structures of government.[45]

It may, then, not only be factors intrinsic to the form of women's *kiba* itself, but also the dependent social relationships in which its performers find themselves inextricably involved, which makes this genre so dependent on sensitive audience reception for its fullest appreciation.

Composers thus situate their criticisms within the context of history. The fragments of older songs may, as in the previous example, provide evocative descriptions of a past way of life in which leadership and area loyalty were sacrosanct. But the existing songs from which fragments are drawn may, themselves, describe more recent situations in which the deprivation, harassment and anxiety of the migrant existence are a feature.

The song *Setimela* (steam train) demonstrates this point. Today performed by a range of women's *kiba* groups, urban and rural, it is presented here in the version sung by the rural-based group *Dithabaneng*:

Setimela sa Mmamarwale	Train of Mmamarwale
Nthshwanyana	Black carrier
Setimela nkabe se rwale buti bokgolwa	Train should carry my brother from *bokgolwa*
Buti e sa le a eya bokgolwa	My brother home from *bokgolwa* (the state of being a migrant who never returns)
Ngwana-mme o tla hwa ese ka mmona	My mother's child would die without me seeing him
Setimela nkabe se rwale	Train should carry women
Se re iseng ka lebowa	It would carry us to Lebowa
khutlong sa thaba	mountain
Ka ntshe gago tsotsi gago mathatha.	Where there are no tsotsis (gangsters) and no problems.

The first part of the song is a fragment which was composed about fifty years ago. The last three lines, recently composed by the leader of a neighbouring group and copied from it by *Dithabaneng*, evoked an elaborate and lively interpretation:

They mean something that can carry them away from the past into the new style of living where there are no problems. I think they also have education in mind, where an educated person can rid his family members of financial problems. We are no longer, as in the past, milling our own crops, today we take them to the mill or get mealie-meal from the shops.[46]

The original character of this song, with its plaintive cry by an individual girl about the absence of her migrant brother, has been transformed through new composition into a self-aware statement of female group identity, linked with notions of nationhood. At the same time, this optimistic view of the benefits brought by the 'new style of living' is mediated by linking it to the deprivation which women have previously suffered on account of migrancy and the modern way. Heartland rural singers, while orienting themselves to progress and the future, regard themselves and their performance as firmly situated within the world of *sesotho*.

Another song which juxtaposes its composer's experience alongside the relatively recent predicament of other women has harassment by police as its central theme. Paulina Mphoka, encouraged by her friends to compose a new song, added new lyrics to the existing ones of *Mosadi wa sepankana*:

Mosadi wa sepankana, mosadi wa diphafaneng	Woman who wears a skin, woman of beer
O rekiša bjala	She sells beer
Mapodisa a ka Lebowa aa monyaka.	The police of Lebowa are looking for her.
Tsodio o otile, mokgwa ntshe ga a robala	Tsodio is thin, he does not sleep
O tshwenya ke malome-agwe	He is troubled by [the ghost of] his uncle
E le go Matšhabataga	Who is called Matšhabataga
Tsodio o bolaile Matšhabathaga	Tsodio has killed Matšhabathaga
Le yena Tsodio o nyakwa ke mapodisa.	He is also troubled by police.
Basadi ba joinile ke masole	Women have now joined the soldiers
Batšea pasa le banna.	They are getting passes just like men.

The middle section is based on a song which, although part of the corpus of *mmino wa setšo*, was itself recently created by *harepa* (German autoharp) player and composer Johannes Mokgwadi, one of the best-known exponents of *mmino wa setšo* in the northern Transvaal. It concerns the molesting by police of Tsodio who, having killed his uncle Matšhabataga, is being both haunted by the ghost of his victim and plagued by the less ethereal representatives of law and order.

This fairly neutral reference to the police is made more pointed by its juxtaposition with the last section, of two lines. This, deriving from earlier female performance, refers to the inclusion of women in the late 1950s within the legislation requiring Africans to carry passes. It records a time when women, moving to South Africa's urban areas, became subject to the same indiscriminate raids and arrests by police which men had been experiencing for decades. Paulina's own, more recent experience of harassment, this time at the hands of the Lebowa rather than the South African police, is recorded in the first section, of three lines. Like a number of other *kiba* singers before they became migrants, she had supplemented her family's income by brewing illegal liquor, and had been arrested by police for doing so.

This combining of three separate incidents lends a weight to each of them which it could not have possessed on its own. None has the links with precolonial rural experience which might be thought necessary to a genre claiming links with the past, but each enshrines a broader view, critical and detached from immediate experience, of such scenarios of harsh persecution. Paulina's addition, here featuring as a new fragment set against an older backdrop, might some years hence appear as part of the collected stock of wisdom passed down from the experienced singers of the past to the novice composers of the future.

But Paulina's song is not only about police harassment. It has also been explained to me in other terms. It is about women's new-found identity as migrants who, like soldiers, form strong collegial bonds, in a disciplined group, with others who share their situation away from home. Another interpretation foregrounds the quality of *botho* (humanity or human goodness), illustrated by default in the story of the murderous Tsodio. *Botho*, described here in the context of other lyrics which refer to the strength and fortitude of women becomes, against this backdrop, a quality especially of women. As with other 'emergent' genres, the audience interprets the lyrics' significance, and even constructs the song anew at different performances through their differing interpretations.[47]

The flexibility enjoyed by an audience in interpreting a song like this one is inseparable from an imprecision about where one genre ends and another begins. The source from which the story about Tsodio comes is not only the wellknown song by Johannes Mokgwadi, often played on the radio, but also a hugely popular radio serial of the same name which has been broadcast by Radio Lebowa. It is the topicality and popularity of the radio serial and the song on which it is based which enables listeners to attach to this brief reference a range of meanings not set down in the text itself.

Genre-boundary blurring, and recontextualising

A blurring of genre boundaries is common within oral performance culture. This, another feature of *oriki*, is closely linked to its character as an emergent form with no apparent closure or fixity. *Oriki* could be seen as constituting a genre in their own right, but are also performed in the context of various other modes or genres, and rely on still further accompanying genres for their fullest understanding.[48]

In the case of women's *kiba*, its very emergence, as a set of previously existing rural genres newly incorporated within a male migrant one, is testimony to this lack of rigid genre boundaries. In addition, the process of composing lyrics and devising actions for particular songs entails a perpetual borrowing or importing of elements from sources apparently external to *kiba* itself.

One source is a series of scenarios from real life, represented in stylised form. Central among these are healing rituals, both divination by *dingaka* (traditional doctors) complete with divination mat and *ditaola* (diviner's bones), and the diagnosis and cure offered by Western doctors, featuring a white coat, a stethoscope, a telephone, and 'medicines' made of commercial soft drinks. There are also dramatic tableaux involving uniformed policemen who perform mock arrests and extract fines.[49]

Kiba also draw from parallel forms of expression within the realm of *sesotho* (*sotho* ways). Among these is a song from *koma* (women's initiation) which, although strictly secret in its original form, has been incorporated into *kiba* in a disguised form as the song *Tšhukutšwane*:

Tšhukutšwane   Female rhinoceros
Mmamogala wa basadi.   The brave one of women.

This comment on the bravery of women, likening it to that of the small but tenacious female rhino, is here taken from its restricted setting within initiation and given a broader relevance. As well as evoking memories of the experience of initiation, the song is thought of in association with the proverb *Mmangwana o swara thipa ka bogaleng* (a mother handles the knife on the sharp side).

Women's *kiba*, as an emergent genre developing within a rapidly-changing social context on which its lyrics reflect, thus draws on parallel forms of *sotho* cultural expression as well as on popular media such as records and the radio as its sources. These elements are integrated within the framework of *kiba* songs, and reinterpreted in the light of singers' contemporary experience. One of the key events around which lyrics are explicated, and which inspires the creation of new lyrics and dance-steps to add to existing ones, is the act of performing *kiba* itself. The apparently domestic concerns expressed by some songs, inherited or claimed by contemporary female performers from their forebears, are overshadowed in certain contexts by the immediacy of *kiba* sung and danced in the here and now.

An example is one of the female equivalents of *monti*:

Ke na le ngwana wa mošemane	I have a boy child
Wena o lefšega	You are a coward

These lyrics reflect in their original version on a fairly common family situation, and one not unknown to *kiba* singers themselves: a woman is boasting about her son, and mocking the inadequacies of another woman whose inability to produce children is proof of her 'cowardice'. But, in becoming a song of *kiba*, these words have been reinterpreted as a statement of boastful pride in the singers' ability to perform, and of scornful disparagement about their rivals' inability to do so.[50]

Another example is the song *Sakopa sa maiesane*, sung and danced to the rhythm of the men's song *kiba* from which the entire genre takes its name. This song was taught to the group Ditšhweu tša Malebogo by Julia Lelahana, who learned it at her rural home.

Sakopa sa maiesane	(Meaning unknown)
Bošego bo ja kolobe	At night pigs are eaten
Mošate gae.	At the home village.
Nna nka senwe bjala	I will not drink beer
Go nwa bo ntage.	As it will make me drunk
Ge ke tagile bo ntira setlaela	If I am drunk I will look like a fool.
Ke melato ya lona lapa le	These are problems of this family
Le tla no šala le e bona	You will see how you solve them when I'm gone.
Le tla no šala lentse le e kisa	You will remain imitating me
Ka gore ge go esa re boya le tsela	Because when the sun rises we will have to go back.

All but the last section of the song consists of remnants from previous songs. While the meaning of the song's title and of the first three-line section was so obscure that none of the singers could explain it, the next section, like a number of other women's *kiba* songs, reflects on the disgrace of uncontrolled drunkenness. The third section, of two lines, speaks of domestic strife in a rural homestead. Julia's composition, the last two lines, follows on in style from the lines immediately preceding it. But it refers to a visit by herself and her fellow *kiba* singers during which they make such an impact with the quality of their performance that local singers copy their songs and dances long after their departure. The idea, imparted by this most recent input, that the song is about *kiba* itself, also affects the interpretation of other lines: hence the specific disadvantage of drunkenness in this context is the fact that it impairs the dancers' ability to perform at their best.[51]

Julia interpreted the song *lekwapa* in similar vein. This, a core song in both men's and women's *kiba*, refers in its original version to a situation of ethnically-based antagonism:

Lekwapa a le bolawe	The Shangaan should be killed
Mamanoko a bo thoka	People of the stick
Tšhagate ga ana taba	Tšhagate is not a problem

The ostensible meaning of the song, still present as an underlying significance in the men's version, is a statement of enmity, set in a warlike context, against a Shangaan who should be killed,[52] and of affinity with 'Tšhagate' (a proper name, here signifying other Sotho-speakers) who can be left to live. But again, in its women's version, the song is reinterpreted as commenting on the rivalry between a competing dance group (equated with *lekwapa*) and the home team (*Tšhagate*).[53]

In these and many other examples which could be cited here, a commentary which contains reference to the domestically-oriented and rurally-based past of *sotho* women is overlaid with new significance. Through a process referred to by performance theorists as 'recontextualising', an older text, incorporated as *kiba* and placed within the new context of migrant women's urban association, starts to offer a commentary on the feeling of fulfilment entailed in being a 'soldier' who has 'joined' other working women and who gains a sense of common identity through performance with these fellow-members.[54]

The home-bound themes of earlier singers have been taken up by women, many of whom had not sung *sotho* music since early childhood, and some of whom had never sung it before arriving on the Reef. Coming from often quite far-flung areas of the northern Sotho homeland of Lebowa, most of these women were pioneer migrants, whose forays to seek work on the Reef were the first, or among the first, made by women from their home areas. When moving into the world of wage labour, they were isolated from others by their situation as live-in domestic servants, domiciled in Johannesburg suburbia. Unlike migrant men from *Sekhukhune* and from other parts of Lebowa, such women had no ready-made groups of *bagagešu* (home people) to turn to for support. Correspondingly, they had little sense of a shared home, or of the shared continuities of *sotho* ways on which to draw.

The capacity of women's *kiba* lyrics to be interpreted as signifying pride in a group's own performance, alongside and simultaneous with these other concerns which derive from the singers' existence as female migrant domestic workers, is what makes this genre particularly adept at carrying the message of a new group identity for migrant women. This capacity enables *kiba* to refer not only to a range of domestic and extra-domestic issues in the lives or past experiences of its singers, but also to itself as a reflexive performative genre. It is through this capacity, too, that women's *kiba* remains firmly linked with the male version of the genre.[55] The themes of self-praise, celebration of performance technique, and friendly disparagement of the inadequacies of rival dancers, are common to male and female performance as they transform heroic and domestic concerns, repectively, into idioms for friendly but fierce competition.

Men's genre, women's genre

Like men, women remake the past through *kiba*. Where men, through dance and music, transform submerged epic themes into statements of friendly competitiveness, women turn domestic themes into commentaries on their success as polished performers. But there is continual ambiguity about whether women identify wholeheartedly with the common projects of *kiba*. On the one hand, as the earlier description of women's *monti* makes clear, there is a unity of purpose with men's *kiba* in enunciating the ethic of competitiveness combined with respectful visiting. But on the other, as can be seen from the lyrics presented above, there is also an independent initiative in which women's *kiba* marks off its participants as the holders of a specifically female migrant identity, pitting their communal sense of skill against that of other women migrants from the north.

Why has a female version of a male genre developed in the circumstances of labour migration on the Reef? Or, phrased in slightly different terms, why has women's music, by adopting the drum ensemble and rhythms of men's, been transformed into a subdivision of men's music? Why have women's migrant songs, so clearly different from men's in many respects, claimed recognition as a part of *kiba*?

In looking for an answer to these questions, it is fruitful to read some of the — still limited — anthropological literature exploring the impact of gender on forms of cultural representation. Recent attempts to understand gender divisions in cultural and musical practice have situated these within the context of other, broader uses of the male/female dichotomy to divide the social world.[56] Based on and simultaneously confirming a division of labour, such divisions also confirm and entrench the differential rights of women and men to exercise public power. They even enshrine the very conceptual dichotomies which are thought to underlie social life: public/private, nature/culture, and the like.[57]

The oppositional division of musical roles between men and women is thus linked, in specific cultural contexts, to other conceptual divisions in the social world. From one perspective, gender-defined musical practices may be seen as complementary and as relying on reciprocal interdependence for their proper definition. But this division may also be seen as serving to separate women's music from the main stream, and as providing women with a socially acceptable but restricted space for musical expression. In this way, a specifically 'women's' music may be one with less of a voice, less of an audience, than that of men.[58]

Despite major disruptions in the form and content of social relationships, dichotomies of this kind are still used to represent gender role divisions in the world of Southern African labour migration. In the northern Transvaal region of *Sekhukhune* in particular, rurally resident and dependent wives/sisters play roles conceptualised as specifically female, and thought of as strongly linked to the domain of *sesotho*. In this rural setting, women's music remains in a separately-defined sphere of female, *sotho* performance. Despite its use by chiefs and homeland elites on occasions of political importance, and despite women singers' use of it, reciprocally, to utter criticism of the holders of power, in everyday settings it is largely ignored by men since it belongs to a domain of things qualified by the adjectival clause *tša basadi* (of women).[59]

Women's music, even that stylistically identified as *kiba*, is thus in rural circumstances generally assigned to a separate sphere and denied a broader audience. It may be in order to escape the lower status of a female genre that its migrant performers, particularly in an urban setting, have sought to make themselves part of men's *kiba*. They 'have begun to "cross over" into the main stream', and have enjoyed a corresponding rise in 'musical status'.[60]

The consequences of a failure to gain such recognition may be seen in the case of the song/poems of migrant women from Lesotho, whose art has remained generically distinct from men's. Lacking a classificatory label of their own, these songs are described by Coplan as having been excluded from the precincts of *sesotho* within which the equivalent male migrant poems are accommodated:

> within the politics of performance in Lesotho, a woman's genre whose texts are often fiercely critical of the behaviour of men and governments is being denied a public identity.[61]

In contrast, the women's songs redefined as *kiba* have undoubtedly gained broader recognition from their inclusion within a previously exclusively male genre. The adoption of the drum ensemble and rhythms of this men's style have allowed women to continue singing and improvising on specifically female songs, under the rubric of an established male migrant cultural form.

If women's migrant song is part of the male migrant genre of *kiba*, and if it evokes an enthusiastic audience response commensurate with that enjoyed by the male version, it is primarily the highly-polished, vibrant and exciting quality of the dancing and drumming which gives it this shared identity. And if, despite its inclusion within *kiba*, it remains distinct from its male equivalent, it is in the importance of lyrics and the freedom to improvise on these that this separateness can be seen.

In the sung and danced aspects of men's and women's performance, there are contrasting variations of restriction and freedom. While men's *kiba*, lacking lyrics, provides fewer opportunities to express comment than women's, the effectiveness of women's ability to do so is curbed by the focusing of the audience's attention away from their lyrics and onto the dancing which is more easily appreciated. On the other hand, while dancing, men have more freedom than women to improvise as individuals, each showing off his own distinctive style. For women, the same rhythmic free flights played on the solo drum prompt a set of movements apparently improvisatory in nature, but carefully co-ordinated as a group.

The creation of a female version for a male genre, or the recasting of a female genre with male instruments and in a male guise, thus represents a seeking of higher status for a style otherwise thought of as being of little account. Within the overarching identity provided by inclusion within the genre of *kiba*, women migrant singers invoke the past experience of rurally-based *sotho* women and recast it in the idiom of urban-based female group membership, while still retaining their links with 'mainstream', male-dominated, northern Sotho migrant culture.

1 I gratefully acknowledge assistance from the Witwatersrand University Research Committee and Mellon Fund, the CSD, and the assistance and support of the African Studies Institute, Witwatersrand University. Thanks to Isabel Hofmeyr, Adam Kuper, and Sam Nchabeleng for comments on earlier drafts. Philip Mnisi, who acted as interpreter, was killed on 5 July 1992, a victim of the senseless violence which characterises life in South Africa. I dedicate this paper to his memory, with gratitude and sadness.

2 For writings which emphasise the cultural making of the migrant experience, see for example H Alverson, *Mind in the Heart of Darkness* (New Haven, 1978); P McAllister, Work, Homestead and the Shades: The Ritual Interpretation of Labour Migration Among the Gcaleka. In P Mayer (ed), *Black Villagers in an Industrial Society* (Cape Town, 1980); Beasts to beer pots — migrant labour and ritual change in Willowvale district, Transkei: *African Studies* 44(2); J and JL Comaroff, The madman and the migrant: work and labour in the historical consciousness of a South African people *American Ethnologist* 14(2) (1987). For writings in this vein which are concerned with performance and aurature, see for example J Clegg, The Music of Zulu Immigrant Workers in Johannesburg — A Focus on Concertina and Guitar. In *Papers presented at the first symposium on ethnomusicology* (Grahamstown, 1981); V Erlmann, Migration and performance: Zulu migrant workers' *Isicathamiya* performance in South Africa, 1890-1950: *Ethnomusicology* 34(2) (1990); D Moodie, Social Existence and the Practice of Personal Integrity: Narratives of Resistance on the South African Gold Mines. In A D Spiegel and P McAllister (eds), *Tradition and Transition in Southern Africa: African Studies* 50(1 & 2) (1991).

3 D Coplan, Eloquent knowledge: Lesotho migrants' songs and the anthropology of experience. *American Ethnologist* 14(3) (1987); Musical understanding: the ethnoaesthetics of migrant workers' poetic song in Lesotho, *Ethnomusicology* 32(3) (1988); Fictions that save: migrants' performance and Basotho national culture. *Cultural Anthropology* 6: 164-192 (1991).

4 For historical and socio-political accounts of changing gender roles in Southern Africa, see the seminal article by B Bozzoli, Marxism, feminism, and South African studies: *Journal of Southern African Studies* 9(2) (1983), and many of the articles in C Walker (ed), *Women and Gender in Southern Africa to 1945* (Cape Town, 1990). Bozzoli's later book with Nkotsoe, *Women of Phokeng: Consciousness, life strategy and migrancy in South Africa, 1900-1983* (Johannesburg, 1991) does examine issues of culture and consciousness.

5 See, for example, E Gunner, Songs of innocence and experience: women as composers and performers of *izibongo,* Zulu praise poetry. In C Clayton (ed), *Women and Writing in South Africa: a critical anthology* (Cape Town, 1989); R Joseph, Zulu women's music: *African Music* 6(3): 53-89 (1983); I Hofmeyr, 'Dikgoro tsa kgale/the Courtyards of Long Ago': Forced Removals, Household Shape and the Performance of Oral History, Chapter 4 of '*We Spend our Years as a Tale that is Told': Narrative in the Changing Context of a Transvaal Chiefdom* (Johannesburg, 1993).

6 The term refers to the fact that the men are resident in Alexandra township, north-east of Johannesburg, and that they come from the area known as *Sekhukhune.* This has as its core, although it extends beyond, a magisterial district of Lebowa called Sekhukhune. It also corresponds roughly to the area known historically as Sekhukhuneland. The area takes its name from the last independent chief of the Maroteng house, who ruled over the Pedi polity before its defeat by the British in the late 19th century.

7 From the verb *go kiba* — to beat time, to stamp.

8 See, for example, Johnston on the music of the Tsonga — The Music of the Shangana-Tsonga, unpublished Doctoral Thesis, Witwatersrand University (1971); Tsonga music in cultural perspective: *Anthropos* 70 (1975) — and Blacking on the music of the Venda — The role of music among the Venda of the northern Transvaal

(Roodepoort, 1956); The Cultural Fondations of the Music of the Venda, unpublished Doctoral Thesis, Witwatersrand University (1964). The exception, for both Johnston and Blacking, was in discussing the music of imported spirit-possession cults whose charismatic leaders attracted a substantial following. See T Johnston , Possession music of the Shangana-Tsonga: *African Music* 5 (1973); Power and prestige through music in Tsongaland: *Human Relations* 27(3) (1974); J Blacking, The Cultural Foundations, pp 64, 333-4. Here, musical change was seen as linked to a kind of social movement: the links between social structure and musical form still gave rise to a logical and invariant stylistic consistency.

9 For unofficial rural genres, see K Barber, Popular arts in Africa: *The African Studies Review* 30(3) (1987); for commoner praises, see E Gunner and M Gwala, *Zulu Popular Praises* (East Lansing, 1991). For *lifela* see D Coplan, Eloquent knowledge pp 414-5. For Zulu guitar styles see J Clegg, Zulu Immigrant workers, pp 2-3.

10 Bafedi Madihlaba, discussion with Deborah James (hereafter DJ) and Anna Madihlaba, Sephaku, 25/1/89; Eva Mogosa, discussion with DJ and Anna Madihlaba, Sephaku, 27/1/89; Mr Makgaleng, discussion with DJ, Apel, 19/7/91; see also Y Huskisson, The Social and Ceremonial Music of the Pedi, unpublished Doctoral Thesis, Witwatersrand University (1958), pp 101-5; 133-6, 140.

11 For detail on the Venda *tshikona* national reed pipe dance, see J Blacking, Musical expeditions of the Venda: *African Music* 3(1) (1962). It is interesting to note that this dance has not undergone a similar transformation into a migrant cultural form.

12 *Sekhukhune* or *GaSekhukhune* is the local appellation, which does not recognise the limits of the magisterial district Sekhukhune, but extends its boundaries to all those parts of the northern Sotho homeland of Lebowa which are south-east of Pietersburg, and even to much of the white farming area beyond.

13 For details on the substantial Pedi involvement in World War II, see P Delius, *Sebatakgomo*: migrant organisation, the ANC and the Sekhukhuneland revolt: *Journal of Southern African Studies* 15(4) (1989), pp 596-7.

14 *Makgakgasa* is an onomatopaeic word describing the sound made by stamping of women's feet with shakers attached. In some parts of the Pedi hinterland, *makgakgasa* has not yet been replaced by *kiba*.

15 Where Sotho denotes a language or a set of musical or other features which have been attributed to a group of people by analysts, it is spelt with a capital and is not italicised. But where, as with the noun *sesotho* or the adjective *sotho*, it denotes a state of being, a way of life or a set of qualities which informants have enunciated or commented upon, it is italicised and spelt without a capital. See JL and J Comaroff (1989), The colonisation of consciousness in South Africa, *Economy and Society* 18(3): 276-296 for a similar style.

16 Since Kirby documented the original few *kiba* songs in the early 1930s, there appears to have been a proliferation as indigenous songs have been included in the genre. The result is a standard core repertoire which, in contemporary performance — as at the time when Huskisson did her research in the 1950s — varies little even between distant areas. P Kirby, *The Musical Instruments of the Native Races of South Africa* (Johannesburg, 1968); Y Huskisson, Social and ceremonial. See Table 1 for core songs.

17 P Kirby, *Musical Instruments* p 257.

18 J Clegg, Zulu immigrant workers pp 3, 7; D Coplan, *In Township Tonight: South Africa's Black City Music and Theatre* (Johannesburg, 1983), pp 362-3.

19 D Rycroft, cited by D Coplan, *In Township*, p 363.

20 Women were acquainted with the drumming patterns of men's *kiba*, and in contexts other than those of compounded labour were often the principal drummers for this genre. But the performers for whom they drummed were male.

21 D James, *Mmino wa setso*: women's songs in a Lebowa village, mimeo, Witwatersrand University History Workshop (1990).

22 See P Delius, *Sebatakgomo* for an account of the changing strategies of Pedi migrants: most moved from employment on mines, where they lived in closely-controlled compounds, into employment in various industries, where they lived in less restrictive accommodation such as municipal hostels, township houses or shacks.

23 Jan Seašane, recorded discussion with Malete Thomas Nkadimeng, Tembisa, 24 March 1991.

24 P Delius, *Sebatakgomo*, pp 589-92.

25 Members of the Lebopo household, discussion with DJ and Philip Mnisi (hereafter PM), Nchabeleng, 19 July 1991.

26 Prince Seroka, recorded discussion with PM, Malebitsa (Moutse), 21 April 1991.

27 I have been unable to establish with any certainty where this name originates. One suggestion is that it comes from the name of Montgomery of Alamein, thus referring, like a number of other *kiba* motifs, to Pedi soldiers' experience of World War II.

28 Prince Seroka, recorded discussion with PM, Malebitsa, 21 April 1991. *Mogobo* denotes both a regimental song of war (the meaning used here by Prince Seroka), and a song sung by initiates who have undergone, and 'conquered' the hardships of initiation.

29 Informal discussions with a variety of informants; and Johannes Mokgwadi, recorded discussion with DJ and PM, GaMasha, 16 July 1991.

30 Members of *Maaparankwe,* discussion with DJ and PM, GaSelepe, 27 July 1991.

31 L Vail and L White, *Power and the Praise Poem: Southern African Voices in History* (London 1991), pp 42, 76-8.

32 The description of this music as traditional has been encouraged by the ethnic music programmes broadcast by Radio Lebowa, originally the northern Sotho division of the SABC's Radio Bantu, in accordance with the official government policy of promoting the separate cultures of separate tribal groups. But it is a designation which has slipped beyond the sphere of control of government planners. The term 'traditional music' has been appropriated by performers and their own audiences in live performance, where it informs their view of the autonomous project in which they are engaged.

33 See P Manuel, *Popular Musics of the non-Western World* (Oxford, 1988), pp 22-3, 85-6, 108.

34 The tendency of *kiba* to retain these features may be explained in the light of an observation made by Blacking that, of all systems of symbolic representation, musical symbols are the most resistant to change. J Blacking, Some problems of theory and method in the study of musical change: *Yearbook of the International Folk Music Council* 9(1977), cited in V Erlmann, *African Stars: Studies in Black South African Performance* (Chicago, 1991), p 11. But this would not of course account for the cases in which, like *marabi,* a transformed and highly syncretic style has arisen in a very short time span. I am grateful to Rob Allingham for making available to me the early recordings of *kiba* in his extensive record collection.

35 Lucas Kgole, recorded discussion with DJ and Neo Phakathi, Sephaku, 3 November 1989. *Lebowa* is the women's equivalent of the men's song *kiba* from which the entire genre takes its name. The popular recording artist and herbalist Johannes Mokgwadi, in discussion with DJ and PM, GaMasha, 16 July 1991, gave a similar account of the origins of women's involvement in *kiba.*

36 Women of the singing group *Dithabaneng,* recorded discussion with DJ and PM, Nchabeleng, 14 July 1991. The name *marashiya* (or *marashea*) probably comes from the name given to the 'Russian' gangsters from Lesotho, whom northern Transvaal migrants encountered on the Reef (Sam Nchabeleng, personal communication).

37 K Barber, *I Could Speak Until Tomorrow: Oriki, Women and the Past in a Yoruba Town* (Washington, 1991) p 15.

38 K Barber and P F de Moraes Farias, Introduction to *Discourse and its Disguises: The Interpretation of African Oral Texts* (Birmingham, 1989), pp 2-4.

39 See for example E Gunner, Songs of Innocence, pp 13, 33.

40 See K Barber, Yoruba *oriki* and deconstructive criticism: *Research in African Literatures* 15(4) (1984), p 504.
41 See K Barber, *I could speak,* p 15; E Gunner, Songs of innocence, p 21.
42 See A Kuper, *South Africa and the anthropologist* (London, 1987), p 187. I am grateful to Adam Kuper for suggesting this line of investigation.
43 L Vail and L White, *Power,* p 42; Coplan, Eloquent knowledge, p 415.
44 L Vail and L White, *Power,* pp 42-5, have borrowed this term from Tracey to describe, with more precision than the term normally has in English usage, the satiric or critical content of much Southern African oral poetry.
45 Lyrics and interpretation from Nkapile Hlakola, discussion with DJ and Anna Madihlaba, Sephaku, 24 January 1989. It is common for women to express their dissatisfaction in this veiled manner with men who hold positions of authority (Sam Nchabeleng, personal communication; see also L Vail and L White, *Power,* pp 248-9). For further information on the co-op, see D James, Kinship and Land in an Inter-ethnic Rural Community, unpublished Masters Dissertation, Witwatersrand University (1987).
46 Lyrics and interpretation from women of *Dithabaneng,* recorded discussion with DJ and PM, Nchabeleng, 14 July 1991.
47 K Barber, *I could speak,* p 15; Gunner, Songs, p 21.
48 K Barber, *I could speak,* pp 1-6.
49 See D James, 'I Dress in this Fashion': Women, the life-cycle and the idea of *sesotho,* paper presented at the African Studies Institute Seminar, Witwatersrand University, 21 September 1992, for a more detailed account of the role of these 'police' in performance.
50 Lyrics and interpretation from *Dithabaneng,* recorded discussion with DJ and PM, Nchabeleng, 14 July 1991.
51 Lyrics and interpretation from Julia Lelahana, recorded discussion with DJ and PM, Johannesburg, 13 October 1991.
52 *Lekwapa* is a Shangaan, or speaker of the Tsonga language. These people lived in areas of the northern Transvaal adjacent to, and even the same as, those inhabited by northern Sotho speakers. Apartheid removals attempted, not always successfully, to separate members of the two language-groups into their respective homelands.
53 Lyrics and interpretation from Julia Lelahana, recorded discussion with DJ and PM, Johannesburg, 13 October 1991.
54 R Bauman and C Briggs, Poetics and performance as critical perspectives on language and social life: *Annual Review of Anthropology* 19 (1990).
55 R Baumann, Performance. In E Barnouw (ed), *International Encyclopaedia of Communications* (Oxford, 1989), p 266.
56 S Gal, Between speech and silence: the problematics of research on language and gender. In M di Leonardi (ed), *Gender at the crossroads of knowledge: feminist anthropology in the postmodern era* (Berkeley, 1991); E Koskoff, An introduction to women, music and culture. In E Koskoff (ed), *Women and Music in Cross-cultural Perspective* (Urbana, 1989).
57 S Ortner, Is female to male as nature is to culture? In MZ Rosaldo and L Lamphere (eds), *Women, culture and society* (Stanford, 1974); S Ortner and H Whitehead, Introduction: accounting for sexual meanings. In S Ortner and H Whitehead (eds), *Sexual Meanings: the cultural construction of gender and sexuality* (Cambridge, 1981); SC Rogers, Woman's place. A critical review of anthropological theory: *Comparative Studies in Society and History* 20(1).
58 E Koskoff, An introduction, pp 8-9.
59 See D James, I dress.
60 E Koskoff, An introduction, p 12.
61 D Coplan, Fictions, p 174; see also D Coplan, Musical Understanding, pp 348-9.

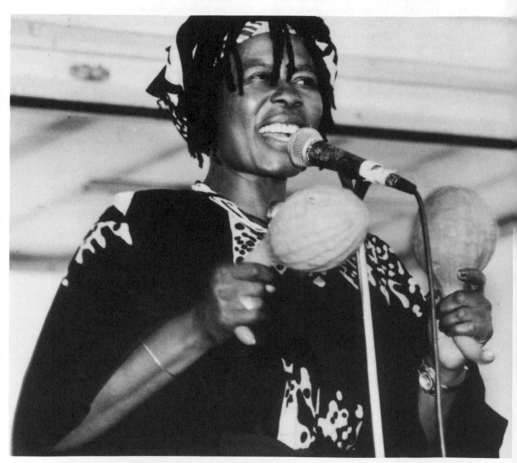

'It is still difficult for women to become musicians . . .' Zimbabwean musician and singer Stella Chiweshe performs at Rusape Stadium, Harare, April 1993 at a Day of Music to raise money for the Zimbabwean national football team's match in Paris against Egypt.

Song, Story and Nation: Women as singers and actresses in Zimbabwe[1]

MOREBLESSINGS CHITAURO, CALEB DUBE, LIZ GUNNER

'If you're a woman, once you decide to become a musician, never, never get married. If you want to sing solo, he'll say "no". People will offer you places to perform and he'll refuse. You'll find all your time has been wasted. Your dreams have not come true.'[2] Such a comment highlights the tensions between performance space and domestic space in the experience of many singers and actresses in Zimbabwe. Women who attempt to move freely as performing artists into the open space beyond the domestic domain are constantly challenged both by their own menfolk and by the dominant concepts of gender roles. 'Loose' was the term used by several actresses and singers when they described the way they were perceived by men (and possibly by some other women). 'At home it is still difficult for women to become musicians. Men accuse them of being loose,' the Zimbabwean musician and singer Stella Chiweshe commented recently.[3] And Harare actress Beauty Zipope, a member of the Glen Norah Women's Theatre, speaking of the group's attempts to challenge the stereotypical depiction of the prostitute in men's theatre, commented on the way the actresses themselves had to contest such stereotyping: 'As women in theatre, we also have to deal with similar attitudes. Many husbands or boyfriends resent us going to rehearsals in the evenings. They say we are "loose". You have to be very committed to cope with such comments'.[4] Women artists, be they singers or actresses are often perceived as 'women of the night' or 'women of the streets'; perhaps this is because they exist in these roles in the unmarked territory outside domesticity and also in urban space which for historic reasons relating both to colonial and indigenous patriarchy has been officially defined as the territory of men.

The messages and images communicated through forms of popular culture have enormous influence in shaping the real language of gender and power relations in a culture.[5] If, in the Zimbabwean context, most of the images transmitted do not in any way disturb the old alliances of colonial-settler patriarchy on the one hand, and indigenous patriarchy on the other, no real transformation of attitudes can be expected to take place. It is in the struggle for space to set out and elaborate a counter discourse, and thus redefine the dominant discourse, that women performers — and in this paper we focus in particular on singers — can have enormous influence and can be seen not only in the old configuration as 'loose' but also, contradictorily, as 'dangerous'. Popular music tends to be music that is urban based even if it absorbs and works with rural and traditional idioms of music and song and moves into rural areas for performances. The question therefore of women in relation to urban space is of crucial relevance to women singers.

This paper will explore the uneasy relations between women as performing artists, in particular singers, and urban space, as well as a second ambiguous and problematic relationship — that of women to the idea of nation, and to nationalism. Its specific focus is on the stories of three women whose lives as singers constantly interrelate with the wider struggle of women to reclaim cultural space within the city and whose careers weave their way through male dominated nationalisms in which women may feature as icons but rarely as active and self-defining agents. A number of recent articles have pointed to the ambiguous interrelations of nationalism and gender. Anne McClintock, writing on gender and nationalism in South Africa states: 'Excluded as national citizens women are subsumed only symbolically into the body politic. Nationalism is thus constituted from the very beginning as a gendered discourse and cannot be understood without a theory of gender power.'[6]

Deniz Kandiyoti has pointed to the contradictions in nationalist discourse on gender, its fluid and ambivalent field of meanings. It is, she claims, both a modern project and a reaffirmation of authentic cultural values culled from the depths of a presumed communal past. The vagaries of national discourse are reflected in changing portrayals of women as victims of social backwardness, icons of modernity or privileged bearers of cultural authenticity.[7] In a recent article on gender, nationalism and women's writing Elleke Boehmer argues that 'the idea of nationhood bears a masculine identity though national ideals may wear a feminine face ... Figures of mothers of the nation are everywhere emblazoned but the presence of women in the nation is officially marginalised and generally ignored.'[8]

The unitary and male gendered form of nationalism has meant that women singers have often operated as emblematic, symbolic figures of 'the nation'. Yet when they have attempted to move away from a normative masculine identity in their narrative of the nation and sing in terms of a plurality of women's experience that is far from emblematic — they may be silenced, or castigated. Women singers — and actresses — like women writers have had to seek out what Boehmer, referring to women writers, calls their own 'strategies of selving'.[9] Through the stories of their lives and the nature of their songs they demonstrate how cultural space is constantly being reclaimed by women and constantly contested by established hegemonies of power. Their stories, and we focus below on three in particular, show that the process of reclaiming cultural space is one that is constantly being negotiated and contested — moments of stasis in such a contestation merely allow older forms of patriarchal control to reassert themselves.

Women artists in Zimbabwe have through a complex of historical forces been squeezed out of areas of social space. The attempts to exclude women from urban space have their roots in the culture of Empire, the specific workings of this in early Southern Rhodesia and its dialogue and dealings with indigenous African patriarchy. As Diana Jeater has pointed out, the Manicheism of Victorian attitudes to race — their belief in the polarity of white and black, the superiority of the former and inferiority of the latter, demanded that 'African systems of sexual behaviour be subject to white control'.[10] Early official policy in Southern Rhodesia was ambivalent about the presence of women in towns. They were — conveniently — seen at first as victims of their own menfolk and in need of protection, much as working class Victorian girls were regarded by the Victorian middle classes as in need of protection from their base and degenerate menfolk.[11]

In the early 1900s the British South Africa Company's initial, and shortlived, attempts at proletarianisation envisaged families of workers living in towns as part of a stable — and docile — African work force. But very little money was ever committed to constructing family accommodation and so very few of the envisaged families materialised. The system of migrant labour which swiftly followed the brief flirtation with proletarainisation may have been the primary force in keeping women out of urban areas but indigenous patriarchy had its own reasons for being wary of giving women a toehold in urban space. Apart from the fact that accommodation in the urban areas was uninviting, African men were not keen to have their wives with them in town for too long, let alone on a permanent basis. Prolonged absences of wives from the rural areas would jeopardise their claims to land and make difficult the harvesting of crops. Neither was it in the interests of the older generation who were fathers as well as husbands to have their daughters absconding to towns where the possibilities of male family heads being able successfully to negotiate bridewealth or extract compensation were slim.

In spite of the hindrances to free movement, and helped perhaps by the paternalism of the 'victims' approach of the Native Administration, women did make their way to towns, sometimes to join their husbands, sometimes to make 'mapoto' (live-in) marriages of convenience, or to make a living brewing beer, or to become prostitutes. Women and young girls seem to have run away from their rural homes for a number of reasons: the increasingly harsh rural conditions and the increasingly heavy work load on the land with their men away, oppressive in-laws, loneliness and frustration as husbands spent longer and longer away at work returning only one or twice a year in some cases. Besides all of these factors there were the alluring consumer goods which from the turn of the century were available from stores such as Meikles in the towns of Gwelo, Bulawayo and Salisbury. Thus women made their way to towns in spite of the difficulties put in their way. Perhaps, for them, town represented an inversion of the more repressive aspects of rural life. Don Mattera records in his autobiography of his youth in violent and vibrant Sophiatown that Johannesburg was called 'Kwa-umfazi ushay' indoda (The place where woman beats her man)[12]. Perhaps there are similar forgotten names by which the urban centres of Southern Rhodesia were known to those who attended 'tea parties' and danced the new dances.

The cosmopolitan life of urban centres with its mix of people, its dances and concerts was recalled with vivid nostalgia by an elderly woman interviewed by Jeater. Her words conjure up a brief sense of the black urban popular culture which must have been springing up in centres such as Gwelo, Bulawayo and Salisbury. The old lady who was interviewed had this to say about such events: 'I never got bored when I first came here, because there were always things going on in the township. There were concerts and dances ... Some of the people from those days were much more interesting than the ones we have today.'[13]

Such new forms of culture must themselves have provided a position on women different both from that of anxious rural patriarchs and paternalist Administration officials. There were, therefore, several colliding discourses on women in this period and in the nascent urban strand women themselves played a more active part in their self-definition. In the new forms of entertainment that seem to have been springing up women were active makers of culture, and participants, as indeed they were — in a more structured way — in the verbal arts of the traditional cultures set in the patriarchal rural areas from which they had removed themselves. Such social gatherings as the one described above did not go unnoticed by whites in the urban centres. As early as 1905 an irritable letter in the *Gwelo Times* complained of Africans hiring unoccupied houses in the townships 'when they wish to indulge [in drinking] under the pretence of tea meetings at 2s 6d per head — ladies 1s 6d'.[14]

The Administration's initial paternalist view of African women as victims who needed protection did in fact allow them some social space in urban areas but this state of affairs did not last long. The Natives Adultery Punishment Ordinance of 1916 was the result of deliberations between the Administration, the settlers and increasingly worried rural patriarchs and it was designed to control the increasing number of 'insubordinate' women who continued to drift into towns seeking emancipation. Although in terms of the law it was the man involved who was deemed responsible (white men were — after pressure from the settlers — omitted from the Ordinance) what it in fact marked was the underwriting of the view of the African urban woman as 'harlot' rather than 'victim' and the closure of the urban space that had previously, in her role as 'victim' been tenuously available to her. By the late 20s and 30s, Jeater argues, urban women were seen both by African men and the Administration as 'immoral'.[15] There may be quite complex reasons for this perception: urban women quite often had no allegiance to a lineage and were thus in a way muddying over a classificatory system, they were weakening and blurring the boundaries between perceived categories — in this case, categories of social relations. Notions of 'daughter', 'wife', 'sister', 'cousin', 'granddaughter' to name only a few were frequently unclear. They thus existed outside demarcated familial spaces and as such they were, to use Mary Douglas's terms in her definitions of purity and danger, viewed as 'dirty, dangerous, unnatural, sinful and threatening'.[16]

If women in urban centres have been viewed by men in this way in the last seven decades — and there is a steady stream of novels in Ndebele and Shona, by for instance, Chakaipa and Sigogo, which continue to underwrite the perceived dichotomy of female rural purity and female urban vice — how have women singers been viewed?[17] Are they even further beyond control and categorisation and have they therefore been set even deeper into the zone of 'dirty and dangerous' than other urban women? This may well be so, and evidence from singers of their being perceived as 'loose' partially endorses this. The category of 'dangerous', however, is more problematic and may link in with the way women artists as agents and effective makers of culture challenge the stereotypes of urban women and domestic space as well as a still dominantly patriarchal discourse. Thus singers contest this gender 'fixing' through their access to forms of song which produce powerful counter images and which often resonate with the power of women's song in traditional art forms. Here too, however, the presence of women's genres and women as verbal artists can still fix and limit their access to expression beyond a certain point. Thus Herbert Chimhundu refers to genres of women's poetry such as *jikinyira* (complaints) and *nheketerwa* (rhythmic utterance of complaints — often uttered by daughters-in-law while grinding flour) but concludes that in general Shona praises and lyrics do little to empower the female voice.[18]

In both rural and urban space, however, the constant making of culture, its fluid rather than static character, allows for the contesting of discourses of domination and the challenging of existing power relations. Singing and poetic discourse in general can be seen as one of the ways of controlling and shaping cultural space and of realigning the relations between dominant and subordinate. The three women singers on whom we now focus have operated either mainly in urban culture using expressive forms which have little or no traditional base, or in forms which combine urban and rural idioms.

Initially we have explored the idea of music and music-making as a means of reclamation of social space. We look, also, at lyrics and the rhetorical and expressive modes that can be used to create that space. We have also looked for continuities between singers, in the same sense that in some African women's writing it is now possible to trace a non-canonic tradition which grew alongside the male tradition establishing itself around Achebe, Ngugi and Soyinka.[19] Thus we can now see links between writers such as Flora Nwapa, Ama Ata Aidoo, Bessie Head and Tsitsi Dangarembga, for instance, in the way in which they establish in their texts a sense of a community of voices, often women's voices, that is unlike the more singular, often nationalist concerns of the male canonic texts. Is there a hidden history of women singers that has been operating in a similar way? Are there 'songlines' which may have been working against a single master narrative or a number of master narratives, songlines which link a number of women singers including Dorothy Masuka and Susan Mapfumo, the first two artists on whom we focus?[20] And is the case of Stella Chiweshe radically different because she is working from a different matrix or are there lines of continuity in her case as well — only different continuities?

'Loose women'

In relation to the question of social control of women and their marginalisation, we found that one of the constant features of women who were singers or actresses was that they felt that they were regarded as loose women, as prostitutes.[21] This point came up time and again in interviews with women artists. Singers, and to a lesser extent women involved in theatre, are seen as in some way even more outside the boundaries of areas of male control and the areas usually covered by 'wife', 'daughter', than other urban women and so, existing in unmarked territory they are termed 'loose' or 'prostitute'. A factor that relates to the 'prostitute' image is the practical question of where women perform and the physical space available to them. Women singers now, twelve years after independence, appear to be far more isolated than women travelling as part of a theatre group and even though women actresses travelling in Zimbabwe with ZACT groups may often be very much in the minority, the new consciousness about theatre as a leavening and vital force in Zimbabwean social and political life, a point made forcefully by Stephen Chifunyise in his article in this book, means that the sexual politics involved tend to integrate rather than isolate the women actors.[22]

Acting itself is still, however, a profession which fathers try to prevent their daughters from following, as Cont Mhlanga's play *Stitsha* which ran to packed houses in Makhokhoba in August 1991 and played again in the March 1993 Inxusa festival emphasised.[23] As yet no recent theatre piece has dramatised the possibly even more stigmatised status of the woman singer. The insecure and — in performing terms — lonely life of most women singers can itself be seen as a metaphor for the marginalised woman artist. Sometimes singers are hired piecemeal to sing with a band at the downtown hotels in Harare, in other cases they have more security and establish a longer term link with a particular band and may tour with them in urban and rural areas. The town locations are likely to be sleazy and the glamour and luxury of performance at venues such as the Sheraton Hotel are not for them — such spots are reserved for foreign artists and tourist audiences.

Take, for instance, the case of the singer Grace who in 1991 was with Ephat Mujuru, the mbira player, and his group. The night we saw them, in late August 1991,[24] they were playing at the Elizabeth Hotel in down town Harare — the atmosphere was steamy, beery and the place was packed with men who sat around, danced alone, or with the very few women who were there who, it seems, were commercial sex workers. For the early numbers, Grace, who sometimes sang lead on her own and sometimes sang with Ephat, wore sexy tight jeans and top and a sports cap and gyrated in the usual hot style as she sang. She then disappeared and came back in a 'woman of Africa' attire — African Java print, long wrap-around skirt and blouse and head tie — she gyrated less and the image she presented was closer to 'wife' or 'mother of Africa' although the music did not change significantly as far as we could tell. The changing between images which gestured in the directions of both the iconic 'Mother Africa' and the stereotypic 'loose' urban woman gave Grace a certain ambiguity of role, and a certain artistic ambivalence. The capacity of the performer to move with a kind of mocking ease between contrasting stereotypic representations of free woman and iconic national Mother showed, perhaps, that the woman singer, however marginalised at one level, has nevertheless the ability to play with collective understanding of gender and question received social wisdom. The urban woman singer, often confined to out of sight down town bars, may like the Basotho migrant women singers of *lifela* of whom Coplan writes be potential carriers of elements of a national culture that is more real than the grand gestures of official national cultural symbols.[25] And the singer as performer has the ability to create a certain aura around him or herself and, as was the case with the singer Grace, to play with and thus interrogate dominant images of woman which are embedded in the nation's discourse on gender. The singer as performer communicates in a way which is coded and formalised — and outside the stream of flowing moving bodies and casual circlings that make up the dance floor above which the singer and other musicians are raised. Performers have a different space, they exist in a charmed circle, and this is part of their power.

'Dangerous' and 'Powerful' women

A second point that came up frequently in our discussions with women singers and those working in the theatre was connected with notions both of danger and of power. As artists they had, they suggested, a kind of power. They were dangerous and that is why men both feared them and wished to control them. They were perceived as 'dangerous' in that they might influence other women to follow their lifestyle, as they were often single or divorced women. The sense of danger was also connected with a sense of their ability to re-vision: through their expressive art they could both reshape and control in a way that was otherwise not possible. This notion of power relates to the acceptance in many African societies of licence, in some situations, within song and poetry — that singers may tell terrible things in song and poetry, set out what is not usually heard and survive with impunity.[26] It is in some cases a combination of the power of sung and poetic discourse and the power of song or poetry in ritual situations which link the singer or poet in a very intense way to forces or influences that may often be present but not tangible.[27]

The lives of the three singers we have taken as examples cover separate but interconnecting periods in Southern African history and in the history of popular culture in the region, stretching from the late 1940s through to the present. Each in her own way can be seen as 'dangerous' and also 'powerful', and each has her own story. Yet they must also be seen as linked and providing a statement that challenges the musical master narratives of their times; their different relations to nationalist narrative highlight, as McClintock argues, the gendered nature of that narrative and their very different experiences and successes question the received wisdom on women in the cities and women as singers.

Dorothy Masuka, 'A musician needs fire'[28]

One of the singers who through her long and eventful life as an artist seemed to demonstrate that kind of power was Dorothy Masuka, now based in Bulawayo.[29] Aunty Dot, as she is often now called, is a contemporary of Miriam Makeba although her career and life have been very different. She grew up in Phumula township in Bulawayo where her father ran a hotel in Seventh Street, and later continued her schooling in Mbare. Even in her early teens her singing talent was clear: 'Singing ripped me off from everything else', she remarked to us, giving a sense of how a singer can, just like a priestess or diviner be aware that she has special powers, that she is marked for no ordinary life. Perhaps the nuns at her Harare school recognised something of this sense of vocation in their pupil from Bulawayo, for it was they who funded her to go to St Thomas's in Johannesburg to continue her education in the late 40s and through to the early 50s. It was not long before her voice attracted the attention of one of the Troubadour Record Company's talent scouts and so at the early age of 14 or so she began her singing career. She became part of what can be seen as a community of women singers who were part of the vibrant black urban culture of the 50s which had Sophiatown as its hub but spread much further afield and was linked through record sales, radio and concert tours to urban centres such as Salisbury and Bulawayo and the towns of the Northern Rhodesian copperbelt.[30] Those who were involved were singers like Dixie Nkwankwa, Masie Hadebe, Mabel Mafuya, Abigail Khubeka, Thandi Klaasen and of course, Miriam Makeba.[31] They were all exploited in financial terms as all black musicians at the time seem to have been.[32] Nevertheless there does for a while in the 50s seem to have been a group of women artists who worked together, interacted and formed what can now be seen as a loose community of artists alongside the male singers and musicians of the time such as Satch Masinga and groups like the African Inkspots and the Manhattan

Brothers.[33] This group of singers — some more than others — drew inspiration from 50s American groups such as the Andrews Sisters as well as from the earlier African-American blues singers such as Billie Holiday and Bessie Smith.

The move from a woman singer working with a male backing group to a group of women singers working together can be seen in Miriam Makeba's progression, singing first of all as lead singer with the Manhattan Brothers and then forming her own female quartet, the Skylarks, with 'most usually' Mummy Girl Nketie[34], Abigail Khubeka and Mary Rabotapa.[35] Another group of women singers who, according to Dorothy Masuka, were seen as lively, less slick and not part of the Johannesburg music scene — 'They didn't perform in Selborne Hall in Sophiatown' — but were nevertheless very popular, were the Dark City Sisters. According to Coplan it was the Dark City Sisters, led by Joyce Mogatusi, who pioneered the new music style with less American influence and more reliance on 'a simplified version of traditional part structure' which became known as *simanje-manje*.[36] There were additional ways in which the Dark City Sisters began to weave a narrative which would be taken up by women singers both within South Africa and across the borders in what was then Rhodesia. They, more than many other popular singers, put astute social comment into their songs thus extending one of the essential elements of traditional song into a new urban context. More than that though, they brought into public song topics from the domestic domain and linked then with broader aspects of black urban culture. In some ways they were thus foreshadowing the kinds of controversial domestic topics that the singer Susan Mapfumo singing in Salisbury in the 70s drew into her songs. They sang about work, about gad-about parents and neglected children, and about husbands who never shared their money and whose wives scolded them continually because of this. One of their songs, 'Emarabini', provides a compact double image of the fast and lively black urban scene of the 50s, and of the strains of domestic life and child-caring. The words (without repetitions) are as follows:

Uye-ye Baba noMama	Ah! Father and Mother
Awu! Awu! Awu! Awu!	Oh my oh my oh my!
Bahlupheka 'bantwana	The kids are having it hard
Bashiywa ngabazali	Their parents left them alone
Bahlal' emarabini	They're at the marabi joint.
Uye-ye Baba noMama.	Ah! Father and Mother.

Another Dark City Sisters song talks about work and the fight against poverty. It is dawn, the cock is crowing and it's time to get to work. Again an image of black urban proletarian and *domestic* life is boldly caught in a few words.

Kikilikiki!	Cock-a-doodle-doo!
Vukani vukani sekusile madoda	Get up men, it's dawn
Vukani madoda siyemsebenzini.	Get up men let's go to work
Nant' iqhude lithi kikilikiki	There crows the cock
Nant' iqhude liphinda, likhala Ma!	Cock-a-doodle-doo!
Isihlalndawonye sidl' ubuphofu!	There crows the cock again Ma!
	The sluggard will eat poverty![37]

Dark City Sisters, less under the influence of American groups like the Andrews sisters, drew more freely on the women's idioms of indigenous discourse and thus easily captured the domestic and grainy metaphors and topics in their songs. They were, however, moving such topics into a far more public space. This slant to their music may have influenced Dorothy Masuka in her own role as composer as she had amongst her compositions a defiant song about marriage and difficult drunken husbands, from the point of view of the wife (see p. 125). Certainly as a group, although the American influence countered this in the case of some, the women singers of the time drew, selectively, on indigenous rural song traditions with their cryptic and frequently hard-hitting social commentaries, moving them into a more public, urban space and reshaping them in the new urban musical idioms of the time, mainly *marabi* and *mbaqanga*. Also, and perhaps equally crucial, the emphasis on topics from what had otherwise been seen as the women's domain became public songs, became part of a subversive counterpoint to more stereotypic and packaged messages of female sexuality, untrustworthiness and so on and established a precedent which was to be maintained both by Masuka throughout her long career and her many travels, and later by Susan Mapfumo operating in a very different social and political climate in pre-independent Zimbabwe in the 70s.

The presence at that time of such a community of women singers existing within a larger group of black musicians who were recording for Gallo and Troubadour, playing live in fixed venues, and touring with African Jazz and Variety could well have been one of the ways of minimising the ever present possibility of the 'loose woman' slur which both indigenous patriarchy and the still new Nationalist government were keen to apply to urban black women. Moreover it created for a time a space within the vital though vulnerable black urban culture for women as vocal artists. Clearly though, if women were present as singers and artists and were, in some songs at any rate, taking on social and political issues showing women as workers, parents and wives, and setting their lyrics to the new beats of the time, other dominant and contrasting images of women were much in evidence. The *Drum* magazine photographs of the period show the new urban woman not so much as 'loose woman', wife and working woman, but as glamour girl and sex object.[38] Yet the energy and talent of the singers themselves, although they were in the minority compared to male musicians and although they may have exploited the ambivalent glamour image, must have offset the tendency to fix women in such limiting terms.

The only film of the period which attempted to show the pain of Southern African black urban life, its links with the countryside and its cultural vigour and fiery spirit was Lionel Rogosin's *Come Back Africa* which was promptly banned on release. Although set in Johannesburg its commentary on racial equality makes it a film emblematic of the colonised experience of the Southern African region and in some ways as true for the Rhodesias as for South Africa itself. This powerful if slow moving film sets two alternative images of urban women alongside the seemingly inescapable polarity of rural mother and urban whore images. First there is the shebeen madam, portrayed not as whore but as strong and independent woman and secondly, very briefly, woman as artist and performer. This is the moment in the film when a young slim singer who turns out to have a voice like honey walks shyly into the shebeen where Can Themba, Lewis Nkosi and others are drinking, and rather self-consciously and with great style discussing the pitfalls of liberalism — and the slim woman with shining eyes begins to sing. The singer is, of course, Miriam Makeba, and she sings a song entitled 'Lakushon' ilanga' which is on the universal theme of lost love, given poignant specificity by the enforced separation of men and women in the context of migrant labour and broader state oppression in the South African situation.[39] Although this image of the woman singer is not part of the narrative line of the film, it has great impact and serves both to undercut and mediate the two dominant and polarising images in the regional narrative of rural mother and urban whore. Thus the presence of woman as singer imposes itself on the cultural text and is in the film a way of publicly acknowledging — or at least suggesting — that a space has been made in South African black urban culture of the 50s for woman as artist and singer.

But the destruction of Sophiatown and the tough censorship laws of the early 60s drastically undercut the fragile base in South African black urban culture which had briefly offered a new freedom, and a new space for women as urban artists. Miriam Makeba left South Africa in 1959 some months before the *King Kong* musical left to tour in England and she did not come back. Dorothy Masuka's departure from South Africa was somewhat different. She was forced to leave in 1958 as a direct result of her activities both as singer and composer, and here perhaps, resonances from groups such as the Dark City Sisters were important.

Composing, politics and trouble

One of Masuka's striking characteristics was that she was not only a superb singer she was also a composer. This side of Masuka's talent is noted by Makeba in her autobiography, 'Dorothy Masuka, the woman whose name tops the list in *African Jazz* has become my best friend ... Dorothy also composes beautiful melodies. Always, she is thinking of a new one. When one pops into her head, she comes to me and says, "Hey Miriam! Take this part". I hum and she improvises by humming another part.'[40] In some cases songs which were often sung later by her sister Miriam once she had gone overseas, were initially Dorothy Masuka's compositions. One such was, according to Masuka, the famous and still popular 'Phata-phata', a song which does not celebrate domestic resilience but describes the street scene from the view of a young and glamorous woman. Masuka recalled that in the walk from Sophiatown to the Troubadour studios in Jeppe Street, Johannesburg, she noticed that young men would not only call out admiringly to her and other glamorous women they would also 'phata-phata' them as they swayed along the pavement and so she composed and recorded the later famous 'Phata-phata' song.[41] Her version, which is on her 1990 release, captures from the point of view of the 'beautiful beholden' the immediacy of the crowded street, the beautiful and smartly dressed women and the young men with their admiring hands as well as voices:

Yo phataphata yoho
Ndithi ndijonge le phataphata!   I look over there and it's phataphata!
Ndijikelele na patpata!   And if I turn around it's phataphata!
Everybody say 'Phataphata'
Yo phataphata yoho.[42]

Masuka had, however, many idioms of composition and moved more openly than the Dark City Sisters into overt political comment. She also commented with ease on thorny social issues as they erupted around her.

Thus she composed a song castigating the Zulu role in the violent gang warfare of the time between the Basotho AmaRasha gang and migrant Zulu workers. She recalled that one day in 1956 in Pimville she was suddenly confronted by the blanketed AmaRasha and the opposing Zulu about to attack each other. And she composed and recorded a song rebuking the Zulu for the destruction they were causing to others and to their own people through their addiction to fighting. There were others as well, which show Masuka using song to record the everyday lives of urban women and the dangers they faced. The song 'Khawuleza!' (Move fast!!) echoed the urban woman's struggle to continue beer-brewing operations in times of harsh legal restrictons and fierce police harassment. Building on the actual calls that would echo from yard to yard when the police were approaching, the song tells the beer brewing women to hide their drums quickly because the police are about to make a raid. So beneath a glamorous image Masuka showed the capacity of the woman singer to engage in sharp social and political comment. But the socio-political comment of such songs and their power to lock in with other forms of political resistance as part of a broad counter discourse was noted by the watchful regime preparing its sweeping laws of censorship. When in 1958 Masuka composed and recorded a song 'UDr Malan unomteth' onzima' (Dr Malan has made a terrible law) her friends decided it was time for her to go. Recrossing the national boundary she returned home to Bulawayo with three of her songs censored in South Africa, with an appetite for political comment and with a reputation at least as solid in South Africa as in her native Rhodesia.

The strong regional links in terms of black musical culture between the Rhodesian centre of Bulawayo in Matabeleland in the west and Johannesburg in the 50s — which are only now being rediscovered[43] — meant that it was not difficult for Masuka to continue almost without a break in her musical career. She quickly became part of the thriving jazz and music scene which was part of black urban culture obscured for years by the dominant discourse of settler culture. Here, however, there was less of a community of women singers than there had been in Johannesburg. There were, Masuka recalled, great musicians like the jazz player 'Khahlu' who moved between Bulawayo and Johannesburg; there was Josiah Hadebe with his stereotypic songs about 'women in the streets', Matzikatire, Jacob Moyo and groups such as De Black Evening Follies, with the singer Christine Dube and the City Quads moving between Bulawayo and the Rhodesian capital, Salisbury which did have more women performers. Masuka was able to hire her own band, the Golden Rhythm Crooners, and so had a degree of economic independence which was of crucial importance and gave her, as an artist, a far greater power of manoeuvrability. In what was to be a brief stay in Bulawayo she continued her dual role as composer and singer, never confining her songs to any safe or soft zone but moving instead into wider discourses of the social and the political. One of her songs, 'UNontsokolo' (The Millipede) fed into the stream of regional migrant experience of the long train journey from home to Egoli (Johannesburg) and joined the body of song, poetry and the written word that has come into existence around the southern African experience of the journey, the train, home and work.[44]

Soon, however, her composing of political songs was to drive her out of the country — with her repuation as a home singer greatly enhanced. Another of her compositions — again touching on an overarching southern African theme, that of dispossession — was 'Sihlal' emhlane njeng' izintandane' (We live in the bush like orphans) — and then, after the murder of Patrice Lumumba, she brought out a song in which she blamed Mobuto for the deed. Perhaps this bold judgement coming out not in confined print but in a melody broadcast to anyone who had a radio or record player, hummed potentially in any and every bar, caught the administration on a raw nerve. Once again song, and the way in which it had the power to challenge and dislocate official authority, was seen as dangerous. Masuka became a marked woman and had to leave Southern Rhodesia. Together with Sketchley Samkange she moved first to Malawi, where she sang for the Malawi Congress Party and then, as she could not return home, she went on to Tanzania where she sang to fundraise for TANU Youth League, in the course of this adding songs in ChiChewa, ChiNyanja and KiSwahili to her repertoire.

Although she was now clearly a singer with a role to play in several nationalist struggles of the southern and east and central African region she never let go of her sharp sense of social, domestic comment. Such songs continued to exist in her compositions alongside those with an explicit political edge which were sharply etched into nationalist discourses. Here the cutting edge of women's domestic experience answered back the tired but ever-popular images of 'beautiful woman', 'unfaithful woman' and so on which were the staple of much popular song. She sang in Swahili one of her earlier Johannesburg songs first sung in Xhosa, in which a woman speaks to her drunk husband and begs him to, 'Leave me alone with my children!' Another of her songs well known in Zambia even in the 70s moves into the domestic domain from the husband's point of view. In the ChiNyanja song 'Osaphika thunyana tun'gonon'gono' with its teasing sexual undertones she scolds a wife who always underfeeds her husband even when he brings home plenty of meat.[45] Essentially, however, Masuka lent her voice and her energies as an artist to the nationalist movements of the region. She made a quick return to Bulawayo for three months in 1965 just before UDI, where her song 'Sihlal' emhlane njeng' izintandane' gained new resonance as the guerrilla war of the second chimurenga was building up its momentum. She then slipped out again only to return in 1980 to a vastly changed cultural and political landscape.

Speaking eleven years after independence, Masuka had little praise for the attitude of the new administration to musicians. She summed up their approach as, 'Music is the business of crooks and prostitutes'. She also noted though, that on some national occasions singers were needed, recalling cynically that she had been offered one hundred Zimbabwean dollars to sing at the April 1991 Independence Day event in Harare. She had refused. Such is the ambiguous and unstable relationship between a central government and those creative artists who can help summon up the symbols by which the nation itself is reified.

Susan Mapfumo, *'I will end up without a home'*

Masuka's long career in which she became a regional figure in the 1950s and 60s, and then a more marginal though still powerful figure within the new Zimbabwe in the 80s and early 90s, in a sense points to the limitations and ambiguities of national boundaries and symbolisms. Yet her story also shows a combination of power and danger in a singer whose voice could weave itself into several narratives of nationalism, and at the same time create a potentially transformative space, in terms of gender stereotypes, outside those narratives. Another Zimbabwean woman singer, of the next generation, was not so fortunate. An obituary notice appeared in *The Herald* of 30 December 1991 with the heading 'Gold disc award winner dies after long illness'. It began: 'Susan Mapfumo, the first woman singer to win a gold disc and form her own backing group in Zimbabwe died last week after a long illness.'[46]

The bland sentence papers over the sorrow and loneliness of Susan Mapfumo's last years which were haunted by her acute problems with drink, her 'crazy' mind. The woman in her gold disc song, Kwa Murewa, sings at one point, 'I will end up without a home/ Staying under a bridge/ and no-one will care for me'[47] — she could almost have been singing prophetically about herself — but certainly she was singing also about many other women both urban and rural whose dilemma and pain her song caught. She was also continuing to air the linked group of topics caught in the lyrics of the Dark City Sister in the 50s and by her — by then far away — countrywoman, Dorothy Masuka.

Throughout the 1970s Susan Mapfumo rode high in popularity with listeners and audiences in what was then still Rhodesia, but she appears to have been fairly isolated as a woman artist. The decade of the 70s, the years of Mapfumo's successes, was noticeable for its lack of women artists — Masuka was by that time long gone and better known on the air waves of Zambia and Malawi than in her native Rhodesia. Joyce Makwenda and Angela Impey attribute this emptiness to the exodus of women singers from the country during 'the repressive years of the Rhodesian regime ... to seek careers elsewhere'[48] Whatever the complex of reasons, the harshness of the UDI regime must have been a significant factor and by the early 70s there was no community of women singers within the country even in the capital, Salisbury. Possibly this meant that the ground gained in terms of challenging the stereotypic images of women and inhabiting a space from which counter images could be produced, was, for the time being, lost.

Nevertheless, Mapfumo's isolation did not at first seem to impede recognition of her as an outstanding singer. She performed first of all with the OK Success Band, gaining her first gold disc with them. Later she moved to the Green Arrows and, according to the scanty information in the *Herald* article, released records which became gold discs while she sang with them. Mapfumo seems to have survived the tense war years with ease. Possibly this was due in part to her participation in the hidden discourse of resistance and nationalism which marked the songs of some groups and individual singers popular at the time. The names of Thomas Mapfumo and Oliver Mutukudzi are often associated with the subtle and allusive songs which were sung in Shona on records and on the radio under the noses of the Rhodesian regime during the liberation war and escaped detection.[49] Another group quoted in Pongweni's invaluable collection, *Songs that Won the Liberation War*[50], is the Green Arrows, and Susan Mapfumo may have sung with them such songs as 'Musango Munehangaiwa' (There are pigeons in the forest) which Pongweni notes as 'a characteristic Green Arrows song in its extensive use of ambiguity'.[51] It alluded to the guerilla fighters in the bush and linked them with the spirit medium Nehanda martyred in the first chimurenga of 1893-6 who broods over the nascent nation like a great guardian spirit. It began like this:

Mwari baba tine zvichemo,	Dear Lord we have requests,
Tiyamurei baba	Help us father

Chichemo chedu, mvura Ngainaye,	We need rain please, Let it fall,
Tiyamurei baba	Help us father
Mwari isanaye musango forest	Lord it must not fall in the
Tiyamurei baba	Help us father
Musango umo mune hangaiwa,	In the forest are pigeons
Tiyamurei baba	Help us father
Hangaiwa dzakatetereka,	The pigeons mustn't be trapped
Tiyamurei baba	Help us father
Hangaiwa idzo ndedzemudzimu	The pigeons belong to the ancestral spirits
Ichokwadi baba	The true father [is Zimbabwe].
Mukadziona musadzibate;	If you see them, don't trap them
Tiyamurei baba	Help us father
Tangai maenda kuna Nehanda.	You see Nehanda first.[52]

Susan Mapfumo sang with other bands besides The Green Arrows, some whose exotic names (like New Tutenkhamen) are all that is left of them and others, such as Harare Mambo and The Real Sounds which are still performing today. After seven years of such piece work she was able to do what Masuka had done with Golden Rhythm Crooners and gain some degree of financial and planning independence through forming her own backing group which she called Fantasy. Mapfumo may well have been part of the resistance songs of the Green Arrows with their resonant allusions to the iconic figure of the female medium Nehanda who was, in typical nationalist fashion, emblazoned (as Boehmer puts it)[53] as a national figure. In fact the real presence of women in the construction of the nation during and after the war was far more problematic and contested.[54]

Mapfumo was, however, also remembered for her beautiful voice and perhaps most of all for the sharp social comment of her songs — commentary which was not in any obvious way part of a nationalist discourse. Possibly these came to the fore of her repertoire when she had the added freedom to choose her own songs and call the tune with her own backing group. Like Masuka, Susan Mapfumo may have lent her voice to the nationalist discourse, but moved beyond it to construct a woman's discourse of gender relations which made the private public. Some of her songs, in a way very similar to Masuka's much travelled 'wife's song to a drunkard husband' bit deep into male patterns of abuse of their wives. In their subjectivity and concern with the crucial everyday patterns of life, and their publicising of the domestic domain, such songs contrasted both with the iconic role often assigned to women during nationalist struggles and with the stereotypes of 'faithless woman' which feed so easily into the wider, overarching image of loose urban woman. Hence the images of the wronged and angry wife which emerge from her songs interrogate and destabilise the supremacy of the symbolic figure of Nehanda in much the same way as women's texts such as Ba's *So Long a Letter* and Tsitsi Dangarembga's *Nervous Conditions* interrogate the static female images in, for instance, the Negritude poetry of Leopold Senghor.[55] One such song by Mapfumo which was very popular, and which is thought to have an autobiographical echo, featured the voice of a wife confronting her husband who is leaving her for a younger, 'fresher' and 'tastier' woman; it was one of her gold discs and is the one to which we have already referred, 'KwaMurewa'. It began like this:

Ndakanga ndakaroorwa kwaMurewa	I was once married in Murewa
Ndine vana vasere	I've got eight children
Zvikanzi amai fambai	I was told to go
Ini ndava kuda vechimanjemanje	Because he now wants the modern girl
Machembera	I was told I was now old for him.

Another of her songs, 'Baba wabhoi' laid out the interior of a marriage from the viewpoint of a beleaguered wife:

Baba wabhoi maita sei?	Father of my child what's wrong?
Munouya nehalf yepay	You bring half of your pay
Munofunga tinokwana here?	Do you think this is enough?
Ini nevana	For me and the kids?
Kupfeka nekudya?	For clothing and food?

Such songs must have played a part in pushing dialogue and debate between men and women over marriage, and a wife's rights, into the public domain in a way that was perhaps not possible with songs on the same or related topics such as the Shona *jikinyira* and *nheketerwa* complaint genres which were sung by women but confined more rigidly within performance conventions in the Shona tradition and which were, moreover, not on record or broadcast over the air but sung among women in the rural areas with few but themselves as audience. In addition, such bold confrontation of marital and sexual politics, with its mention also of economic anxieties, contrasted with the stereotypic and 'safe' depictions of women in men's songs. As Stella Chiweshe remarked of Mapfumo as she reminisced almost twenty years later, at that time it was 'As if she was fighting a war with men. Men were singing about loose women who go out with other men. There she was singing about the men who didn't bring anything to the house and what did they think she was going to use with the kids?'[56]

Presumably, as 'KwaMurewa' was a gold disc, it was bought and listened to as avidly by men as by women and may have provided a means of openly engaging in a relatively new urban discourse on marriage where women were openly asking questions which custom would not so easily allow them to ask. Perhaps, however, for some listeners and particularly men, the charm of the singer's voice and the sweet rhythms softened the blow of the message. On the topic of social inequality, Mapfumo also sang of poverty and — by implication — poor wages, and wove into the message of her song 'Mari' an appeal against conflict and violence:

Ndiyaniko akawunza mari	Who invented money?
Ndiyaniko pasi pano	Who can it be on this earth?
Munongedzi! Ndiyaniko?	Show me! Who is it?
Ndimubaye baye! Ndiyaniko?	So I can murder him/her. Who is it?
Nekekana kangu	Murder him with my small axe.
Kuvengana kwanyanya	Too much hatred
Kurayana kwanyanya	Too much killing.

The ironic complement to Mapfumo's superstar status was, however, her isolation. The songlines between her and a singer such as Masuka who could have underwritten her beautiful but disturbing songs on men, marriage, children and money were too thin to be of any effect. Essentially, she was on her own.

At first this did not appear as a burden but rather part of her 'star' quality. Mapfumo's independent stance in the production of her music and in the management of her own band seems to have astonished some, at least, of her male fellow musicians. In a 1979 interview, at a time when she may have been at the peak of her form and influence — and economic strength — with her own band and with Gallo as her recording studio, the interviewer quoted below made it clear that such independence was not, in his view at any rate, the norm for women.

In a 1979 interview, West Nkosi said of Mapfumo that she was one of the best woman vocalists and the only one in the country with superstar quality ... 'One thing that surprises me is that she writes her own songs and arranges the backing by herself. No one else gives her a hand in her songs ... What I like especially,' said Nkosi, a record producer, 'is that she is not a copycat. She is original in her music.'[57]

In spite of her independence and the acknowledged 'originality' of her music — which may have been a passing gesture of surprise at the public-domestic nature of some of her best known songs — Mapfumo sank swiftly from public view in the early 80s. Was this because her songs were sometimes too uncomfortable for her audience, in spite of the golden voice and the beat? Or was her demise related, in addition, to a new phenomenon: to the rise of nationalist musicians at the time of and after independence, and the positioning centre stage of a certain totalising discourse around male imaged nationalism which drove out other kinds of music and other kinds of singers? Together with the euphoria of independence came singers like the ex-combatant Comrade Chinx with the macho image of the male guerrilla-fighter, the spear, the gun — what happens to an 'original' woman singer in such a climate of national ecstasy? Do her messages become, like the name of her band, a mere 'fantasy'?

Stella Chiweshe

You know it happens that when I play mbira, sometimes I end up not knowing if I'm the one who is playing, and then I'm just enveloped by the sound and I'm just taken and then it's hard if someone says, 'Ah, change the song and play this one'.

Stella Chiweshe has travelled through several terrains in her journey as a woman musician. Yet one dimension which she always carries with her is the liminal space of the spirit medium and the sense that her music, however popular and commercial it may now be, resonates with the experiences of earlier voices which register their presence in and through the mbira music.

Whereas other mbira players and groups — such as that of Ephat Mujuru — may have tried to free the instrument from its deep associations as an instrument tied closely to spirit possession,[58] Chiweshe has carried these associations with her and is at the same time a populariser. She is a woman who seems to have thrived on difficulties — and she has had many. She was pointed out as an mbira player by the spirit of her great great grandfather, a fighter in the first chimurenga of 1893-6 who, through her mother who is a spirit medium, announced that he wanted four mbira players for himself. This was in 1961 when Chiweshe was nineteen but for two years after that nothing happened. 'After two years it came, a great pain when I heard mbira again.'[59] She then began to play for herself and after a time her mother's uncle took, what Chiweshe stated emphatically, was the unusual step of teaching a woman mbira, and he taught her her first two songs, 'Maururu' and 'KwaTente'. It was another few years before she played in public with other mbira players and in those early appearances she was censured by men and women alike. The men who were mbira players squeezed her out of her place in the middle of the group so she would often have to go and sit in front — and so, ironically, ended up in a more prominent position than she would otherwise have had. Nor were the women spectators sympathetic. For them too, she was a transgressor, breaking down the norms of gender behaviour. 'They would say: "Just look at her! Just look at where she's sitting in the middle of the men! What kind of a woman is she?" Really, they were blaming me ... Now they admire, admire what I did to learn mbira.'[60]

For many years Chiweshe would be invited along with others to events such as the completion of training of spirit mediums, the ceremony to bring home the spirit of the deceased, and rain-making ceremonies. She recorded her first song as early as 1974 and so was in a minor way, a performer during Susan Mapfumo's years of success and the singers knew each other.

Yet the crucial transition from woman mbira player existing within the ambit of Shona music and belief, to popular commercial performer with an urban base was not a simple matter. Nationalism, and more precisely the wave of cultural nationalism of the early post-independence years provided the necessary passage between the two. In 1981, a moment when singers and artists were of crucial importance in creating an image of the new nation (unlike the moment ten years later mentioned on p. 126 by Dorothy Masuka), the Ministry of Education and Culture assembled over two hundred dancers and musicians and then selected ten men and ten women to form the National Dance Company. Chiweshe was one of the ten women selected to work on a play which was to tour numerous countries including China, India, North Korea, Germany, France, Bulgaria and Switzerland. The play, called *Mbuya Nehanda*, charted the history of the liberation struggles of the new Zimbabwe — the war of 1896 and the second war of independence from which the country had just emerged. It was in a very direct way a nationalist narrative and also one that was meant to identify the new nation of Zimbabwe through its history of struggle and through its culture, all encapsulated in the play. Chiweshe played the lead role of the rebellious spirit medium, Nehanda, who was executed by the British during the first chimurenga.

At first Chiweshe danced and acted but did not play the mbira on stage. Her present style of performing on stage may have been formed during this period and it is another way in which she keeps at bay the stereotypes laid at the door of women singers in urban popular culture. Chiweshe strides restlessly around the stage like a woman possessed. There is nothing sexually enticing about her singing and performing style, nor does she fit easily into the 'Mother Africa' model. She is more priestess or prophetess and comes from the liminal area beyond sexuality and fertility. She is in a way in a space beyond male control, at the same time she harnesses an area of power which has until now been claimed by men, she is both transgressor and innovator. Her style contrasts with that of other popular women singers such as Katerina or the South Africans Yvonne Chaka Chaka and Brenda Fassie, and also sets her apart from the macho and phallocentric performing style of singers such as Lovemore Majaivana and Comrade Chinx.[61] To arrive at this point though, she moved through cultural nationalism, playing the reified chimurenga heroine Nehanda in the national drama which toured so many countries and so writing herself into the narrative of the new nation. Only in 1984 did she begin to play mbira on stage and was invited to Germany to perform on her own. In 1987 she added two young musicians who played marimba and then she added a bass player and drummer, 'I thought of the bass as the male voice and the drum is like the heart beat and it helps me when I'm dancing, you know, stepping hard — so I added the drum kit.'[62] Her band, Earthquake, was formed when she played in Germany in 1987 as part of the Beat Apartheid concert. Now she, like Mapfumo and Masuka before her, has her own band and thus, far more than many of the country's male musicians, controls her venues, and her making of music.

A community of artists? A counter narrative?

Both Dorothy Masuka and Susan Mapfumo seem to have gained an area of control for themselves as artists by composing some at least of their songs and this became an important part of their power as artists. It is also a part of their ability to mark out a path contrary to what the stereotype demanded, chart a counter discourse, answer a master narrative. They constructed a discourse around their songs rather than slotting into an existing set of images, feeding into the loose lost woman in the twilight zone of urban life and permanently on the margins. Chiweshe's attitude to composing has some points in common with theirs but she stresses the continuity with existing songs which she shapes to suit the new performing mode she has evolved. Thus she sings songs which an urban Zimbabwean audience might recognise for their rural roots, which resonate very directly through a rural-urban continuum, as well as through a time continuum. Take, for instance the hunting song, 'Machena', the war song 'Baya wabaya' (Kill and kill indiscriminately) and the courting game-song, 'Sarura wako' (Choose your own) — the latter also used by Chenjerai Hove in his latest novel, *Shadows*. When asked why she does not sing copyright songs, Chiweshe replies, 'I don't want my elders' songs to perish ... What I'm doing is enough. I *am* singing copyright'.[63]

Yet in spite of such protestation Chiweshe does compose new songs. Sometimes, she says, she hears a tune in her head and the words follow. Thus the lament for the death in 1985 of Samora Machel, 'Ndinogarochema' (I always weep) began as a guitar tune played by her husband, to which she fitted words. In the area of composition too, therefore, she is ready to push ahead and use the strands of a validating 'tradition' while weaving new patterns with them. There may, however, be ways in which Chiweshe's strengths are also chains. She draws on 'tradition', remoulds and composes herself, yet she may not be able to move outside what is a confining cultural nationalism. She find the persona — real though it may also be — of the singer/spirit medium beyond gender a profoundly limiting one. She can popularise known and loved songs such as 'Chemtengura', about the man with the scotch cart who would travel all around Zimbabwe singing his only song, 'Chemtengura' so people called him that. But the question remains, can she move out of the nationalist mode? Can she move away from the powerful and animating shadow of Nehanda? Does she need to?

The dream and its function as a validator for otherwise unlikely or inexplicable action may serve as a crucial vehicle for a change of focus for this innovative and increasingly popular artist. Chiweshe uses the dream as a medium by which to validate the continuities in the journeys she has made and the place she has come to. When she was seven, she told us, 'I dreamt I was on a high platform and the people were on one side and I was on one side alone ... So I realised when I was with the National Dance band that this was what I wanted. I even found in 1987 the material I was wearing in my dream when I was young.'[64]

She may find that the dream returns again to underwrite new journeys. What is indisputable is that she is a striking cultural presence within a popular culture which is still dominated by the norms of patriarchy.

There are few other strong women performers, and the image of 'loose urban woman' and 'loose singers' is very current. The enlightened laws of sexual equality of the post-independence government of Robert Mugabe have been severely undermined by the police operations of 'cleaning prostitutes off the streets', which, like a deadly giant vacuum cleaner, swallowed up women from the pavements of Harare and other towns in 1982 and again in 1990. Women in towns are, it seems, in the new nationalist discourse still loose and still dangerous.

There are fascinating interconnections between the three singers on whom we have focused who cover different if overlapping periods in Southern Africa's history. The differences are in part created by the climate of the time. Perhaps Masuka has shown herself to be the most resilient, Mapfumo, perhaps the most gifted and the most vulnerable, the one who was erased from an active life both as a musician and as a commentator. Chiweshe embodies new trends and could become embroiled in the icons of nationalism or could show herself to be yet again an innovator who continues to thrive on difficulties, who maintains crucial rural-urban continuities concerned with health and healing as much as entertainment and who has the capacity to topple taboos and dislodge stereotypes. Certainly viewing the three as a line of singers set amongst others makes the landscape of Zimbabwean and Southern African popular music and the narratives of nation and gender very different, and far less unitary. They bring a changed landscape, and suggest possibilities for a different discourse.

1 This paper is based on work in progress started in August 1991 and is part of a larger project on Women and the Verbal Arts in Zimbabwe. It was presented by Caleb Dube and Moreblessings Chitauro at the University of Zimbawe in an earlier version as Women musicians, actresses and preachers: How did they get there? in the seminar series run by the Women's Studies Association and the Department of African Languages and Literatures on 1 November 1991 and by Liz Gunner in June 1992 at the Britain-Zimbabwe Society Research Day on Civil Society in Zimbabwe, St Anthony's College, University of Oxford; also at the New Literatures in English Annual Conference at the University of Bayreuth, and to the Postcolonial Literatures Seminar of the English Institute of the Free University of Berlin where it was presented by Moreblessings Chitauro and Liz Gunner. We would like to thank friends and colleagues who helped in various ways when we were collecting material for this article: Dr Herbert Chimhundu and Dr Anne Jeffries of the University of Zimbabwe, Tsitsi Vera and Tisa Chifunyise in Harare, Sheila Cameron of the Zimbabwe Union of Musicians for setting up meetings with actresses and singers in Bulawayo. Also thanks to Anne McClintock and Rob Nixon who commented in London on a draft of the paper. Part of the research was generously funded by the British Council and for that we thank them.

2 The words of a Harare woman musician who prefers to remain anonymous, quoted by Joyce Mukwenda and Angela Impey in the September section article on Women

Musicians in Zimbabwe: Past and Present in the *Diary of the Zimbabwean Women in Contemporary Culture*, Harare, 1991 (referred to in future as *Diary ZWCC*).

3 *Diary ZWCC* March 22/23.

4 *Diary ZWCC* July Theatre photo caption.

5 For an overview of the increasing recognition of the role of popular culture as shaper of social text see Chandra Mukerji and Michael Schudson, Popular Culture in R.H. Turner and J.F. Short (eds.) *Annual Review of Anthropology* 12, 1986, pp. 47-65.

6 A.McClintock, Family Feuds, Gender, Nationalism and the Family, *Feminist Review* 44, 1993, pp.61-80.

7 Deniz Kandiyoti, Identity and its Discontents: Women and the Nation, *Millenium: Journal of International Studies* 20, 3, 1991, pp. 429-443.

8 Elleke Boehmer, Stories of Women and Mothers: Gender and Nationalism in the Early Fiction of Flora Nwapa, in Susheila Nasta (ed.) *Motherlands: Black Women's Writing from Africa, the Caribbean and South Asia*, London: Women's Press, 1991, p. 6; on women and nationalism see also the Introduction to Nira Yuval-Davis and Flora Anthias (eds.) *Woman — Nation — State*, London: Macmillan, 1992, pp. 1-15.

9 Boehmer, Stories of women, p. 9.

10 Diana Jeater, Marriage, Perversion and Power: the Construction of Moral Discourse in Southern Rhodesia 1890-1930, Doctoral Thesis, University of Oxford, 1990, p. 95. The following discussion relies heavily on Jeater whose work focuses on Gwelo (Gweru) although she also draws on evidence from districts such as Makoni in the east and events in Salisbury (Harare).

11 See the account of the connection between notions of degeneration and progress in the emerging self-definition of the Victorian middle class in Anne McClintock, Maidens, Maps and Mines: *King Solomon's Mines* and the reinvention of patriarchy in colonial South Africa, in Cherryl Walker (ed.), *Women and Gender in Southern Africa to 1945*, Cape Town: David Philip; London: James Currey, 1990, pp. 96-125.

12 Don Mattera, *Memory is the Weapon*, Johannesburg: Ravan, 1987, p. 69.

13 Jeater, Marriage, Perversion and Power, p. 182.

14 Jeater From the correspondence column of the *Gwelo Times*, 14.10.1905 quoted in Marriage, Perversion and Power, ibid.

15 Jeater, Marriage, Perversion and Power, pp. 390-393.

16 See Mary Douglas, *Purity and Danger*, referred to in Sara Delmont and Lorna Duffin (eds) *The Nineteenth Century Woman: her Cultural and Physical World*, London: Croom Helm; New York: Barnes and Noble, 1978, p. 14.

17 See for instance the following novels by N.S.Sigogo: *Akulazulu Emhlabeni* (There is no heaven on earth), Gwelo: Mabo Press and Rhodesia Literature Bureau [RLB], 1971; *USethi Ebukhweni Bakhe*, Gwelo: Mambo Press in association with the RLB, 1970; Gudlindlu Mntanami, Gwelo: Mambo Press in association with the RLB, 1967 and Chakaipa, *Dzasukwa Mwana Asina Hembe* (You wash the clothes of a naked child), Salisbury (Harare): Longman, 1967; *Garandichaiya* (Hold on, I'll be back), Salisbury (Harare): Longman, 1963. See also R. Gaidazanwa's wide-ranging critique of the representation of women in Zimbabwean fiction, *Images of Women in Zimbabwean Literature*, Harare: College Press, 1985.

18 Herbert Chimhundu, Sexuality and socialisation in Shona praises and lyrics, paper read at the Power and Marginality in Oral Literature Conference, School of Oriental and African Studies, London University, January 1991.

19 For an illuminating account of this process see Florence Stratton, Manichean Aesthetics Reconsidered: the Politics of Gender in Contemporary African Literature, Doctoral Thesis, University of London, 1991.

20 See for instance the ongoing work by Joyce Makwenda: Research and Recent Traditions, Zimbabwe Contemporary Music of the 1940s, paper read at the AVA-90.

21 Interviews conducted in Harare and Bulawayo in August and September 1991.

22 Interview with Batsairnai actresess; also Julieth Kurebwa, interviewed by Caleb Dube, 2 and 29.9.91, U. of Zimbabwe.

23 See *Vox Populi: Township Theatre News*, [Bulawayo] Vol 1, 4, p.1, Inxusa Festival Launches Amakhosi's season in Makokoba Township.

24 Caleb Dube and Liz Gunner 27.8.91.

25 See David Coplan, Fictions that Save: Migrants' Performance and Basotho National Culture, *Cultural Anthropology* 6, 2, 1991.

26 See for instance E.Gunner, Songs of Innocence and Experience: Zulu Women as Composers and Performers of Zulu praise poetry, in C. Clayton (ed.) *Women and Writing in South Africa, a critical anthology,* Johannesburg: Heinemann, 1989.

27 Kirsten Alnaes, Singing with the Spirits: Song and ritual among the Bakonzo in Western Uganda, paper presented at the sixth Satterthwait Colloquium on African Ritual and Religion, April 1990.

28 Dorothy Masuka to MC, CD and LG Bulawayo, 26.8.91.

29 All the details about Dorothy Masuka's life and careeer come from an interview the writers had with her in Bulawayo on 26 August 1991. Further references will be to D.Masuka Interview.

30 Miriam Makeba describes one of these tours, with the Manhattan Brothers in *Makeba: My Story*, Miriam Makeba with James Hall, London: Bloomsbury, 1988, pp. 55-57.

31 For Makeba's account of those vital but hard years see *Makeba: My Story*. pp. 46-74.

32 Makeba recalls that Gallotone paid performers two pounds fifty a day and no royalties, Story, p. 52.

33 David Coplan, *In Township Tonight! South Africa's Black City Music and Theatre,* Johannesburg: Ravan, 1985.

34 See the review of the ZMC African Heritage collection Volume 1 Miriam Makeba and the Skylarks in *Horizon* February 1993, p. 45.

35 *In Township Tonight* lists Letta Mbulu as one of the Skylarks, not Mummy Girl Nketie, see p. 168.

36 *In Township Tonight*, p. 177; D. Masuka Interview.

37 From an unmarked recording, transcribed by Liz Gunner and Mafika Gwala.

38 See Jürgen Schadeberg (compiler), *Finest Photographs of Old Drum,* Lanseria: Bailey's African Photo Archives, Distributed Penguin, 1987; see also Dorothy Driver's work in progress on *Drum* and women.

39 Makeba attributes the composition of the words of the song to Mankhewekwe Dvushe and calls the song a 'Xhosa tune'. *Story,* p. 52.

40 *Story,* p. 66.

41 Masuka Interview Bulawayo 27 August 1991.

42 Masuka spent some time in Port Elizabeth visiting relatives and quite often uses Xhosa in her songs, as here.

43 See Echoes of a Lost Era, Joyce Makwenda and Tarcisio Adolfo, *Horizon*, June 1992, pp. 34-36. The article focuses on music in the old Mbare township of Salisbury in the 30s, 40s, 50s through to the early 60s.

44 See for instance V. Erlmann *African Stars: Studies in South African Peformance,* Chicago: Chicago University Press, 1991; Oswald Mbuyiseni Mtshali, *Sounds of a Cowhide Drum,* London: OUP, 1972 especially, Amagoduka at Glencoe Station.

45 P.comm Jerome Hachipola 30.3.93 Harare.

46 *The Herald,* Harare, 30.12.91, Gold disc award winner dies after long illness, by Jimmy Salani.

47 Stella Chiweshe quoted these words translated from the song in an interview in Berlin on 23 June 1992.

48 Ibid.

49 See for instance Matiregera Mambo (Lord you have abandoned us) by Thomas Mapfumo and the Acid Band and Ndipeiwo Zano (Please give me advice) by Oliver Mutukudzi, in Alec Pongweni (compiler), *Songs that Won the Liberation War,* Harare:

College Press, 1982, pp. 103-5 and 107-9.
50 Alec Pongweni (compiler) *Songs that Won the Liberation War*, see pp. 124-7; 140-8; 158.
51 See Pongweni, *Songs*, pp. 140-3.
52 Pongweni, *Songs* p. 143
53 Boehmer, Stories of Women; Irene Staunton's compilation of autobiographies, *Mothers of the Revolution,* Harare: Baobab Press, 1990 attempts to write on the presence of women in the war; see also Caroline Rooney's review article of Staunton, Mothers of the Revolution: Zimbabwean Women in the Aftermath of War in *African Languages and Cultures* 4,1 (1991): 55-64, Special Issue on The Literatures of War, ed. Theodora Ezeigbo and Liz Gunner.
54 See Staunton, *Mothers* and Rooney, Women.
55 For discussion of gender and nationalism in African writing see Florence Stratton's Manicheism Reconsidered: The Politics of Gender in African Literature, Doctoral Thesis, School of Oriental and African Studies, University of London, 1991 and Boehmer, Stories of Women and Mothers, and Mothers of Africa, Doctoral Thesis, University of Oxford, 1990.
56 Stella Chiweshe Interview with MC and LG Berlin 23.6.92.
57 *Herald* obituary 30.12.91.
58 Interview, Ephat Majuru with CD and LG, Elizabeth Hotel, Harare August 1991.
59 Chiweshe Interview.
60 Chiweshe Interview.
61 Our thanks to Lucy Duran for pointing out the difference in her performing style and its significance.
62 Chiweshe Interview.
63 Chiweshe Interview.
64 Chiweshe Interview.

Traditions of Poetry in Natal*

ARI SITAS

We have been facing a 'brilliant chaos' of words, for the last few years
have been tremendous for poetry in Natal. But we have also been reeling
from collisions between two poetic traditions, a scripted and an oral one.
And both traditions have been colliding in the context of political and
labour initiatives in the area.

The two primordial poles of the 'oral' and the 'written' stand opposite
each other drenched in prejudice: after all, a hundred years of work in
plantations, in sugarmills, on the docks and inside factories have torn the
traditions apart, leaving little room for interaction. For example, Lawrence
Zondi, the most 'natural' and 'oral' of contempory labour poets — one of
the most rooted political and labour leaders in the Midlands, the area's
oral historian and intellectual — pours scorn on all those 'Englishmen' in
his orations: those black scribes who have been *distanced* from the people.[1]
For example, Alfred Qabula, another labour poet, also orates against
education that emasculates traditions. He insists that he only praises
'rough hands that hold the plough' in his work.[2] On the other hand, our
educated scribe shrinks away from the vernacular noises of oral poets,
responding against something 'tribal', something 'apartheid-induced',
something that is narrower than a wholesome national spirit. What both
traditions are in danger of missing is that they share an 'unconscious
surplus' of creative energy. I shall proceed in the pages that follow to
offer a more *conscious* assessment. And I will venture later a further
argument: that unless these territories are understood, we cannot even
begin discussing the strength of 'people's poetry' in Natal and its own
internal criteria of excellence.

The fate of oral as against scripted creators was separated, parcelled
and dispatched down different emotive paths. The former followed
ordinary people from the countryside to their hostels and compounds;
from there, to the townships and back. It followed the trials of the Zulu
Royal House, of the chiefship system, of rebellions; it disappeared and
reappeared revitalised by Ethiopian and Zionist sermonising; it continued
to speak and communicate with ancestral shadows; it buried kin; it

influenced song-cycles. It led a peculiar existence in the nooks and crannies of an advancing industral economy in South Africa. It has in short a complex career in the lives of people to whom paper was as good for rolling cigarettes as it was for words.

The scripted sign had a different career; it was elevated through mission schools, it was made scholarly and initiated to the many currents of English literary traditions. It learnt how to be patted on the back by liberal institutions. It learnt to admire imperial culture and came to accept its criteria of excellence. By the time it found itself in print, it had been accustomed to 'cultural dominants' which were established through imperial networks. Such preoccupations led many black poets to aspire to the status of *black* Shakespeare, Keats or Shelley, and through trans-Atlantic connections to aspire to become a Langston Hughes. The life of H.I.E. Dhlomo is a rich source of some of these tendencies,[3] some of these 'acceptances' of literary criteria, but simultaneously his was the first significant rejection, which marked from 1941, the origins of a 'resistance poetry' whose impulses race down the years through poets like Mazisi Kunene, Mafika Pascal Gwala to the present. The turning point is the *Valley of a Thousand Hills,* the poem about a world that surrounds us.

Dhlomo

Dhlomo broke away from the 'dictatorship of a small group of Europeans', that is, liberal control, by *imagining* himself a 'bard', a 'people's poet', an *'imbongi'* of the black population. Such an 'imagining' allowed him to write as if the connection between his pen and the people was unproblematic. Although unschooled in the dynamics of 'oral' lore or poetry, traditions he repressed in favour of civilised imperial culture, he manged to utilise such an unconscious surplus to transform his project. 'My creative work', he asserted, 'is the greatest thing I can give to my people, to Africa. I am determined to die writing and writing and writing.' From his new role, his creative project became the desire and ambition to write genuine 'black classics' of literature, in the service of his community.[4]

Such an ambition and the writing it inspired was seen by Dhlomo to be in the services of the *'New African'*: a 'class' which consisted of 'organised black workers — who are awakening to the issues at stake and to the power of organised, intelligently-led mass action and of progressive thinking intellectuals and leaders'.[5] Despite such Africanist impulses, his 'writing and writing' was in English — an English pregnant with archaic affectations and a style which was caught in a peculiar imperial timewarp.

The tension between his imagined poetic role and the poetic language available to him, produced the *Valley of a Thousand Hills*, his flawed masterpiece of African-ness: the poem is about the beautiful 'playing-ground' of gods, where, 'wild visions crawl and tear and mock (his) soul' and where, 'sweet hill and hill piles high to form and mould/ this swift dimensionless god-wrought ingot/ this spirit-teasing sparkling miracle'. The most un-African idioms and descriptions are deployed to express one of the most profound statements of Africanist sentiment of the 40s. Nevertheless, the valley with its old men, those ancestors who 'sit with visions and unspoken thoughts/ deep in their eyes and countenances grave; and they remember and remember but/ all dumb their tongues'; the valley with its peasants toiling away in song and with its echoes of Shaka and Dingane, becomes the creative source, the wellspring of a poetry of protest against oppression. For this valley is also an emotional heritage of beauty which was throttled as it was turned into a place where 'Wealth and Power and Blood Reign Worshipped Gods', where, for 'hills we find mountains of strife;/ for rills deep streams of blood and sweat'.[6]

This break from prior artistic shackles coupled with his burning ambition to create his masterpieces found Dhlomo becoming the 'bard' of the ANC's Youth League; and in Chief Albert Luthuli he found a carrier of Shaka's mantle'; and, as the revitalised ANC of the late 40s and early 50s was exercising its emotional adjustments for an era of mass action, Dhlomo's poetry, still in English, still distant from the murmuring of the lower classes, continued to echo national and class sentiments: 'Everywhere I am haunted/ by the wailings of the wounded/ by the groans of the frustrated/ by the people daily hounded/ by fear and by hunger/ by man-made danger/ ... By the vested interests of the Powerful Class' which also closed all eyes to beauty and to truth. Yet alongside his social commitment his verses continued to be marked by the melancholy notes of an urban abjectness as the poet gazed at a pale wan moon, at the ocean and the lights of Durban's Esplanade.[7]

Nevertheless, he was gifted enough to understand his own predicament as a bard of the people, but distant enough to misunderstand the people's. In his 'People's Poet Lament', he sums up his anguish with remarkable clarity: 'Must ever I remain unheard? Attempting/ in vain to get/ through mighty grind of printed/ word — a hearing?' and he implores his 'Sweet Muses fair', to make him, 'the poet of the Masses mute/ ... That I may dare/ their storms to raise'. Unheard by the people, imprisoned by the printed word, he is yearning for the creative impulse that would inspire these mute masses to action. One is caught in a predicament that can cut two ways: either these masses are deficient in their recognition and understanding of the printed word and art, also of their political mission, and are in need of the Dhlomo-like intelligentsia; or Dhlomo's craft is deficient in reaching their ears. The power of the poem is that it cuts both ways simultaneously. Dhlomo has been identified as an articulate member of the progressive black *petit* bourgeoisie in South Africa in search of a new national spirit; he has also been seen as an exponent of an African nationalism with little space for the aspirations of Natal's Indian community and so on. What is crucial for this argument, though, is that he opened up, together with poets like B.W. Vilikazi, a clearing, a little territory for further poetic launches.[8]

Kunene

Mazisi Kunene's project begins from the territory peg-marked by Dhlomo and Vilakazi. But Kunene knows how to be 'heard' as his poetry is cast in Zulu, the language of the majority in Natal. Indeed, his whole creative effort has been a reinvention of Zulu tradition and its heritages, and further: the remapping of the place of Zulu-ness in the broader African aesthetic geography. But his lines flowed after the 60s crack-down — a crack-down that has forced him into exile and away from his natural audience. So despite intentions, and despite the linguistic accessibility of his verse, exile has placed obstacles between his words and the people's ears in Natal: obstacles, and a new distance. Furthermore, his versatility in both oral and written genres allows him to imagine himself *within* the lineages of Zulu *izimbongi*. He is the tradition's inheritor but also its critic: 'Had you, by your wisdom, narrated the whole tale', he tells his ancestral prophetic poets, 'our children's children would have been spared the / humiliations',[9] as truth always outlasts its prophets. Yet words orated in Zulu could not reach their presupposed audience; they also fell on deaf ears in exile, so they found themselves in print, on reams and reams of paper. Still unread, they frustrated the author to translate them into English. Through this Kunene has found a receptive international and Pan-African audience, but not a local one. In Natal, the black population has remained ignorant of his contribution — a contribution that has attempted to rid itself of every influence that has arrived in Africa under colonial flags — religious or military.

There is not enough scope here to examine and to do justice to Kunene's shorter Zulu poems, or his enormous heroic epic of Shaka, his equally enormous and primal 'Anthem of the Decades', or his shorter recent poems. Single-handedly, he has created new perspectives on Zulu nationalism, with Shaka a revolutionary emperor and nation-builder; with the same bravado he has recast all Zulu mythology — of the origins of the cosmos, of the earth and of its people — in the 'archetypal' cycles of the 'Anthem'.[10] Of course he offers an easy target for people who are against the revival of Zulu ethnicity as a foundation stone for homeland independence, and his work could be used for such conservative ends. Despite such treading of danger-zones, his work is larger than that: it is, according to him 'a cosmic address, a prayer to life, a celebration of the great accomplishments of man'.[11] If Dhlomo gazed at the pale, wan moon at the edge of the ocean, Kunene from the red sand by the 'white tail of oceans' commands all the little crabs to follow him, which they do as he announces to them: 'we don't need a dream, we do not need a paradise/ we are the dream'.[12] Following him into orbit, through some of his later shorter poems, we shall be able to scan his humanist project, his sense of tradition and resistance.

Kunene's is also poetic argument: 'We erred too, we who abandoned our household gods/ and raised theirs with soft skins and iron flesh/ ... then to follow helplessly the babblings of their priests/ we emulated their ridiculous gestures and earned their laughter'. Against Christianity or Western civilisation he asserts historical and indigenous roots: 'we are not the driftwood of distant oceans/ our kinsmen are a thousand centuries old/ only a few nations begat civilization/ not of gold, not of things, but of people'. And it is precisely this humanist heritage that has been severed through colonial domination, by the 'strangers', the 'foreigners': 'the feet of strangers pass our house/ trampling our ground with fierce footstep'. He observes that, 'the madman has entered our house with violence .../ claiming the single truth of the universe'. He has stampeded over all indigenous culture: 'the reed of my flute has been broken .../ the feet of strangers have crushed my flute'. These feet have initiated the age of tears and have brought with them the 'night' of oppression as people are exterminated in the darkness of the mines for gold, for profit: 'those who waited in the night of the earth/ until their eyes succumbed to darkness/ until they bellowed with mocking laughter/ until they lived the illusion of escape;/ they were our fathers, our husbands and our children'.[13]

Kunene invites people to follow him on a journey through the night, this darkness into the morning — a journey that of necessity takes one through the wisdom of the ancestors to find that: 'they were breaking the long ropes of the night/ setting the world loose, turning it at will to their east/ I saw them stand unafraid, as the earth hurled into the void;/ and I knew then that the vision of a new era is born of the nightmare'. In this journey the ancestors' wisdom, the past dignity they have been preserving, become important components for freedom. It is through them, argues

Kunene, that the harvest-basket finds the homesteads and it is through them that tradition survives: they are 'the great voice that carries the epics/ ... for indeed life does not begin with us'.[14]

From them one draws both the heritage of liberation and the dreams of the festival. For as, 'the women of our village/ like a travelling herd of giraffe/ their heads thrust against the blue afternoon' as they stride on the ridge of the world like shadows,[15] and as the seeds of childhood are scattered by violence, Kunene, enriched by his communications with the ancestors, assumes the elders' role and hands over the heritage of weapons to generations to come in stunning simplicity:

Since it was you who in all these thin seasons
Gave to our minds the visions of life,
Take these weapons for our children's children
They were ours.
They broke the enemies' encirclements.
So let our children live with our voices
With all the plentifulness of our nightmares
Let them bury us in the mountain
To remind them of our wanderings
The sunset steals our youth
We must depart.
We must follow the rails of the killer-bird
Or else sleep the sleep of terror
To generations thereafter.
May they inherit the dream of the festival
We who watched the eagle roam over our heads
We who smelt the acrid smell of death
We who saw the vultures leave our comrade's flesh
We bequeath to you the rays of the morning[16]

Kunene bequeaths to the post-1976 generation, not only weapons but also a dream of the festival, indeed, liberation *is* the festival, it is 'the old dancing arena', filled with festival crowds. It is the beauty of the dancer, a metaphor for culture, ecstacy and abandon. 'I the son of the son of the sun/ I, the dancer of the south, pupil of the mountain shadow/ ... I am all movements, I am the caterpillar/ I am the twisted horns of the sacred ram/ I am the sound of ecstacy returning/ I am the cluster of white cranes in flight/ ... Like this we dance to the limits of the universe'.[17] It is also a vision of a long embrace of a traditional communalism which is at one with the wisdom of the cosmos:

There is a heritage of wisdom in the sky:
The continuous succession of suns and moons
The furtherance of love through the souls of the clouds.
The inverted bowl pouring out the abundance of stars
The fierce encounter of our truth and their truth
The suspended rivers churning out into the sea
The earth, our earth falling slowly into sleep.
Her eyes closing into the darkness of the rains
The vision of the green plant in her hand.
The preponderance of the dreams of tomorrow
The magic reawakening of our lives
The coalescence of our minds beyond the mountain
The rediscovery of our clansman
The long embrace, the tears of joy across the desert[18]

And such an eventuality is a cosmic imperative, as change and movement are of the essence of the universe and its 'strange powers of endlessness'. A cosmos 'created by the cracking of shells and the meeting of light with night, by the ultimate discord and order of things/ by the whirling beam of violent light, by the coagulation of substances in the eternal movement!' After all, the poet has become a visionary, a seer, who will 'lead you into the valley of tranquillity/ where you shall learn the anthems of the universe/ to speak finally the secret languages of the cosmos'. Through them you shall learn that, 'all the joys and pains are a single grain in the cosmos/ As so are all the peoples and children of the earth'. And by implication, the pains of colonial and capitalist domination are minute transitory forms to be swept by the triumph of rivers, 'dragging the former masters of the earth/ into the ocean, into the myriad aspects of the universe'.[19]

Here, then, is the burning ambition of Dhlomo to create black literature of note. In Kunene it takes the form of an Africanist affirmation, rather than an anti-white, anti-imperialist statement. And within that, an affirmation of a Zulu epic culture and poetry. Here too, there is a similar assumption of the *imbongi's* role. In Kunene there is also the attempt to provide his poetry with its own aesthetics of beauty and in many introductory comments, with its own philosophical foundations. It is a poetry that has purged itself from any reference that resembles the *contents*, the 'truths' or structures of the 'stranger' or the 'foreigner'. Both aspects of his poetry act in unison to create a poetry of remarkable strength and dexterity; but at the same time a poetry of peculiar limitations.

The distance of Kunene's poetry from the actual *contents* of oppression and exploitation, the refusal to treat the minutiae of these 'grains of sand' in the cosmos, provides him with a privileged perspective, and an assumption of wisdom that is impervious to everyday errors of judgement; it also allows him to develop a declamatory assertiveness and to weave lines of intense simplicity. Yet at the same time that very distance separated the work from the directness of everyday experience and social reality. The result is a poetry dislocated from the immediate structures of feeling and the rhythms of resistance of a modern day industrial proletariat, a 'grain of sand' as oppression remains *general*, metaphoric or symbolic. Indeed, since the Shaka epic which was a great historical reconstruction, his poetry's reference to people, nature and things has become symbolic, with a symbolism which registers spiritual reference points. Words are about their secret sacred meanings: not *this* or *that* hill, with these or those social meanings, but Hills, Valleys, Ancestors, Cosmos have become archetypal, primordial concepts. In this sense Kunene is aspiring to the role of Zulu praise poet in a context that cuts across the boundaries between the written and the oral. He can be viewed as a poet who leads the way toward the spiritual preoccupations of the black consciousness movement. But it is in the latter movement's reflection of Zuluness that we are to encounter Mafika Pascal Gwala's project.

Gwala

Gwala, from *Jol'iimkomo* through to *No More Lullabies* and finally the few but remarkable poems which have appeared in *Exiles Within*, has exhausted the creative limits of the scripted word here: beyond his poetry lies an unknown, an untested terrain, for every subsequent poet in Natal has been consciously or unconsciously writing in his shadow. From the gutsy exuberance of the first work, to the tortured lines of the second, to finally the authority of the line, rhythm and sound of the third we are faced with a complex inheritance.[20]

Part of its complexity has to do with the fact that most black consciousness poetry in the years of its origin in the late 60s and early 70s, to its later late 70s decline was *performed* poetry; initially performed only among small groups of black militants, it moved in larger and larger concentric circles outwards attempting to reach the black working class. Yet only a few voices, and Gwala's is one of them, reached that far. And although it developed a rhythmic vibrance and an orating quality of its own, it was unable fully to confront and interact with a popular, black working class audience. So what was written for performance remained bound by the printed page, affirming rather than enacting orality.

Jol'iimkomo is a distorted echo of Kunene's call; it is distorted and 'polluted' by the shack worlds of Mpumalanga and the grit of Durban and it is written in English with the rhythms and lexis of Zulu pressing heavily on it. There are other pressures as well which make Gwala's a very different English, it is consciously 'donnered' (as he insists) by people's everyday speech-genres, machine rhythms and localisms. Still Kunene's echo is there, fanned further by the rising tides of the black consciousness movement in South Africa, in which Gwala had a formative yet peculiar role to play. A poem like the 'Children of Nonti' is an Africanist affirmation of pride and dignity with few equivalents in the 70s; but it is a black consciousness soaked in working class grit.[21]

With him the universe shrinks; it is hardly a 'cosmos' — it is a space of urban grime. The moon hangs palefaced from the jet-infested sky where 'skylabs bid for power'. His lines do not walk on the 'red beachsands' commanding crabs to follow (as they do in Kunene's) — they step over pebbles from eroded valleys, gashed rocks and chipped hillsides. There is no festival — but rather all night gigs, drunken stokvels and lovemaking under gum trees with one's backside pierced by mosquitos — amassing from the nearby pulp factory's industrial waste swamp. There is no ecstacy or abandon — just being 'jazzhappy'. We are faced with a world where 'Blackness blacktalents/ Blackness echoes the real blues/ Blackness chucks out the death and fear in our streets'. But within this oppressive cosmos, there is *resilience*, there is *struggle*, there is 'bliksam vim' in the children of Nonti. Gwala takes one through the everyday struggles of poverty in 'Gumba, Gumba, Gumba'; he engages with the hassled lives of communities like Clermont, and argues despairingly with the soul of urban streets like 'Grey Street' in Durban. And it is this constricted cosmos of tin, of clocks and machines, of black struggle but also of class struggle that haunts any reader — where middle class 'non-whites' have become a 'fuckburden' to blacks. Within this world, Gwala assumes the role of an urban *imbongi* of scripted letters.[22]

If *Jol'iimkomo* teems with gutsy exuberance, *No More Lullabies*, his second collection, is a disturbing mixture of poems: angry, human, and *transitional*, it feels like a work of anticipation rather than arrival. The poems continue being the sounds of the township that service apartheid's factories; they are marked by the wastelands of Hammarsdale and Mpumalanga and they grind on with their, 'spindle now/ ... machine blues' as the black working class is pummelled with the deceiving comforts of Castle Beer, Wimpy Bars and Kentucky Chicken in this age of 'plastic' and 'robot man'. Gwala writes from the 'visceral monotony of the surroundings', pounded by Natal's sun, 'its glowing heat gnawing like/ wild dogs at us' and haunted by the sounds of so many fathers who 'wobble through the night/ piss drunk, who do not even know their names'. He writes from the danger-zone, the 'moment of Rise or Crawl/ where this place becomes Mpumalanga'.[23]

But there is also unresolved restlessness in the poems, which strikes out at targets with different moods, or with the same ones striking over and over again. It is ironic, angry, humane and prophetic. His jabbing at the black middle class intensifies as we see it emerging 'from behind stockpiles/ of books/ now clad in Afro-style', wearing dashikis manufactured in Hong Kong. His frankness also intensifies as he asks aggressively, 'what's poetic/ about shooting defenceless kids/ in a Soweto street?' Anger is mixed with analysis and references to the political figures of Lumumba, Fanon and Cabral tempered slightly with the 'jazzhappy' horn of a Charlie Parker solo. But not enough to stop him from ranting against class leeches and oppressors.

Gwala is caught between a deep affinity with the sounds of the street and one with the defiant growth of the mulberry tree in the backyard of his ghetto. And further, there is warmth and compassion when he whispers that 'there is with all the odds against/ a will to watch a child grow', knowing at the same time that the dockers in Durban's harbour are 'waiting for a tornado/ or something to snap'. Then, 'history will be written/ on the factory gates/ at the unemployment offices/ in the scorched queues of dying mouths'. There is compassion, but no more lullabies for the children of Africa after the Soweto insurrection. In this work Gwala can still self-deprecate his art by calling himself a 'sharpwitted writer/ far better on essays than on poems', but by 1985 the poetic essays he develops in *Exiles Within* are of a breathtaking intensity.[24]

In a poem like 'New Dawn', Gwala creates a remarkable sense of rhythm within his 'donnered' English, so that each line rolls out with tremendous authority to deliver what is in essence a castigation and a diatribe against the real trends of black middle-classism — its spurious consumerism, its new 'academic drawl' in a 'New Dawn', where the 'Fuehrer wears a black mask'. Gwala is caught in the night fighting against such a dispensation, but it is a night of also crawling as he waits, 'my belly to the grassy ground', and in this state and from this darkness he dreams of another dawn, as the Casspirs haunt the township. Listen to the night:

> Tonight, this echoless night
> Like a dried cistern,
> A night so quiet;

It's the dry quiet of a pod
Shed of its seeds by the wintry winds
But I have seen carnations of Truth before,
Sniffed the red roses of hope
As my country bends
With the grey dawn wind
I hear hisses of the mamba
As the browning leaves rattle
Like a kettle on the boil.
The Afrika wind smiles at me
And kisses the willow tree
So full of red bloom promises:
By the summer the red blossom
Will cast my ears to whispers
Of a future wrested[25]

Unbeknown to him at that particular moment, Mi Hlatshwayo, Dunlop's *Ucingo obunameva* — the taut barbed wire, *olahlaba amaphoyisa alulahla*, whom the police seize only to have their hands torn, like a 'kettle on the boil' was orating about the rise of a Black Mamba; and the old and wise 'Feathered Mamba' of the Midlands, *Indlondlo enophapha'ekhanda*, Lawrence Zondi was urging poetically his BTR Sarmcol co-workers to smash through the walls of Jericho with their bare hands: and Jeffrey Vilane, *Ingqhudulo engezananimpondo bathi iyahlaba*, (The Hornless Buffalo who carries the rumour of powerful horns), 'The Rhinoceros who devours machines' — all these, were beginning to initiate a revival and renewal of *oral* political poetry.[26]

But before we descend into the sounds of this other tradition, we ought to retrace the peg-marks and look at the creative impulses that have accumulated over time. A common argument is that black poetry or 'people's poetry' in South Africa is the poetry of angry commitment.[27] It is that and more: Dhlomo's, Kunene's and Gwala's poetry is often very angry and very committed to a variety of social causes. But it is *more* than that: anger does not exhaust its wealth, nor do the statements of commitment give it its only life-force. It is not an accumulated bundle of slogans or resolutions, it is not merely a statement of correct principles. It is also a peculiar event *in* and *through* language: it is an imagined oral language — communication trapped in print. It is an event which attempts to orate through writing. In this lies both its value and its limitation. It is the product of an imaginative act that permits creators to assume the mantle of an *imbongi* or a 'people's poet' and to assume that the linkage between them and the people is immediate. And the oral grassroots poets are wrong. Although many black middle-class writers, 'Englishmen', or people who have abandoned the plough assume this role, yet at least in the three poets above, a surplus remains, as their poetry is a unique event in 'language', and each text desires an oral communion with people. The tragedy is that they remain, particularly in the case of Dhlomo and Kunene, 'unread' by the people. And even if Gwala is known and quoted far more widely than the other two, it tends to be largely in the bars and shebeens but recently also the stadium of his own in Hammarsdale. There is a double tragedy — none of these poets will be 'read' unless their works become 'orally' accessible, and the people will not 'read' until conditions that make reading possible prevail in their lifetime.

Vilane, Zondi, Hlatswhayo and Qabula

Over the last few years Natal has emerged as the cradle of a robust cultural movement within democratic labour organisations. In all major industrial centres black workers are asserting their creative powers whilst demanding at the same time control over them: 'We have been singing, parading, boxing, acting and writing,' asserts a 1985 document of the Workers' Cultural Local in Durban, 'within a system we did not control. So far black workers have been feeding all their creativity into a culture machine to make profit for others ... This makes us say that it is time to begin controlling our creativity'.[28] The trade unions sceptical at first of this newly-found zest, are beginning to place such work on their agendas very seriously; new institutions are emerging: cultural locals, joint worker-community and youth projects; *izimbongi* are pacing up and down orating their 'words of fire' in mass gatherings. From Richards Bay to Ladysmith in the North, from Howick to Durban and as far south as Port Shepstone, a multifaceted cultural contribution is growing. Oral poetry has emerged as one of the most powerful means of expression. Labour poets like Qabula, Hlatswhayo, Ntanzi, Zondi, Vilane and many more have revived the oral poets' craft and traditions.

The oral traditions of poetry have had their own complex trajectory of experiences which cannot be fully addressed here either; suffice it to say that in polite dashiki-clad society they are seen as the domain of two social forces — of traditionalists (and therefore uneducated) and of the black underclasses (and therefore uneducated) — they are a fragment of tribalist survivals. It would be ridiculous to defend the prowess of formal Zulu praise-poetry, its imagery and its performance qualities. It is a powerful medium for words, despite the fact that most of it, to quote Gwala, has lost its 'bliksam vim'. The praise-poetry of the royal houses of the Zulu kingdom, of prominent chiefs and so on, after surviving from mouth to ear, to ear from mouth for generations, has for some time now found itself recorded and in print through the efforts of some pioneering researchers/individuals. But with the development of homeland policy, KwaZulu's education departments and Inkatha's cultural curricula, most of this praise-poetry has turned into *scripted* textbook material. It has been canonised as a poetic-literary tradition, to be learnt off by heart, to be recited and tested in exams. Furthermore, with the importance of chiefship and ritual in the KwaZulu homeland still enshrined, it has also spawned its own official *izimbongi* whose task is to be the performing storehouse of all the main kings' and chiefs' praises. But beneath the surface of this more official poetry now, the craft has survived in multitudes of ways in the lives of ordinary black people. From church sermonising to family rites, a more *ad hoc* and improvisatory dimension of the craft has remained, particularly marked and enriched in Ethiopian 'nativist' or lay-preaching performances. It has led through the years to a subterranean existence as black working class life continued to subsist on oral modes of communication and celebration.

When Alfred Temba Qabula started in 1984 to orate his *izimbongo*, his praise poetry, he released an untapped source of popular energy which, without warning, exploded everywhere in Natal. What was latent, what has remained subterranean, poured out in volumes and volumes of sound in the context of labour struggles and their mass. Ordinary black workers with performing and rhetorical power began orating their poetry in Zulu, using all the elements they could gather from their cultural formations to express a new sense of self-identity. Hundreds of workers have been performing their poetry since 1984 — some of it vibrant, some of it an index of assertiveness and defiance, some of it written first and then recited, some of it totally spontaneous. This oral polyphony and its growth has continued to this day. The distance between this poetry and what the *izimbongi* of the scripted word have unleashed is great. Yet the point is not that this is some kind of 'purer' genre or a 'superior' one: rather it is a question of understanding their differences and seeing what positive renewals can occur in both through their encounter. But also since the publication of *Black Mamba Rising* (and indeed sice FOSATU Worker News started publishing these poems in two languages for national consumption) many of the oral poets imagine themselves in print. They have become, limping at first, but with more rigour later, both readers and in some cases writers of poetry. In tracing briefly the contributions of Vilane, Zondi, Hlatshwayo and Qabula, a clearer idea of the phenomenon and its grassroots prowess can be developed. This is necessary in order to show how these people and their vernacular noises, their pushing outwards of the expressive resources of poetry in Zulu, are no apartheid adjustment, nor are they tribal embarrassments. There is a surplus here too, another terrain that needs peg-marking.

Another powerful voice stretching Zulu language in new and unexpected ways is Jeffrey Vilane, recognised as a formidable praise-poet in Northern Natal/KwaZulu. He is versed in all the formal praises of the pantheon of Zulu official praise poetry. In earlier times (pre-1985) he was to be invited again and again to orate such praises from Jama's to Shaka's from Cetshwayo's to Buthelezi's. His oral abilities and his rhetorical dynamism have placed him in one of the central leadership roles in Northern Natal's worker communities. He has been the leader of the region, a shop-steward, bus boycott leader, and the national president of his union. In 1986 he was shot at, injured and his house gutted by anti-COSATU vigilantes. The year before he had spent long periods in detention. Vilane, a devout Christian, a Zulu nationalist and an advocate of workers' control, has left his imprint on the form and substance of every mass gathering in the north.

But in his case the discovery of tradition, pride and dignity occurred not through oral sources but through school books and texts. In reading the heroic poetry of the Zulu people, a desire to learn all about it, to collect it and perform it was awakened, was activated. So from the scripted gathering of these traditions we move again once more to their performance. According to him:

> I used some of the Zulu kings' poems like Shaka's izibongo in public gatherings. But my favourite has always been, among all the chiefs and the royal people, Cetshwayo. He was the first one to be handcuffed and accused of defending his land and his people. I respect Shaka; he was our national mobiliser, the nation-builder, but now for us, for me as a worker in the struggle, I admire Cetshwayo's heroism; not because he was a chief or a chief of the Zulu people, but he was a hero in the struggle against colonialism, he was detained, sent over into exile, he suffered so that his people would not be exploited and their land would not be taken over by the foreigners.[29]

These days he uses some of Cetshwayo's praises to begin his orations, then he stops in his tracks and asks them how do they feel their struggle features in such heroic scales? And then he orates about their struggles. For him the working class is sometimes a cow without calves, always milked dry for the benefit of others; it is the naked tailor of clothes it never wears, but it is also the child of a brilliant snake, the black buffalo which routed the *amabutho*, the regiments, who came to castrate it, to stop the spread of its seed. It is this 'snake' that he describes in his *izibongo* which borrow freely from folklore and other worker poets like Hlatshwayo and Qabula:

And they wondered whether it was a snake
or whether a mole
digging, digging away by the ocean
near Thekwini.
It resurfaced again further north in the lands of the Zulu
the oppressors did not see it at first
but when the men saw it they lost their imincento (traditional
 'underpants')
panic-struck they chased around asking
what species of snake is this?
And at night all the men lay awake from fear
and during the day they would spot the Ndundulu mountains
covered by dust storms from the din of digging.

Through such constructions, Vilane recreates the history of labour organisation in Northern Zululand: how Ulundi reacted to the growth of unions, how the employers started squealing, how he a 'foreigner', a 'Shangaan' (he is from Ingwavuma) was called in to account for himself; how the workers responded and what metaphorical steps were taken to organise the unions in South Africa. He attempts to describe, explain and educate, using the elevated language of the *imbongi*, interspersed with call and response sequences, songs and chants. The power of his poetry lies also in his performing skills and the vibrant rapport he creates between his words and any mass-gathering.[30] He is in the words of Gwala, 'resurrecting oral poetry from the tombs of the past' and he is beginning to construct a robust Lazarus.[31]

Lawrence Zondi, in contrast to Vilane, is completely 'spontaneous' as he is not formally educated. But at the same time he is a carrier of oral traditions from the nineteenth century to the present. He comes from chiefly lines, related to Bambatha and to chief Msiba — his clan had been wandering the spaces between Umvoti, Underberg, Pietermaritzburg and Lions River for a century. Now as agriculturalists, now as labour tenants, now as dispossessed and landless wage-labourers. His poetic abilities, but also his singing ones, his deep knowledge of folklore and biblical stories match his political experience as a worker leader since the 50s in the Howick area. To quote from Bonnin's work:

> Baba Zondi (is the) imbongi of the 970 striking Sarmcol workers. The struggle of the Sarmcol workers is full of bitter experiences which form the material for his poetry. His style of oration is spontaneous, an event or a word unleashes him. Grabbing a stick, he strides up and down, words pouring out. He calls up images of Zulu culture, past experiences and struggles of the Sarmcol workers, but also of other oppression; his style is a mixture of the traditional imbongi and the lay preacher.[32]

Moreover, any public gathering, large or small is decorated with his rhetorical powers of story-telling, call and response orations, analyses and bursts of ecstatic poetry. His language is bereft of the formal praiseology that Vilane thrives on, although he knows many of these praises, it is rather seasoned in the gatherings of workers on the farms, in the lay-sermons of wandering preachers from the seditious Sibiya of the turn of the century to Cekane of the last two to three decades. But unlike Kunene he does not feel these as 'the babblings of *their* priests', but as a source of deep and resonant metaphors that cut through the ancient symbolism of suffering, oppression, exile, wanderings, slavery and emancipation. With him the working-class is a 'black creature of many wheels', but also the class that is reliving the emotional states of Nineveh, Sodom, Egypt and Jerusalem, It is the total communism of primitive Christianity together with the communalism of a worker's soviet. It is the harshness of mechanical motion but also the feathers of the loerie, for which his grandfather was killed. It is many centuries of linguistic development, of elevated heroic speech trapped among the oil-cans of a factory's belting department.

After 1985, it was Zondi who amazed Hlatshwayo and Qabula with his 'performances'. Their cultural work kept on taking them to Mpophomeni where they would experience his prowess and then, in vain, attempt to get him, after the meeting to repeat his lines. He could not perform out of context, but through such exposure two new lines of development opened up: the increasing search by Hlatshwayo to find a total acoustic context for his poetry and in Qabula a narrowing-down of his symbolic storehouse to religious millenarian metaphors. In both there is a growing, simultaneous reverence for the total orality of Zondi and for texts they are beginning to discover.

Since the publication of the *Black Mamba Rising* book, Hlatshwayo's poetry has travelled down two paths: the first involved an attempt to develop the natural powers of the poet's voice in the contexts of mass-meetings. He consciously sought all traditional methods of performer-audience communication to achieve a totally acoustic poetry. This took him down the way of children's boast praises with their own rhythms and call and response mechanisms; to chanting and to formal oral poetry. This was combined with his reading of Dhlomo's *Valley of a Thousand Hills*, which ignited an ambition to create a total polyphonic oral poetry, with many *izimbongo* coming forward each adding all of value in their tradition, in an all embracing, experimental poetic performance. In the former case, poem-chants like 'Two Shelleng' were developed, in the latter only a fragment with Qabula and Ramaegkele, 'People's Salutations' which involved Zulu, Xhosa and Sotho poetry. This search culminated in Hlatshwayo's powerful combination of the imbongi's craft with a toyi-toyi subterranean rhythm to produce a tribute to Dunlop workers, 'the Workers' Trail'. Some of its inner rhythms can be felt in the English translation:

There:
  Follow the trail
    that leads through the thicket
    the trail
    that has flummoxed
    armed,
  columns of men
    the trail
      that has eluded
        Botha on a Casspir
      the trail
      which baffled
        Capitalists from England
      but
      which also baffled
  Sons and Daughters of this land
And has even confused sometimes
    veterans of our political dreams.

  Follow this trail
      it leads you
      through Congella

    The whirlwind Inkhanyamba blows through

        this thicket
    here: through it runs the true track
    here: we quarry the granite
    to found the South Africa of
    tomorrow ...[33]

This extract points to a poetry that is beginning to be both rhetorical and musical, and rooted in the symbolism of Hlatshwayo's early 'Black Mamba Rising' poem. Nevertheless, his poetry has moved on a second path, where as a cultural coordinator for COSATU he is increasingly playing a more national, a more script-related and propaganda role. He is also the movement's obituary chronicler. Here his poetry is beginning to experience strains, as he has not yet found the simplicity that can elevate it beyond slogans: it does occur in his tribute to his comrades from Sarmcol after their assassination, expressing deep sorrow for their loss. It works less well in his poem about the Pietermaritzburg violence and collapses into a series of programmatic statements in the Living-Wage Sermon.[34]

As the crisis has deepened, and the problems facing COSATU have escalated, the cautious triumphalism of Qabula's earlier Zulu poems declined and praise-poetry grew leaner in its imaginative symbolism. Indeed as cultural activists' lives were put on the 'line' as well, a haunting poetry of death and redemption was born. 'Death' in the *Black Mamba Rising* anthology is a transitional poem, as liberation becomes tantamount to *overcoming* the physical routing of death. From then on, Qabula's poetry turns to the Bible for its symbolic labour and, given the anxieties of these times, it is imbued with a new millenarian determinism. This is particularly marked in his 'Dumping Ground' poem, composed under conditions of extreme hardship and threat:

Wherever
he has placed his creatures
on the day of his calling
they shall respond
even at the dumping ground
— where filth is piled-up high
alongside humanity's rejects and rubbish —
they shall respond ...

Am I dreaming?
What do these eyes of mine see?
The world is beginning to blur in front of my nose

I can see
the mountains, the valleys and hills coming together
the sun, the moon and the stars are amassing
you cannot separate the sea from the rivers
and waterfalls
everything is blurring together and spinning
Am I mad or am I dreaming?...

at the dumping ground
they have dug a deep hole
they have chopped all the trees to tiny pieces
they have poured paraffin and set them alight
they have dumped and buried them in the deep hole
they have stacked broken bottles
old and rusted pieces of metal and iron rods
and broken bricks on top
to make sure they are never to grow
ever again.[35]

He is also beginning to enhance the everyday speech-genres of ordinary
people through his lines and to work more on the theatricality of his
poetry, on its dialogues and discussions. It is beginning to move in a
peculiar way closer to Mafika Gwala's poetry of urban wastelands as
opposed to the rhythms of the countryside. It is also a vision from *within*
the contents of everyday oppression and violence. All these new elements
find a peculiarly powerful presence in his stunning new poem about a
'Small Gateway to Heaven':

Tall brown walls crowned
with barbed wire fences
Walls that hide what lives inside
from all outsiders.
And inside them, the inmates never see
the world outside
they hear sounds
rumours of lives
they hear stories.
And on these walls: two gates.
A small and a big gate
just as it was told in the
histories of custody

but also in the stories of the entrances to Heaven ...

And we joined the queues through the small gate to Heaven.
And I have seen this prison of a Heaven
this kraal which encircles the slaves
and I saw it as the heart of our oppression
and I saw the walls that separate us from the life of love.[36]

Far from being the product of colonial domination, or a sigh of
backwardness, the poetry of Vilane, Zondi, Qabula and Hlatshwayo, and
many more is a very important event in South Africa's languages. It is the
consummate result of a struggle by people who have a large, immediate
audience, a clear organisational project, to create a popular poetry that is
of the people, as the people are changing themselves and the world
around them. They do not have to worry about 'proper' English, they
compose in the language they know best, which is in the main Zulu, and
trust the translation of their work in most cases to others.

They also have a clearer view of what it looks like, feels like and sounds
like in amongst the broken flutes, the houses invaded by madmen, the
factories, the hostels that so many poets use as symbols of oppression.
Their reliance on an oral granary of symbolic traditions, indeed their
revival in a new context, has immense advantages but inevitable shortcomings. In trying to capture the new contents of experience through the
old poetic language, they have created a peculiar new vision around
worker struggles.

But still, we are caught in Kunene's, Gwala's and Qabula's night, and it
is difficult to trace peg-marks in this darkness exactly. Nevertheless, in
conclusion, I would like to put forward five basic co-ordinates that
capture the contribution of both traditions.

The 'people's poetry' that has developed in Natal stretching from
Dhlomo through to Zondi and Vilane which is both oral and written, in
Zulu and English, has developed around five common principles. First, it
is marked or haunted by an 'aura' of hope, a promise however distant, of
redemption — a scent of the red blossoms of Gwala's dawn; Qabula's
wheels turning, grinding on forward proclaiming the morning; Kunene's
ancestral wisdoms that there are mornings born despite nightmares; of
Hlatshwayo's decrees that no stone remains unturned for all eternity.
Second, it is haunted by death or deaths, and the violence the current
society unleashes. It is a constant encounter with death, obituaries and
transcendence; a funerary poetry with or without tears. It informs both
the authoritative comfort that Kunene masters in the face of it, and

Qabula's liminal anxieties. Third, it is a poetry that happens *despite* the harshness; it states that there is defiance and that *it* is defiant. It is sometimes angry, sometimes playful because there is pride and complex emotions dammed-up in the children of Nonti. Fourth, it claims for itself total familiarity with the people. It aspires to orality even though in Dhlomo and Kunene's case this is a gesture not a fact. It is of the people, it communicates to them; but it does so through the 'unfamiliar'. It renames the world, it invents new ways of comprehending, of seeing. Natal looks different after Gwala has redescribed it, so do the institutions Qabula and others touch with their words.

Finally, it is at its best moments self-reflective and critical of popular organisations and popular habits and practices. It has been capable of developing these through two mechanisms: a metaphoric and a metonymic one. Both the bold imaginative relocating of self vis-a-vis the black past and the nationalist present, as in Dhlomo and in a more intimate way with Kunene, has forced the two earlier pathbreakers to move closer to the praise poetry of African orature. Gwala too, situated in the raw, strong sensibility of the ghetto and the tough remembering of generations of Zulu history has searched for a voice close to that of the *imbongi* — a new, urban ghetto *imbongi*. And metonymically, to *be* an *imbongi* in a new political context, as is the case with the trade union poets, has liberated oral poetry from its traditional role. Both the expansive inclusive positions of the first three poets and the more closely situated poetry of the present worker poets share the five principles outlined. It is the *way* they have expressed them that each tradition can teach the other new perspectives, and it is in this resonance across the two traditions that the criteria of 'excellence' need to be sought. The reasons why the complex of principles have predominated demands a sociological answer, but the way these are articulated as events in language, demands aesthetic argument.

---

* This paper was compiled from a series of talks for performers and writers in the labour movement. The merging of the talks necessitated many omissions. Another omission is the intellectual debt that this owes to a series of scholars: Liz Gunner, Jeremy Cronin and Kelwyn Sole, whose ideas I have raided in many an instance. In the background also, these talks were haunted by the scholarly work of a further troika — Tim Couzens, Jacques Alvares-Pereyre and Jacques Sevry.

1 Cf D Bonnin's, We Went to Arm Ourselves at the Field of Suffering: Traditions, Experiences and Grassroots Intellectuals, Workshop on Regionalism and Restructuring in Natal, Durban, 1988, p 28.

2 AT Qabula, *A Working Life, Cruel Beyond Belief* (Durban, 1989), see chapter 1.

3 See T Couzens, *The New African: The Life and Work of HIE Dhlomo* (Johannesburg, 1985).

4 Ibid, pp 211, 213.
5 Ibid, p 33.
6 T Couzens and N Visser (eds), *HIE Dhlomo, Collected Works* (Johannesburg, 1986), pp 211, 223, 233, 229.
7 Couzens, pp 255, 325.
8 Couzens and Visser, p 365. BW Vilikazi, *Zulu Horizons* (Cape Town, 1962).
9 M Kunene, *The Ancestors and the Sacred Mountain* (London, 1982), p 72.
10 M Kunene, inter alia, *Zulu Poems* (London, 1969); *Emperor Shaka The Great* (London, 1979); *Anthem of the Decades* (London, 1982); *The Ancestors and the Sacred Mountain*.
11 Kunene, *Anthem of the Decades*, p xi.
12 Kunene, *The Ancestors and the Sacred Mountain*, p 32.
13 Kunene, in *Tri-Quarterly*, 69 (1987), pp 323-4; *The Ancestors and the Sacred Mountain*, pp 12, 26, 32, 20, 30.
14 Ibid, pp 64, 12, 74, 40, 3.
15 Ibid, p 27.
16 Ibid, p 1.
17 Ibid, pp 56, 5-6.
18 Ibid, p 11.
19 Ibid, pp 71, 37, 22, 71.
20 MP Gwala's work: *Jol'iinkomo* (Johannesburg, 1977); *No More Lullabies*, (Johannesburg, 1982) and, in *Exiles Within* (Cape Town, 1986).
21 *Jol'iinkomo*, p 46.
22 Ibid, pp 47, 35, 32, 52, 22ff, 38, 21.
23 *No More Lullabies*, pp 23, 26, 38, 82, 51, 8.
24 Ibid, pp 8, 10, 50, 77, 1, 12, 61, 44, 77, 67.
25 *Exiles Within*, p 20ff.
26 Praise-names, by Alfred Qabula.
27 See Mlungisi Mkhize's Poems of Anger are Taught by Oppression, *Echo*, 30 October 1986.
28 Worker's Cultural Local Durban. Principles and Aims: Talk for FOSATU Education Workshop, 1985, in AT Qabula et al, *Black Mamba Rising: South African Worker Poets in Struggle* (Durban, 1986), p 69.
29 J Vilane, Interview, Durban, 1987.
30 Ibid. During the Interview Vilane orated two poems; they are kept with the Culture and Working Life Project. There are also two pieces of video footage in the project which capture Vilane'a oral prowess — singing, speaking, chanting at Currie's Fountain Stadium.
31 M Gwala, *Staffrider*, 7,1 (1988), a review of Mzwakhe Mbuli's *Before Dawn* (Durban, 1989) and of *Black Mamba Rising* (Durban, 1986).
32 D Bonnin, p 2. It has been particularly difficult recording Zondi's poetry. SAWCO in conjunction with the Culture and Working Life Project, attempted to have a constant recording of all his public 'performances'. Phineas Sibyia, the chairman of SAWCO, started recording, but after his assassination in 1986 only one tape was recovered and that was lost in the process of translation. The only existing pieces are Zondi opening the MAWU AGM proceedings in a stadium with a prayer/chant and what Debbie Bonnin recorded during two worker gatherings in Mpophomeni in 1987. In short, the task of recording and preserving his contribution has not even begun.
33 The poem is translated by the author and is in the Culture and Working Life Project's files. Sections of the Zulu original appeared in *Natal Arts Quarterly*, 1 (1988).
34 There are seven of this kind of poem in the Project's collection. The three mentioned here have inter alia appeared in translation in the *South African Labour Bulletin* and on Living Wage Campaign posters. The performance of Hlatshwayo, Qabula and Ramaegkele's 'People's Salutations' is captured on video, May Day 1986, Currie's Fountain Stadium.

35 Qabula's work appears in English as part of the autobiographical book, *A Working Life*, The Dumping Ground, pp 1-5.

36 Ibid, pp 49-52. Qabula has only composed one 'praise-piece' since 1986: 'The Black Bufallo [sic] of Africa' which is about Nelson Mandela, pp 110-111.

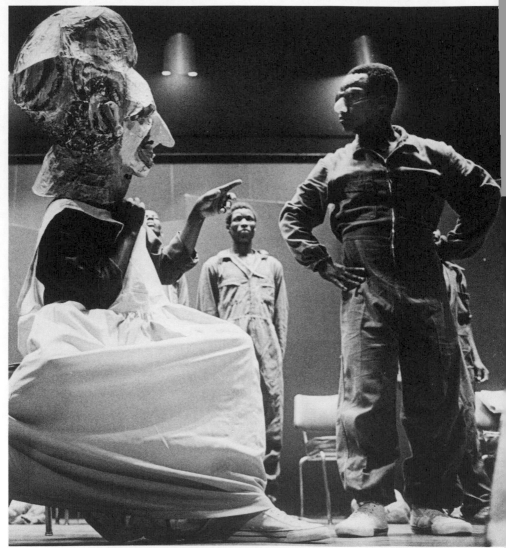

Picture: Paul Weinberg/SouthLight

'Maggie Thatcher' makes an appearance in *The Long March* performed by workers from Sarmcol at the History Workshop at the University of the Witwatersrand in February 1987.

Political Autobiography in Search of Liberation: Working Class Theatre, Collaboration and the Construction of Identity[1]

PAUL GREADY

Working class theatre in South Africa is perhaps an unlikely autobiographical subject: it forms part of a cultural groundswell aligned to the progressive trade union movement; it is a tool for education and mobilisation, unequivocally preaching the message of working class unity and advancement; and the plays are essentially oral forms of cultural expression, often devised through collaborative workshop, and explicitly for performance.

This chapter, looking at the worker theatre movement in Natal in the mid-1980s, essentially between 1983 and 1987, will argue that it revolved around the conventionally autobiographical issues of life experience and identity but was organised through the political collectivity of class rather than the individual personality.[2] In trying to understand worker theatre as autobiographical, adjustments can be made from external literary assumptions and theories to those of more local relevance which might be brought to the service of other cultural and literary readings.

Worker theatre is an interesting case study in the generic complexity and elusiveness of cultural forms from within predominantly oral cultures. It jars with many interpretive categories such as theatre, literature and, perhaps particularly, autobiography. But as Elbaz has argued the construction of genre is itself an ideological and hegemonic exercise which restricts literary practice to approved forms of expression. Initiatives that transgress and thereby demystify the generic structure or 'horizon of expectancy' with reference to what (in this case) is autobiography, are either banished to its periphery or the concept of autobiography is changed. In such ways old genres die and new genres are born, the new imbricate upon the old and 'horizons of expectancy' are reformulated.[3]

Autobiography as a cultural category is shifting ground and its imposition on a range of cultural production has implications not only for the cultural product but also for the genre itself. Assumptions governing the production and reception of conventionally conceived political autobiography, the sub-genre in which worker theatre most logically resides, are challenged by its inclusion.

Autobiography has come to be conventionally conceived as a prose genre, the power of which resides in its capacity to delineate certain kinds of lives and personalities. The hallmarks of the genre are a 'relentless individualism' and tendency to aggrandise the self. The dominant ideologies of the self do not exist in a vacuum, but comprise one component and product of the way in which political systems of thought permeate modern daily life. Autobiographical ideologies of self are chiefly grounded in the tenets of liberalism and capitalism. For example, the idea that the individual is free, among other things to write about him/herself, inasmuch as they 'own' themselves and their capacities and achievements.

Certain commentators have argued that this generic individualism poses more of a problem for some ideologies than for others. How to situate an individual life and achievement with reference to an ideology and/or institution which gave the individual prominence becomes the central dilemma of the radical political autobiographer of the left.[4] Doherty argues that political autobiographies have a 'tendency to weaken the force of a revolutionary critique made through the prism of personal experience'. In essence autobiography will give prominence to the ideologue at the expense of his/her ideology.[5]

This narrow theory of political autobiography is predicated on a number of assumptions that lack universal validity. It proposes too stark a divorce between the personal and the political, negating the capacity of autobiography to integrate the two successfully.[6] The autobiographical interface between personality and ideology is far more fluid than the inevitable ascendency of the former over the latter. Ideologies are not fixed abstractions but evolve over time influenced by, among other things, adherents and their autobiographical writings. Perhaps most importantly, the theory assumes a certain kind of society and/or individual product of or aspirant to such a society — literate, permeated by secular individualism, profoundly influenced by the practice and ideas of liberalism and/or capitalism — and the resulting prose genre of autobiography that epitomises its conception of personal worth.

In truth, autobiography can be either a conservative or a revolutionary document/practice, and indeed can be both simultaneously. It is an almost infinitely elastic genre, open to a diverse array of appropriations. Autobiography has been described as the most democratic of genres as it does not depend on publication, is available to everyone and is wedded to no particular form and so can take its imprint directly from experience. In addition, it is a great cultural enabler: it can become the door through which the marginalised enter into the house of a non-familiar tradition of literature or culture, often irreparably modifying it in combination with other cultural forms.[7]

To confine autobiography in South Africa to the conventional would be to neglect its potential to produce a whole range of formal and other experiments and to construct the majority of the population in terms of their invisibility. As the marginalised in South Africa have assumed agency by working both within and against the rules of a range of genres, the tensions introduced into autobiography — for example by race, class, ideology, orality and performance — have led to new forms and dispensations and new 'horizons of expectancy'.

Much South African autobiography, particularly of an oppositional nature, proclaims an ideological and cultural message that challenges apartheid, liberalism and capitalism, and related notions of literary convention. This revolutionary autobiographical mission has not always been achieved successfully,[8] but its widespread application has far-reaching implications for the genre itself.

Elements within the working class in Natal appropriated the somewhat unlikely form of theatre, synthesised with more familiar cultural forms, to tell of their life experiences. Worker theatre was the performance of a revolutionary autobiographical subject. The 'lives' were those of strikes and factories, 'lives' translated into public documents, as well as those of a particular class and its representatives. A previously downplayed and silenced world view, one which 'educates people about our struggle and puts across a true picture of things — our picture',[9] was given voice. The movement represented an act of repossession and reconstitution, as much a political as a cultural act. Black workers acquired greater control over the means and content of their own cultural self-representation. This enabled them to forge an autobiographical space in which they could critique their own experience and give creative expression to the conditions of their lives, thereby gaining access to hitherto inaccessible powers of self-definition.

Self-definition is a creative process involving selection and omission, exaggeration and fabrication around a desired purpose. Pascal has argued that autobiography 'imposes a pattern on a life, constructs out of it a coherent story'. Coherence is a function of having a 'meaningful standpoint' from which to interpret life, a present position which enables life to be seen as something of a unity, something that may be reduced to order.[10] Using the terminology of Laclau, autobiography is an attempt to manage and force coherence upon a diversity of 'subject positions'. One or a selection of subject positions are privileged at the expense of others. A person can only be reduced to one or a subset of such positions through the surgery of the creative act. In the process diversity is censored, structured and given direction in pursuit of order and in accordance with an evolving purpose.

Worker theatre was a self-consciously collective and ideological form of autobiographical expression. A characteristic of this movement in the mid-1980s was what Doherty calls 'the certainty of the ideological mind',[11] a conviction that 'our picture' was the 'true picture', which underpinned the autobiographical construction. The collective ideological mind mandated a coherent world, a survival adaptation, made possible a measure of control and order that was lacking in daily life and attempted to control a diversity of identities and discourses towards a particular end. It attempted to comprehensively constitute itself — encompassing all aspects of its internal organisation, cultural production and performance and self-presentation — around the unity and solidarity of worker life experience and a class identity. The impulse towards unity was especially powerful largely because of the particular socio-political context of Natal.

Such an identity construction obviously had national and international dimensions since it was, in part, a response to both apartheid and capitalism, but it was perhaps most significantly a response to the ways in which these and other socio-political factors manifested and still manifest themselves in Natal. Natal continues to be engulfed in political violence as Inkatha and the ANC (along with affiliated organisations in the unions and elsewhere) are locked in conflict, essentially over issues of control and power. Worker theatre emerged in the early 1980s to become a participant in the fraught political and cultural environment of Natal. It engaged in what was virtually a war situation on the side of those elements which were trying to redraw the map with reference to ideology and identity and to move away from race and ethnicity towards a focus on class and, in time, a more general oppositional unity.

Identities simultaneously became more polarised and more focused. An ideological identity is often a bulwark against disunity and uncertainty, or what Erikson has referred to as 'identity confusion'.[12] For the class-based movement in Natal, the prevalence of certain aspects of 'Zulu-ness' was perhaps the epitome of 'identity confusion'. Natal worker theatre became a participant in a localised race-class complex and confrontation where identities and ideologies have been manipulated, simplified, silenced, polarised and entrenched: they are a matter of life and death. Identity became so certain precisely because it was so contested, so uncertain.

And yet the existence of layers of identity and selfhood cannot totally be silenced, or are vocal due to their very silence. Nowhere was this more evident than in worker theatre's multi-dimensional collaborative orientation. At one level of collaboration, cultural activists involved in worker theatre tried to underplay their role in an effort to align themselves politically to and empower the working class. Such a position was in line with worker theatre's organising principle of working class unity and advancement, but it was ultimately misleading and obfuscatory. The collaborators in worker theatre — including unions, intellectual activists, worker activists, performers and audiences — were often wrongly presented as participating in a seamless collaboration.

Collaborative cultural practice is a transaction on many levels between different cultural practices and forms, languages, races, classes, agendas and so on. As a result cultural meaning, despite efforts at conflation into one undifferentiated voice, inevitably resides in a multi-voiced, hybrid product. What becomes important is the tension between the desire for a single voice and the ways in which multiple voices make themselves heard. Such tensions simmer unresolved beneath the surface, raising their heads as fractures, discontinuities and contradictions within a projected self-image.

Worker theatre represented many things beneath its cloak of uniformity. It was a precarious coalition of participants and identities which simplified internal divisions, collapsed distinctions over a broad front and suppressed the appeal of competing identities. This unilateral declaration of near one-dimensional self-representation was a distortion of shifting and contested relationships, an announcement of growing cultural independence, and a political response to a political context which sought to mobilise its constituency and challenge the structures of power. Worker theatre externalised and accentuated the fact that subject creation in autobiography is the site of contending discourses, normally contained within the autobiographer's head and the written page but in this case, in a real sense, played out on a stage. Simultaneously a rigorous attempt was made to channel, manage and censor the discourses towards a particular end. In the context of the above discussion new 'horizons of expectancy' can be seen to emerge and the outline of an alternative theory of political autobiography takes shape.

Working Class Theatre and the Context of Self-Definition

The apparent clarity of the theatre movement's self-definition privileged, masked and silenced a number of issues relating to the way in which worker culture contextualised itself culturally and politically: within oppositional culture; in the particular political dynamics of Natal; the 'terms of involvement' with reference to engagement with broader political and social issues; and so on. Often the uniqueness and particularity of worker culture was stressed at the expense of dissecting complicated and evolving relationships within the context in which it evolved. Contextualisation formed part of the wider discourse of self-definition. A good example of this was worker theatre's interaction with the labour movement, and the way the two together negotiated the political situation in Natal.

The collectivisation of identity had many rallying points, but perhaps most importantly, worker theatre's claim to a community of believers was institutionalised by its affiliation with the progressive trade union movement, specifically since 1985, with COSATU. The consolidation of the progressive labour movement as a major catalyst in the South African political arena facilitated the emergence of new cultural fronts, including worker theatre, but in creative conjunction with poetry, dance, music, choirs and other performance based forms. Plays and other forms of worker culture were officially sanctioned and supported by the progressive labour movement. This support assisted access to a variety of resources and facilities such as an audience at gatherings and meetings, publishing facilities and other forms of wider dissemination. Working class theatre gained its identity from the fact that it was the self-conscious cultural articulation of a political movement. In its ideal realisation each performance was 'a renewed affirmation that the struggle of the working people for their liberation has found an expression in dramatic form'.[13] Cultural influence within the life of the union was identified chiefly as its ability to consolidate, expand and mobilise its constituency, as well as to promote the related aims of education and unity.

The institutional basis for worker theatre's political agenda and unified identity was both unambiguous and empowering. There was union support for the creation of what are known as 'cultural locals' within union structures which provided a structural base to try to ensure that workers had control over the creative process as well as their own cultural production and promotion. The dominant institutions of culture had served workers poorly, denying them control and access, and diluting or misrepresenting their message.[14] In part cultural structures were intended to address the drought of resources and facilities in working class communities.[15] By trying to address issues of practical and political control, cultural structures sought to provide what Kirkwood has described as the 'infrastructure of ... cultural momentum',[16] and manage culture within the trade unions:

> [the DWCL was formed] to coordinate, encourage and redirect cultural work among workers in the unions (interview with M). Cultural structures are perceived as relevant to the degree that they enable workers to intervene at the appropriate conjuncture. Such structures or formations would ensure that the cultural work that was mushrooming from the ranks of the workers is not lost to the labour movement.[17]

There were various landmarks in the theatre movement's initial momentum. The *Dunlop Play*, initiated in 1983 to contribute to pressure for the recognition of the Metal and Allied Workers' Union (MAWU), became 'the root of an enormous cultural tree'. It 'created a space within the labour movement for cultural activity over and above union struggles' and fed directly into the formation of the DWCL. Cultural work spread horizontally through 'imitation-effects'. Von Kotze, Workers' Theatre in South Africa, *New Left Review*, 163, May/June 1987, p 84. The objectives of the growing number of cultural locals were epitomised by, and largely reflect, the 'Aims and Principles' of the DWCL formulated in 1985 and described as 'one of the most important pieces of writing ever put down by a group of workers and activists'.[18] In them, the DWCL declares: 'We are a movement that announces a real democracy in this land — where you and me can control for the first time our productive and creative power. That is why in Durban we formed within the unions a Workers' Cultural Local'. The document goes on to look at the difficulties faced, why culture has an important role to play in the workers' struggle and how cultural work is strengthened in the worker movement. If worker theatre as autobiographical practice were to have a single autobiographical text this would be it. It is one of many documents in South Africa, of which the most significant is the *Freedom Charter*, that attempt to write a country into being. The author(s) translate themselves into the texts in such a way that they become their totally public 'lives'. Such texts can be seen as the authors' definitive autobiographical statement.[19] The theatre movement, in part as the result of such landmarks and structures of cultural momentum, achieved impressive if uneven growth during the mid-1980s.

Another factor furthering cultural momentum emerged at the level of worker leadership. Performance and performers gained stature within public gatherings. Those who occupied and controlled the foreground created, over and above the democratic process of election and decision making within unions, 'leadership, hegemony, consent, identity-formation, solidarity and so on ... in the public world of mass gatherings'. In Natal, workers began to combine their cultural creativity with very public forms of leadership.[20] Partly as a consequence, cultural activists also acquired worker leadership positions through democratic means. Some, for example, were elected as shop stewards. The affinity and overlap between grassroot leaders and cultural activists has been unique to Natal and has facilitated the continuity of the cultural movement.[21]

The relationship between worker culture, its accompanying structures and the trade union movement was not without its tensions. There has not always been agreement about the priority given to culture. The Comment in the 1989 special issue of *Staffrider* on worker culture noted: 'We are constantly pressing our unions to take culture more seriously ... Our political leaders should be taking a greater interest, giving more time, participating in debates and giving more guidance'.[22] On a more general level the assumption that trade unions and associated cultural structures could automatically realise the interests of workers oversimplified the difficult dynamic of organisation, particularly within the political environment of Natal.

The labour movement itself was not a homogeneous entity but was the subject of intense and often violent contestation. The political landscape was largely simplified within the worker plays to demands for union recognition (*The Dunlop Play*, *The Spar Play*, *The Long March*); the condemnation of liaison committees and in-house unions (*The Dunlop Play*); and the juxtaposition of *impimpi*s (sell-outs) with a united workforce (*Gallows for Mr Scariot Mpimpi*, *You're a Failure Mr Mpimpi*). Other elements of the labour and political context received less attention. For example, there was little recognition that competition for union membership between the UDF/ANC-aligned COSATU and UWUSA, launched by Inkatha in 1986, has been a major site of conflict, or that the related political struggle has entered union structures. As Sole commented in a review of *Organise and Act*, 'a full discussion of the problems this form of theatre (and, indeed, COSATU) have had in their attempts to forge a unified working class consciousness in the strife-torn regions of Natal ... are rather lightly touched upon'.[23]

In an exception to this omission Sitas has outlined how cultural momentum and continuity have been plagued by various factors, some of which relate to the political tensions in Natal. An initial 'optimism epidemic' was crushed by the 1985 declaration of a State of Emergency, and the subsequent explosion of violence in the Natal region. The conflict between pro- and anti-Inkatha groups entered the cultural locals creating division and 'the social fabric and dynamic of the locals was torn to shreds'. By 1986 cultural activity was thriving again as typified by *The Long March*, a play which centred on the strike over union recognition and subsequent sacking of British Tyre and Rubber (BTR) Sarmcol workers in Mpophomeni/Howick.[24] Sitas claims that 'despite or because of the COSATU vs UWUSA/Inkatha conflict cultural activity was spreading like wildfire'.[25]

At the centre of political conflict were the interrelated issues of ethnicity and violence. It has been variously argued that there is no one conception or appropriation of notions of tradition or 'Zulu-ness' in Natal. Worker culture involved struggling within existing cultural formations with 'sturdy non-class forms of articulating experiences' and 'sometimes strong racial and gender insensitive connotations'. The key issue was that of transformation, or how such energies were harnessed.[26] Revealingly, the actual reality and complexity of ethnicity, its role at the heart of political and cultural conflict, and the means and degree of transformations of consciousness and ideology required to address 'identity confusion', were largely absent, particularly from the plays themselves. Political conflict could not, however, be avoided. Perhaps the most poignant way in which it made its impact on the theatre movement was through township violence in which activists soon became caught up and of which they were, on occasion, the targets.

The play, *The Long March*, for example, was updated to include the killing in December 1985 by Inkatha vigilantes and men in KwaZulu police uniforms of four residents of Mpophomeni. One of them was Simon Ngubane, a shop steward, cultural activist, performer and driving force behind the play. Several incidents left unanswered questions about the extent of the political and ideological cleavages being faced. Little has been said, for example, about the worsening political violence and political divisions which caused the collapse of the *KwaMashu Street Cleaners' Play*.

Usually the autobiographical agenda silenced the main sources of identity competition and 'confusion', and of fractures in the projected solidarity, as a central demand towards the coherence of worker unity. The management of contextual self-definition was a component of the construction of identity. Identity was an arena of contesting articulations and transformations and worker theatre's packaging thereof was only one of a number of realities engaged in fierce competition. The aim was to consolidate and mobilise a constituency, principally for COSATU and its allies and against all the forces ranged against them.

The union/culture interfaces of leadership and structure, and strength through unity in the progressive union movement — the factors which bound culture in its multi-layered collaboration with the trade unions and thereby most clearly assisted in giving theatre its identity — were persuasively articulated in plays and/or analyses of the movement. On the other hand, factors which contested or undermined identity — differing attitudes to culture within and between unions, difficulties of union organisation and competition between unions for allegiance, and the related issues of ethnicity, violence and political conflict — were usually silenced or used in ways in which, or to the extent to which, they could bolster the cohesion of the theatre's autobiographical strategy. Thus an inevitably flawed attempt was made to create order from chaos. Worker theatre was a political response to a political situation. Regional politics played a very particular role both in undermining its very existence and generating the necessity and motivation for its continuation.

Working Class Theatre and the Dynamics of Cultural Production

Performance and Audience

The message from within the theatre movement was and remains clear: it is the act of performance, the practice of theatre, the interface between performance and audience, that is of primary importance. The audience has contributed crucially to the emergence, recognition, official authorisation and composition of worker theatre. Theatre was both embedded in and constitutive of an interpretive community.[27] Worker theatre on the whole addressed other workers, and established a working class audience within the black community. In the words of von Kotze: 'Emergent worker plays are not meant for a consumer public ... they are created and performed within the perimeter of working-class leisure time — and space.'[28] Plays were performed for working class and union audiences, not in established theatre venues, but in what Sitas has described as 'cultural spaces': 'material environments, institutional or non-institutional, that act as physical and social carriers of events in popular or working class culture'.[29] These could be any place where people and workers met. Cultural presentations took place at various kinds of events from the specifically cultural to 'spaces' where people had already gathered for some common purpose, such as union meetings or political rallies, where they could 'slot into' the event. The interaction between performance venue/context, performance, and audience influences audience responses and has, therefore crucially shaped the theatre movement itself.

Sitas has argued that worker gatherings, and particularly performance within such gatherings, are the most potent ways through which public identities, solidarities and the fabric of mass movements are created.[30] The audience participated actively in a process which was essentially collaborative. It was in such gatherings that Natal's working class cultural revolution was launched. Worker theatre was, therefore, initially trying to generate identity through culture and to mobilise a constituency not in the comfort of a living room but within mass worker gatherings. Such a performance context obviously contributed to the genre's didacticism and focus on unity. Within these gatherings prior to 1983 performance genres existed which had their own dynamics and patterns of audience expectation and participation dictated by life experiences. People brought with them 'pre-coded' a series of 'rules or "tropes"', and aesthetic models, that influenced the ways in which they participated in mass events.[31]

The role of performance in worker gatherings was appropriated and transformed by the introduction of plays whose emphasis was not as much entertainment as education and mobilisation. Theatre challenged expectations and modes of participation.[32] Worker expectations about meetings and performance were jarred and new performance genres struggled to gain acceptance at mass gatherings. Performers and activists, facing the challenge of how to capture worker imagination and interest, started to borrow from one another. As already noted, worker culture had to work within existing cultural formations. The result was a 'tremendous collision' of performance modes. The constant transference and flux between performance modes and audience expectations created an accumulation of contradictions. The generic complexity of cultural forms becomes clear, as does their potential to liberate familiar interpretive categories.

Sitas has identified theatre as a 'plurimedial' event in which tensions exist between the old established forms like song and dance and the new strategic function demanded of them within a play.[33] It would be interesting to know the enthusiasms and resistances voiced by performers and audiences to the revision of performance forms to serve new purposes, and more about reactions to the overall formal construction presented within the framework of a 'play'. Some performances failed because of an unconvincing jarring quality, others brought about successful innovations and genre combinations which engaged with audiences and created new aesthetic models.[34] Sitas is careful to point out the enormous potential but also the limitations of this process of innovation and performative cross-fertilisation, with reference both to the public life of events and the strains running through the cultural formations.

Theatre practitioners were faced with the dilemma of how to win over and engage their audience. In their efforts they used a range of devices from aspects of familiar cultural convention to direct appeals to the commonality of life experience. Call and response techniques and the singing of union songs were participatory devices which were frequently used. Audiences could intervene in the act of performance by, for example, asking for portions to be repeated, suggesting different endings or soliciting improvised responses through their interventions. As Peterson has asserted with reference to the play *Ziyajika*, performance becomes multi-dimensional:

> the plot also serves as a catalyst for embarking on *another* performance, involving the audience ... Dramatic conflict is thus located both within the performance (as interpreted by the actors) and in the audience, depending on their contributions.[35]

At an earlier stage, fellow workers fed constructively into the formation and evolution of plays, often vetting and commenting on them before official performances took place.

Tomaselli has gone as far as to argue that there is no distinction between 'actor and viewer, stage and life or performance and reality', they are all part of a whole which connects art and life. Sitas's response to the notion that 'all the world's a stage' is an 'emphatic NO'.[36] Clearly the relationship between performance and audience is highly complicated and requires further research. It extends beyond simplistic notions of spontaneous identification. Working-class audiences, for example, differ. Touchstones of the familiar within plays, governing the ability to relate and participate, include class related issues — dominant forms of work experience and work disputes, union affiliation — and non-class or less overtly class issues — fluency in relevant languages, knowledge of cultural forms used and degree of comfort with the uses to which they are put. While class does not totally condition audience participation it does obviously have a role to play. Sitas notes that the more blacks are exposed to school education, missions or churches, the less audience participation there is.

The interaction between performance and audience helped shape the identity of worker theatre. Facets of this interaction included the role of performative contexts such as mass gatherings and performance genres within them; the creative tensions between interacting performance modes and the new roles such modes were expected to perform; the relationship between changing performance function and aesthetics and audience expectations; and the interaction between the overall play and audiences of varying compositions.

The relationship between performance and audience was a formative area of collaboration between worker theatre and its broadly defined constituency. As one example, there was a contradiction in achieving the intimacy required for audience/performance interaction when theatre was 'slotted', often unbeknown to the audience, into other events, and where identity formation was attempted and seen as being most effective within mass gatherings. Kromberg in fact states that plays were abandoned at mass rallies because the distance between performers and audience was too great for facial expressions and gestures to be seen. Theatre struggled to 'work' in such a context, and the ultimate judge of this was the audience. Worker poetry proved a more effective medium in large gatherings.[37] Therefore, the site where performance venue/context, performance and audience intersected in the cultural process was an important determinant of worker theatre's identity, crucially influencing the direction of its evolution.

The Troika of Content: Life Experience, the Workplace and a Vision of Freedom

The content of worker theatre drew largely on a troika of seminal formative features: the reflection of worker life experiences; the centrality of work and the production process; and the political projection and attempted cultural realisation of a vision of the future. Sole has stated that, 'Of performance-orientated literature, theatre is possibly the medium most conducive to presenting situations, episodes and sequences which together most immediately constitute an approach to lived experience'.[38] According to one commentator, for the worker participants in *Ilanga*, 'performing in this play was more than manifesting acting skills, it was a question of bringing their daily-life experiences to the stage'.[39] Constructions of life experience were of crucial importance.

The Dunlop Play was a clear example of life experience and life story within a theatrical production. The play begins with a *bekezela* party given by the company on the twenty-fifth anniversary of some of their workers. Amidst great congratulation, a worker is presented with a huge gold papier mâché watch. The play then sets out to show what he really got in return for his labour, and the hardship of his first day at work is depicted.

The old man returns to narrate the 'cranky' (unfolding tableaux) scene which links his first day at Dunlop to the present by depicting important events and moments over the twenty-five year period. He tells of his responses to important labour and political issues over the years. The workers detect an *impimpi* and call for the manager. The old worker intercedes and again turns narrator. What follows indicates the failure of a liaison committee, which in turn feeds into a lunch hour scene in which workers discuss the need for effective unionisation. The police arrive, called by the *impimpi*, but the group transforms itself into a mock religious gathering. The *impimpi* reports talks of unions to the management which responds by trying to set up an in-house union. In the resulting conflict between members of the in-house union and MAWU, the bosses are called to arbitrate. They ask the workers which union they want, and the support for MAWU is loud and unified. The play ends with the *impimpi* joining MAWU and the audience participating in a song.

The play combines the story of the working life of one man, clearly seen as representative of all workers, with insight into issues of relevance to workers such as work conditions and demands for union recognition. In addition, its content reflected and participated in an actual situation at Dunlop in which an in-house union had been set up in opposition to MAWU and there were demands for recognition of the latter.[40]

The Dunlop Play was designed for mobilisation. Von Kotze has categorised plays into those for 'mobilisation' — which are conceived quickly to contribute to the impetus of worker actions and generate support for workers and a specific struggle or conflict within their workplace among an audience that can extend beyond the working class; and those for 'education' — which contain a moral message, often focusing on a single central theme (migrancy, exploitation of women, conflicts between generations, unemployment), with the aim of imparting knowledge and understanding of issues.[41]

Both categories draw on life experience. Mobilisation plays seek to capture an immediate and ongoing event, issue or grievance such as a strike, when the organising principle of worker theatre is in its element.[42] In such circumstances identities are polarised and entrenched and class divisions are most apparent. Identity is seen through the intense prism of such events and resides in unity and solidarity, the collectivity of the moment. Otherwise the worker is categorised as the enemy. As strikes and other labour actions are retold, workers construct a picture not simply of the act of protest but also of themselves. Educational plays are an attempt to impart knowledge about a broader range of issues. Worker theatre had to try and achieve continuity and coherence as an ongoing process. Educational plays extend worker theatre beyond the most obvious arenas where labour conflict and mobilisation would tend to prioritise class unity above the morass of competing identities, and attempt the much more difficult task of making class a permanent, 'natural' medium of self-identification.

Plays shared a didacticism, presenting a definite and consistent interpretation of the structures of oppression and exploitation. However, the categorisation of plays is based upon an understanding that worker plays 'work' in different ways.

Those within the theatre movement have often emphasised the importance of realism. Several of Sitas's 'contradictions'[43] relate to this question. The first is that the centrality of representing the reality of production and work as the site of exploitation and oppression creates enormous aesthetic problems — 'how do you portray steelwork and foundrywork with their furnaces smelting away at 1 800 degrees Celsius, the noise and the dust, the looms and shuttle sounds of textile factories or the rubber plants with their giant mills, presses, extruders?' Another 'contradiction' refers to the tension between mythological aspects of portrayal, which abound in working class culture (and, surely, in all other forms of culture), and real aspects of portrayal, typified by worker attempts to show their situation realistically. A final 'contradiction' lies in the conflict between cognitive and cathartic moments. To communicate lessons and engender thought the audience should not confuse certain aspects of the play with reality. Audiences should not substitute for themselves victories shown on stage as the definitive statement of the play. Cathartic moments — worker victories, the singing of well-known songs — most easily stimulate thought but also create emotional identification with those on stage. Thus the involvement and participation of the audience needs to be tempered by a kind of critical distance.

These 'contradictions' raise a range of questions: if there is a predisposition for the 'mythological' where does the desire to tell life experiences realistically originate and why; what transformations in content and formal assumptions are required; and how does realism intentionally and unconsciously combine with other elements present in the plays such as symbolism, irony, and parody? Realism in the heat of mobilisation or given the didacticism of education can only be seen as a construct of the autobiographical agenda: 'our picture' is the 'true picture'. Worker theatre depicted life experience, but life experience was a construction and cannot be equated with uncomplicated notions of realism.

Secondly, within the more general emphasis on the experiences of the working class, cultural expression designated centrality to the work process and workplace conditions, to the relationship between culture and production. This enabled the injection of a class specificity and prioritisation of worker issues previously unknown within anti-apartheid culture. To have acquired such a capacity for self definition was enormously empowering. As worker culture's focus on class experience and the workplace became less absolute, a characteristic which was fairly generalised by the end of the 1980s, its gaze extended increasingly into the community and beyond, but significantly, largely on its own terms.[44]

Finally and more generally, working class theatre also encompassed the construction and projection of a liberated future:

> M (interview) points out that the importance of working class culture 'is to make the vision of a new South Africa which will not know oppression and exploitation. Through culture this world can be lived and seen ... culture must be a mirror and a medium. It is from this mirror that we catch a glimpse of the new liberated society free from oppression and exploitation. A working class culture has to do with this vision.'[45]

Here again any simplistic conception of worker plays as realism is inappropriate. The construction of a desired future did not reside in the realm of realism but, like the construction of realism itself, was a function of a pervasive autobiographical agenda. However, this political vision of the future was not simply a projection, worker culture attempted to ground its political vision within its internal social organisation and theatrical practice with a rigour unique in South African cultural history. There were many examples of this rigour within worker theatre: the alliance with the trade union movement; independent structures of cultural control and production; the relationship between performance and audience; the emphasis on play-making and performance, the collaborative workshop method employed; and the worker bias in play content. Worker culture achieved its aim to an unprecedented degree but inevitably tensions remained.[46] Nevertheless, culture was both 'a mirror and a medium' through which the vision could be 'lived and seen'.

Worker theatre's formative troika represented a highly selective representation of lived experience and a vision of the future, designed to serve specific ends. At the level of content, as at all other levels, tensions remained: at the junction of aesthetics, realism, life experience and the autobiographical organising principle; between different categories of plays; in the division between that which was given expression and the significant amount of life experience which was not articulated; in the negotiation of control over content selection; in devising the ways and the terms for extending theatre's gaze into a strife-torn community; and in interactions between past, present and future, culture and politics, dream and realisable vision. These tensions were all part of the formulation of identity, of the one 'voice' containing many 'voices'.

The Workshop Process

There is a long tradition in South African oppositional theatre of using the collaborative workshop method. As Steadman claims it is one of the lasting legacies of theatre from the apartheid era. Workshop theatre is a political act which is a movement towards an essentially democratic production process and communal vision. It empowers its participants both creatively and politically — workshop plays can be made by all regardless of race, education, or ability to write or speak any one privileged language — and has elevated the practice of play-making into an end in itself. The benefits gained from the workshop process by participants cannot be negated by the lack of, or a poor, final product. It emerged as theatrical form in conjunction with broader developments, typified by the emergence and doctrines of the UDF and COSATU.[47]

In working class theatre strenuous demands have been placed on the workshop method. Kirkwood has remarked, with reference to *The Long March*, on the 'depth' of the workshop process.[48] The method has had to mobilise the creativity of often non- or semi-literate participants to whom the concept of a 'play' is sometimes completely foreign. Of central importance to access to workshop theatre is the fact that plays and play-making draw on the overwhelmingly oral forms of everyday expression — 'the roots of plays are found in story-telling and traditional forms of culture'[49] — and the belief that everyone has a story to tell:

> [Cultural structures] embarked on a systematic campaign of producing plays, poems and songs on the lives of working class people. All these tell the stories of ordinary people's struggle. And importantly, they show that each person has a story to tell, that you do not need to be well-educated or specially gifted to tell a story or to write.[50]

Fleischman argues that workshop theatre is essentially an oral form of cultural expression and it is this orality that makes it oppositional to dominant trends in theatre practice. He illustrates this through a study of workshop theatre as form conducted on three levels: production, structure and social process. In the production phase improvisation is 'particularly close to the act of oral composition'. It takes the form of spontaneous composition around a structure or theme, drawing on observation and life experience to make play segments or episodes in what is in essence a communal and participatory act (it is also true that performances can take on a similar form, allowing for improvisation around set structures and themes).

At the level of structure Fleischman argues that the repetitive and formulaic nature of workshop theatre, the repetition of actions and themes and the formulas through which they combine, is influenced by a tradition that goes back to oral storytelling forms. Some of the formulas he identifies are of particular relevance to worker theatre, for example, the infliction/defiance/consequence/assertion sequence.[51]

Finally, at the level of social process, workshop theatre like oral forms documents contemporary history. The oral basis of workshop theatre raises questions about the cultural repertoires workers brought to workshops and the ways in which these were used in theatrical production and performance.

Von Kotze in *Organise and Act* mentions numerous participant skills constituting, and in addition to, those from the realm of orality: these include proficiency in music/singing, poetry, dance, self-defence, boxing, soccer, and so on.

> Each person brought in their special skills and interests. Some people might think that these skills have nothing to do with making and performing plays, but this is the training these people have.[52]

In dynamic multi-form productions the incorporation of such skills was often part of the essence of the plays. As has already been mentioned, the cultural potential and limitations of cross-fertilisation between cultural forms were widely explored. Many forms were oral in nature, and these lay at the heart of the broader process of formal transformation and appropriation.

No commentators have explored the oral strategies and understandings brought to workshops by participants of different gender and ethnic groups, social and class backgrounds, different degrees of exposure to urban and rural cultures, levels of education, and so on. What oral forms were the most prevalent; who were the carriers of these forms and what status did they have among performers; were oral forms perceived as being 'true/historical/ realistic' or more 'fictional' in nature; what patterns of transformation and appropriation affected oral forms; what was the impact of workshop participants' speaking different languages and to varying degrees of fluency? In some cases oral forms would already have been influenced by such media as television, radio, newspapers, and by other affiliations such as that to various forms of religion. A range of questions needs to be addressed in relation to attitudes to the refashioning of oral forms to meet the needs of the particular context of worker theatre.

Oral narrative forms and structures were clearly put to uses which are both familiar and new and unconventional, within workshopped worker theatre. An example of oral transformation took place within the play *Ilanga*, whose genesis lay in the arrest of a group of strikers. Halton Cheadle, the lawyer representing the arrested strikers, found it impossible to take meaningful statements or to cross check the different versions of what took place. He set up a role-play and the workers collectively reconstructed the events in a way which consolidated the narrative, provided reinterpretations of events and uncovered new information. The workers had originally misunderstood what was required of them. They knew nothing of courtroom procedure, the significance of corroborative evidence, accurate statements and the importance of actually having witnessed the events in question.[53] The result of the process was an indication of one way in which oral narrative could be transformed within the workshop context.

Though narration and monologues in plays were considered 'untheatrical', they were used to supplement and link dramatic and other action and to impart information such as background and history which was both crucial and difficult or impossible to portray in another way. Where possible they were supplemented by other cultural forms. In *The Dunlop Play* one of the old man's narrations was supplemented in various ways: a cranky was used to illustrate historical process; a song was sung softly as background; and short sketches were devised to bring some of the images to life. According to one commentator the final scene was an 'exciting multi-media presentation'.[54]

Sitas places orality at the centre of two of his creative 'contradictions'. One contradiction lies in the tension between the 'spoken' and the 'acted' in a play. Much is contained in the actual telling of a story which is difficult to recreate in acted sequences.[55] A related contradiction is the uncomfortable relationship between the subtle dynamics of oral communication and the frequent need in a play to narrate uncomplicated information to explain and construct 'reality'. Oral narrative was therefore transformed, appropriated and interacted with other cultural forms, not always successfully, in order to meet new demands within workshopped worker theatre.

It is important to note that not all worker plays were workshopped and that the composition of workshops varied. Critical literature from within the theatre movement gives a complex picture of play-making which belies any simplistic assumption that all plays were, or indeed should have been, workshopped. In workshops themselves the balance and interaction between cultural activists and workers varied; plays and story lines conceptualised or scripted by individuals sometimes stood on their own while at other times they formed the basis for improvisation in workshop; and some plays had a more informal genesis. The flexibility to harness diverse creative energies was surely one of the movement's strengths.

It is, however, often implied that play-making was synonymous with the workshop process and that this process was an intrinsically superior method of cultural production. Von Kotze rightly acclaims *The Long March* as a workshopped play in which the workers had a minimum of formal education, spoke little English, and had next to no experience with and in the theatre. Her evaluation of the play *Once Bitten Twice Shy*, is less flattering. Qabula had the story in his head and simply told participants what to do, thus it was less of a collective project. According to von Kotze this method was not as successful (intrinsically?) as full participation at every level of creation and production by all members of the group.[56] Attitudes to individual authorship vary. Von Kotze claims that such a categorisation is unproductive as what is finally expressed 'is not so much the work of one mind but rather the experience — both in the content and the actual making — of a collective'. However, members of the Durban FOSATU cultural local noted elsewhere the need both to work collectively and to allow space for individuals to develop, so plays have been both 'written by one person' and 'workshopped by all the participants'. The emphasis on individual writing has actually, and perhaps inevitably, increased.[57]

A final point needs to be made about the workshop process. It cannot simply be assumed to be inherently or totally democratic. Like all such collaborative forums it has its own power dynamics which struggle to undermine those characterising the wider social formation. The 'depth' of workshopping and the sympathetic attitude and approach of cultural activists may reduce but will not eliminate their formative influence. Luther has highlighted the ambivalence of collaborative theatre, which both facilitates progressive elements within plays and reflects in microcosm the inequalities between the groups of which its participants are representatives.[58]

Nevertheless, the prevalence of the workshop process was another manifestation of worker theatre's collaborative basis. As a complex collaborative enterprise workshopped theatre inevitably captured and reflected many influences and perspectives. Numerous formative relationships and interactions took place within the workshop. For example, performance modes, notably oral forms, were engaged in a series of unique interactions within workshops and performance. Other tensions within the creative process included the balance of power between participants in the workshops and tensions between individual and more collective models of creativity, and between the oral and the written. All these dimensions of the creative process contributed to identity formation. The theatre movement was the product of layers of discourse and collaboration. One of the most important agents in this process was cultural activists, the ghosts in the autobiographical machine.

Working Class Theatre and the Ghost in the Autobiographical Machine

The Dynamics of Control and Power

There was inevitably a role for cultural activists in worker theatre. As Sole has stated, 'there are few possibilities in South Africa and elsewhere of workers gaining access to the dominant culture's world of "drama" and "literature" which are not mediated by some form of patronage or outside technical assistance'.[59] Generally, the criteria for cultural involvement by activists have been the subject of some debate.[60] White middle class activists in worker theatre have depicted themselves as 'participant observers', seeking to downplay their role by aligning themselves politically with and trying to empower, the working class. There are, however, problems with such unselfconscious alignment and the ensuing lack of analysis of the nature of the evolving relationship between intellectual cultural activists and the class on whose behalf they speak and in whose cultural production they participate. This alignment is in some ways admirable, and coincides with worker theatre's organising principle, but it unhelpfully obfuscates the debates and dynamics of control and power within worker theatre.

The position of the working class cultural activist as worker, performer, cultural enabler and often worker leader is perhaps even more complex.[61] Orality, performance, and the cultural enabling of others is linked to status and power. For worker activists access to skills and education such as role-play and greater language proficiency was enabled through the workshop and performance process; actors toured with plays both in South Africa and abroad and some participants gained professional mobility within cultural structures and the unions. Culture has arguably been enabling, albeit in very different ways, for all activists. Lives have gone in new directions and taken on new dimensions through participation in cultural activity. In the light of these issues it becomes imperative to formulate an understanding of what exactly it is that cultural activists do.

In *Organise and Act*, von Kotze acknowledges that activists perform a large variety of functions. An important example was *The Long March* which activists helped to 'shape and direct'. Key input was required in certain scenes: for example, the scene representing the production process and the 'brainstormed' Maggie Thatcher scene which placed Sarmcol in an international context. Activists found and paid for a venue for a week-long retreat which facilitated concentrated and uninterrupted work on the play. Later, activists expended considerable energy on organising *The Long March*'s tour of South Africa.

Activist intervention can be identified in the following areas: the provision and sharing of technical and other skills denied to worker participants (for example, the training of participants to act rather than simply tell their story); the shaping of life experiences into an aesthetically grounded theatrical product ('shaping and structuring'); and the provision of linkages, knowledge and facilities outside the realm of worker experience and access. Von Kotze, in conclusion, makes the distinction between 'participation' and 'overriding intervention'.[62]

Analyses by cultural activists of their role in the process of working class cultural production lack specificity. Instead, words such as 'shape', 'structure' and 'direct' are used repeatedly. Little has been documented, for example, about the patterns of responsibility and function taken on by different kinds of activists, or about the evolving relationship between activists of various kinds and the worker community. Sitas has talked of worker poets being 'yanked out of their initial impulses', and of changes in worker poetry influenced by a change in status, but also external factors ranging from deteriorations in the political situation — particularly violence — to written texts.[63] What were the implications of worker theatre activists, who, to a significant degree were also worker poets, being 'yanked out of their initial impulses'?

An uneasy feeling persists that activists are engaged in 'impression management', trying to control perceptions of the cultural movement and their position within it. This is exacerbated by anomalies that occasionally undermine their self-presentation as 'participant observers'. Actors in *The Long March* replied to audience suggestions about changing the play by saying, 'Together as actors we decided not to change things without the advice of our organisers'.[64] Collaboration is not a seamless process, but one consisting of discourse and contestation. At stake are issues at the heart of the working class cultural movement: control, power, cultural decentralisation and dissemination. The presence of a ghost in the autobiographical machine asks of this autobiographical project the most challenging of questions in relation to the dynamics of control and power: whose story is this?

'Shaping' and 'Directing': Ideology, Theory and the Contours of Criticism

The utterances and writings of cultural activists have crucially shaped perceptions of the worker theatre movement. Much of the analysis of the movement has been theirs, and to a significant extent it is through them that the outsider must negotiate a passage towards new angles of analysis. In order to facilitate this it is important to identify some of the areas in which cultural activists have most significantly wielded influence. Intellectual and worker cultural activists also bring to the play-making process cultural and political repertoires, which inevitably influence patterns of intervention and the nature of the cultural process and product.

Activists, it will be argued, have critically moulded the process and image of worker theatre by elaborating and systematising its ideology, grounding it in a theory of form/production and through their influence on critical debates. The emphasis on the 'event' and the practice of theatre at the expense of these factors is part of an attempt to render the activist invisible and empower the working class. However, it is ultimately counterproductive and misleading. Activists involved in working class culture need to be far more aware and publicly vocal about the exact nature of their participation.

Are we to assume, for example, that the consistent ideological thrust of the plays was arrived at 'organically', that radical consensus was somehow inevitable? It is incorrect to assume that the working class is spontaneously anti-capitalism/apartheid, or that all its struggles are immediately political or revolutionary.[65] Sole has noted that the nationalist and popular symbols and traditions that make up part of black worker identity are available for a variety of political ends. This is particularly relevant in Natal. In part taking issue with cultural activists, he goes on to say that they can have some effect on the rearrangement and use of such symbols and identities for progressive ends 'but an acceptance of socialism cannot be ensured once and for all by such vanguardist means'.[66] There has been no self-consciousness in the theatre movement either about possible 'vanguardism' or its potential long term implications for the worker culture movement.

It becomes necessary to ask how, in Gramscian terms, 'inherent' ideas — those based on direct experience, oral tradition or folk memory — were transformed into 'derived' ideas — those borrowed from others, often taking the form of more structured systems of ideas. The transformation from 'inherent' to 'derived' is not politically neutral, but carries connotations of control and power. How was the ideological identity of theatre constructed: how were aspects of worker subjectivity which were not encapsulated in notions of struggle, solidarity and unity reformulated or silenced; what problems and resistances were encountered; and how permanent were attitude changes? Furthermore, how and why did 'slippages' occur, creating ideological discourses within the plays themselves and appearing all the more glaring against the remaining backdrop of formidable consistency? Why for example in *You're a Failure Mr Mpimpi* was Mr Mpimpi's humiliation cemented, after he lost his job, by his having to stay at home, do the housework and look after the baby? Was embarrassment at male participation in such activities really the kind of attitude worker theatre wanted to perpetuate? Perhaps such attitudes actually represented the intrusion of non-'politically correct' but nevertheless widely held attitudes within the worker community. The formative role of the cultural activist was, in different ways, central to all these questions and issues.

The reasons why ideological formulation was generally so watertight, why selection and censorship were so rigorous, have already been discussed. Crucially, however, in the context of this discussion, the elaboration and systematising of ideology by cultural activists was part of the process of worker theatre's self-construction, of the creation of identity. Ideology, importantly, formed part of a wider theoretical malaise facing the worker theatre movement.

In emphasising the primacy and seriousness of practice, Sitas has argued that the need to theorise the 'event' has not been an 'instinctual desire', and that 'theory and critique is always a postmortem examination'. Elsewhere he acknowledges 'a screeching content in search of theoretical forms' with the proviso: 'but not yet, there can't be, a conceptual baggage of aesthetic values that necessarily flows out of a working class position in society'.[67] Form is somehow not yet ready for theorisation and Sitas is highly critical of theorists in South Africa for foisting imported theoretical models upon 'events' which show an 'acute insensitivity' to local artefacts. He argues that the universality of worker alienation is handled through unique local forms — defensive combinations — in which similarly unique cultural formations proliferate. Any theory of performance has to be situated within such combinations:

it is only through the exploration of theatre as an event in popular culture that [a] theory of aesthetics begin[s] to make sense of what takes place in the cultural spaces of the working class ... Whether a new aesthetic shall arise within popular culture linked to theatrical performance is a point of speculation and/or cultural struggle.[68]

However, Sitas does provide his creative 'contradictions', several of which have already been mentioned. The remainder are summarised below. A clash of 'moral orders' emerges between the new seriousness of a moral order based on forms of worker association and old cultural formations and practices, both in workshops and in performance/ narrative.[69] A related contradiction exists between attempts to show heroic collective action and the vibrancy of individual characterisation. Another contradiction is the clash between the need for rapid dramatic time and 'an obstinate correlation between pride, dignity and time in the worker performances'. Stories and performances unfold in their own time, lacking customary 'time discipline'. What Sitas provides through his 'contradictions' are perhaps thoughts or notes towards a theory of form and performance which shows a sensitivity to local artefacts. The extent to which these contradictions and their cultural manifestations are 'unique' rather than composed of overlapping systems of similarities and differences both with other cultural enterprises in South Africa and with working class culture around the world, has not, however, been illustrated.[70]

It is unquestionably the case, as Tomaselli and Muller have argued, that intellectual cultural activists brought to their interventions a theoretical consciousness, and that theoretical intervention was not post hoc but intrinsically part of the process of cultural production.[71] A theory of production emerged which was linked to the political movements and ideas to which theatre was aligned. Consistent strands of theory permeated all facets of what worker theatre was and did. Theory therefore, informed content and form, play-making and performance, and was, at all levels interconnected with practice. Plays, and indeed Sitas's 'contradictions', testify to the existence of an implicit theory of dramatic effectiveness and praxis. Von Kotze's assertion that there are no 'recipes' for playmaking fits poorly with what Sole has described as an 'imperative and teleological tone', which applies equally to procedures for content and form.[72]

There was undoubtedly a specific approach to cultural production and form which can be summed up in a few keywords and phrases: independent cultural structures; collaborative workshop method; working class participants and audience; multi-media/form presentation; worker life experience, and so on. It does, however, await comprehensive formulation and a greater exploration of subtleties and nuances. Cultural activists were key movers in the articulation of this approach, which again formed part of the process of identity creation.

Why, with reference to the interrelated fields of ideology and the theory of performance, have cultural activists failed to detail their function? Perhaps for similar reasons to those which explain the nature of their incursions into the field of criticism.

The analysis by cultural activists of worker theatre generally emphasises what the theatre movement does and has done. Internal criticism has generally served the wider goals of the theatre movement: 'The difference is that we don't criticise in order to divide workers but rather to do the opposite: to strengthen the unity of workers, and make leadership accountable to us'.[73] Criticising to unite potentially facilitates what Doherty calls a suspension of investigatory inquiry.[74] The absence of an environment of thorough-going self-criticism and analysis can lead

> to an overstressing of the need for a unified culture of resistance and an understressing of the simultaneous need to allow cultural variety to flourish, and for critical comment and democratic discussion.[75]

The only really rigorous critical dissection from within worker theatre has come from Sitas's 'contradictions'. He looks at the overlapping contradictions and discourses between desired method and message, the capacities and limitations of the theatrical form, and the complexity of worker participants who simultaneously encompass characteristics and preferences that work with and against the desired theatrical process and product. As contradictions are worked through creativity is generated and weaknesses/limitations are revealed. For example, Sitas acknowledges that difficulties in representing the reality of the factory production process in *The Dunlop Play* 'haunted' the workshops and performances, while according to von Kotze in *Organise and Act* 'a lively and descriptive image of an assembly line' was created.[76] Why did such critical inconsistencies occur? The tendency to submerge and pass over problems in order to promote working class unity and advancement was, clearly, not universal. It was a further example of the fractures and contradictions in projected self-image, of the many 'voices' contained within the one dominant 'voice'.

Sitas has claimed with reference to worker poetry that an 'examination of what the standards ought to be in this kind of poetry hasn't appeared'.[77]

The same applies to worker theatre. The approach to cultural production and form outlined above suggests the kinds of parameters that the theatre practitioners used to evaluate themselves. A play was 'good', for example, if it was the product of collective collaboration in workshop or if it empowered previously disadvantaged workers.[78] However, it is ultimately inadequate for the movement itself, and its political and cultural evolution, to suggest that a play is good simply because it is workshopped with non-literate working class participants. While the benefits gained from the process of play-making cannot be negated by a poor final product, such considerations should not eclipse evaluation of the final product. There must be greater evaluation of whether and how plays 'work' as theatre. Why, for example, are all workshopped plays not equally good?

One obvious avenue for research would be to analyse audience responses. Kromberg's work on audience evaluation of worker poetry, in particular in the context of mass rallies, has revealed specific and consistent criteria used by audiences in their appreciation or otherwise of the poetry. He also found that outside the context of the rally, individuals expressed a far more critical appreciation of the poetry than was discernible in the mass response. In an attempt to explain the disjuncture between individual criticism and mass appreciation Kromberg states:

> The events ... are ... part of the oral mobilisation of different cultural formations and individuals into a broader interpretive community. The rallies therefore function to express common interests and unity. Criticism is either suppressed in the interests of the larger aim of solidarity and unity, or it is less consciously forgotten amid the excitement generated by this sense of community ... both audience and poets are acting as agents in the consolidation of an interpretive community ... In the context of the mass rally an aesthetic value is placed on unity that could be said to overwhelm other criteria of assessment.[79]

As has already been discussed, the audience contributed crucially to the emergence, composition and evolution of worker theatre. What does the fact that plays were introduced but subsequently abandoned at mass rallies tell us about the audience response, and how, why and where such plays 'work'? To answer such a question more research is required as to what criteria were/are used by audiences in the evaluation of plays, and whether and how such criteria vary between different performance contexts.

By focusing attention on theatrical practice — play-making and performance — activists highlighted the participating working class. But as Sole has argued in another context: 'The desire of a more privileged and better educated stratum to align itself "downwards" can be seen in the insistence in the literature on performance and direct communication with an audience'.[80] To have concentrated on ideological construction, the theory of production/form/aesthetics, or to have revised the contours of criticism away from its primary unifying function would, in part, have placed the spotlight on crucial axes of cultural activist influence. It would have revealed the part played by activists in the construction of the theatre movement and the nature of control, status, and power in this collaborative autobiographical act, thereby revealing the ghost in the autobiographical machine. For worker theatre to serve its purpose activists have felt they must become virtually anonymous. While cultural activists stand between audience/reader and the autobiographical subject as a kind of ill-defined absent presence, the overlapping layers of selfhood and identity within worker theatre will remain elusive.

However, activist participation, while significant, was primarily concerned with the packaging and promotion of working class lives. The process and product were collaborative in nature encompassing a multiplicity of voices, but one voice predominated, that which reflected worker lives and hopes for the future. Ultimately activists sought to empower workers culturally and politically so that they could control the means and define the content of their cultural self-representation. But this was an exercise fraught with difficulties. Worker theatre and worker culture more generally, were always characterised by both dynamism and frailty. By 1989 the Comment in the special issue of *Staffrider* on worker culture was sensing 'the dangers of stagnation' and warning that unless cultural workers took urgent action 'the momentum and energy created will simply drift further into the past'.

It is important to analyse who or what has been empowered and enabled through worker theatre and, more generally, worker culture. For example, it has generally been easier to secure the status and advancement of individual worker cultural activists than the continuity and unity of structures such as cultural locals which were needed if plays were to flourish. For this and various other reasons, some of which have been touched upon, there has been a marked slow down in the production of plays. A study conducted in 1990 of how workers in Durban used their leisure time found that only 6.5% were involved in drama, but 37.8% had heard about worker plays, 33.7% had seen worker plays and 18.3% had read worker plays.[81] In essence worker plays have struggled to find a broad based worker constituency and to maintain the momentum generated in the mid-1980s; the reasons for this require more comprehensive research. Ultimately generalised cultural empowerment and independence for the working class will only be achieved by greater critical self-consciousness on the part of activists about what exactly they do and the shortcomings as well as successes of their various initiatives and overall approach, and more particularly by structural changes such as improvements in education and the acquisition of political and greater industrial democracy.

Conclusion

Worker theatre in the mid-1980s was the performance of a revolutionary autobiographical subject. The emphasis on class, the workplace and associated concepts of unity and solidarity became less absolute, but during this initial period worker theatre imposed a pattern on worker life and gained its standpoint from an allegiance to these concepts. The need for a rigid central core — the certainty of selective clarity — was a conscious statement of identity within Natal's backdrop of 'identity confusion' and uncertainty. As in all autobiography this collocation of identity was a construction, the product of an autobiographical strategy. However, it remained irretrievably riven with the many dimensions of identity and collaboration.

Within the dynamics of worker theatre are enduring pointers towards an alternative theory of political autobiography. Sidonie Smith argues that autobiography has played and continues to play a role in emancipatory politics.[82] Using the basis of, and expanding upon, definitional aspects of what Smith calls the 'autobiographical manifesto' it is possible to outline a framework for a theory of political autobiography of relevance to worker theatre, and other arenas in South Africa and elsewhere. Such an autobiographical act is an appropriation and the contestation of sovereignty with reference to identity, motivated by an alienation from the historically imposed image of self. Marginalised experiences are exposed and the legitimacy of a new kind of knowledge is publicly announced. Identity is often radically political, asserts that life is political and is formulated around oppositional contours of self, notably a collective orientation. In addition, this autobiographical performance educates and mobilises towards a particular end, the pursuit of a vision of a liberated future. While such autobiography will document the past and present it also gestures forward to the possibility of change. This vision of the future is not simply a projection but is grounded in the cultural practice of the present, thereby attempting to forge the link between present and future. Tensions and discourses normally contained within the mind and text of a single writer are both multiplied and externalised by the context, content and form of such autobiographical initiatives which simultaneously try to manage and channel these tensions and discourses towards a particular end.

Participants do not necessarily construct their narratives in ways that are conventional: the packaging of the life story and experiences is determined by different consciousnesses and cultural forms. Beyond the conventional prose text, space is created for the communication of life stories, or parts of life experience, in the form(s) of the participant's choice. Attention must therefore be paid to indigenous cultural modes, largely the oral and performative, and the way in which these interact with each other and external forms. Autobiography is a practice, an evolving process, rather than an isolated product. The creative process is likely to be both individual and collective/collaborative in nature. Where appropriate, there must be greater awareness and analysis of the role of cultural activists and enablers: what do they do, how do they do it, and what are the implications for the final product and ongoing cultural process? These notes towards a new theory of political autobiography provide the genre with a revised 'horizon of expectancy' in pusuit of both political and cultural liberation.

Worker theatre illustrates that autobiography can be virtually all things to all people. Ways need to be found of enabling the marginalised, working class and others, to communicate directly in the mode of their choice the nature of their lives under apartheid. The life story will inevitably take on multiple forms, sometimes in the most unlikely cocktails. Through worker theatre and other seemingly unconventional autobiographical initiatives, the 'horizon of expectancy' of a genre that has become constrained within the individually written prose text can be liberated. Such an explosion of expectations will be destructive, creative, define new limits and in the words of Halton Cheadle, be 'really hell of exciting'.

1 I would like to thank the Leverhulme Trust for providing the financial assistance which made the research for this article possible.
2 Worker theatre began in Natal after the arrival in Durban of two former members of the Johannesburg-based Junction Avenue Theatre Company (JATC), Ari Sitas and Astrid von Kotze. Their involvement grew from participation in *The Dunlop Play*. Prior to worker theatre developments in Natal some worker plays had been devised elsewhere, including *Ilanga Lizophumela Abasebenzi (The Sun Rises for the Workers)*, involving members of the JATC. For further details on the context on which the Natal worker theatre movement drew, see M Orkin, *Drama and the South African State*, Witwatersrand University Press, Johannesburg, 1991 (chapter 7, Khalo, pp 180-208);

A Sitas, Culture and Production: The contradiction of working class theatre in South Africa (henceforth, Culture and Production (1)), *Africa Perspective* 1 (1-2), 1986, pp 84-110; K Sole, Black literature and performance: Some notes on class and populism, *South African Labour Bulletin (SALB)* 9(8), 1984, pp 54-76; K Tomaselli, From Laser to the Candle, *Ilanga Le So Phonela Abasebenzi* [sic]: An Example of Devolution of Theatre, *SALB* 6(8), 1981, pp 64-70; and The semiotics of alternative theatre in South Africa, *Critical Arts* 2 (1), July 1981, pp 14-33; K Tomaselli and J Muller, Class race and oppression: Metaphor and metonymy in 'Black' South African theatre, *Critical Arts* 4 (3), 1987, pp 40-58.

3 R Elbaz, Autobiography, Ideology and Genre Theory, *Orbis Litterarum* 38, 1983, pp 187-204 (pp 189-90, 199-200).

4 Horowitz has asked, 'how do those who believe in the masses create a legacy of their own good works?' He goes on to question whether totalitarian systems (and others?) with an emphasis on mass participation and identification will come to find the autobiographical genre intolerable. In a similar vein, Doherty has suggested that for those of a particular political persuasion, 'the autobiographical act itself borders on ideological heresy'. See I Horowitz, Autobiography as the presentation of self for social immortality, *New Literary History*, 1977, pp 173-9 (pp 176-7); T Doherty, American Autobiography and Ideology. In A Stone (ed), *The American Autobiography: A Collection of Critical Essays*, Prentice-Hall, Inc, New Jersey, 1981, pp 95-108 (p 105).

5 Doherty, op cit, pp 103-4.

6 Many forms and presentations of autobiography are more complex and subtle in this regard. For example, memoir, which is frequently political in nature, presents a personality intimately entwined with history, with the public world. See F Hart, History Talking to Itself: Public Personality in Recent Memoir, *New Literary History*, 1979, pp 193-210; and J Cox, Recovering Literature's Lost Ground Through Autobiography. In J Olney (ed), *Autobiography: Essays Theoretical and Critical*, Princeton University Press, Princeton, 1980, pp 123-45.

7 See A Stone, Introduction: American Autobiographies as Individual Stories and Cultural Narratives. In A Stone (ed), *The American Autobiography: A Collection of Critical Essays*, Prentice-Hall, Inc, New Jersey, 1981, pp 1-9 (pp 2, 7); J Olney, Autobiography and the Cultural Moment: A Thematic, Historical, and Bibliographical Introduction. In J Olney (ed), *Autobiography: Essays Theoretical and Critical*, Princeton University Press, Princeton, 1980, pp 3-27 (p 15). Olney argues that Black Studies courses and programs in the US have been organised around autobiography, in part because black history was preserved in autobiographies rather than in standard histories and because black writers entered the house of literature through the door of autobiography. As such it has been and is 'the mode specific to the black experience'. A similar argument could be made for the role of black autobiography in South Africa.

8 There is a seductive lure to the aggrandising pull of autobiography, particularly prose autobiography. The Ravan Press Worker Series, for example, illustrates the ambiguity that while 'the story of one tells the struggle of all', the story of one is also exemplary, or at least becomes so in the telling.

9 Interview (with FOSATU Cultural Group): Culture and workers' struggle, *SALB* 10 (8), 1985, pp 67-74 (p 72).

10 R Pascal, *Design and Truth in Autobiography*, Harvard University Press, Cambridge, Mass, 1960, p 9-10.

11 Doherty, op cit, p 103.

12 E Erikson, *Life History and the Historical Moment*, WW Norton and Co Inc, New York, 1975, p 258.

13 A von Kotze, *Organise and Act: The Natal Workers' Theatre Movement, 1983-1987*, Culture and Working Life Project, University of Natal, Durban, 1988, p 100.

14 Durban Workers' Cultural Local (DWCL) — Talk for FOSATU's Education Workshop, 1985 (Aims and Principles), states the following: 'we have been culturally

exploited time and time again: we have been singing, parading, boxing, acting and writing within a system we did not control. So far, black workers have been feeding all their creativity into a culture machine to make profits for others ... This makes us say that it is time to begin controlling our creativity ... At the same time, in our struggle we must also fight against the culture profit machines.' In A Sitas (ed), *Black Mamba Rising: South African Worker Poets in Struggle*, Culture and Working Life Publications, Durban, 1986, p 60.

15 The barriers and obstacles to be faced and overcome have been and remain enormous. Transport costs, distance and safety were major problems. A combination of work and wider social demands meant that culture took place at odd times when workers were tired and time constraints were prohibitive: 'Never once, therefore, could a full run-through of the *(Dunlop)* play be achieved before performances' (A von Kotze, Workshop Plays as Worker Education, *SALB* 9 (8), 1984, pp 92-109 (p 95). Performances were often hampered by poor staging and technical equipment. Of all the worker cultural forms, theatre was the most equipment-, facility-, and time-intensive and the attempt to be self-sufficient was inevitably costly. Overcoming constraints in one area could simply create tensions in another. For example, family and social tensions surely arose from long anti-social hours spent engaged in cultural work. Cultural work in this context was an act of sacrifice and attrition as much as one of imagination and creativity.

16 M Kirkwood, Literature and popular culture in South Africa, *Third World Quarterly* 9(2), April 1987, pp 657-71 (p 659). This is not the first time that a politically allied theatre movement in South Africa has found 'structural expression' (see, for example, Bheki Peterson's paper in this volume).

17 M Ngoasheng, 'We Organize and Educate ...': Cultural intellectuals within the labour movement, *Staffrider* 8(3 and 4), 1989 (Special issue on Worker Culture), pp 29-38 (p 34).

18 Von Kotze, *Organise and Act,* op cit, p 66.

19 See Cox, op cit. This article discusses Thomas Jefferson's authorship of the US Declaration of Independence, and the presence and weight of the original text of the document in his autobiography.

20 A Sitas, The Voice and Gesture in South Africa's Revolution: A Study of Worker Gatherings and Performance-Genres in Natal. Paper delivered at History Workshop, University of Witwatersrand, February 1990, pp 1-17.

21 A Sitas, The Flight of the Gwala-Gwala Bird: Ethnicity, Populism and Worker Culture in Natal's Labour Movement, unpublished paper, pp 1-41.

22 F Meintjies and M Hlatshwayo, Comment, *Staffrider* 8 (3 and 4), 1989.

23 K Sole, Review of *Organise and Act, Review of African Political Economy* 48, Autumn 1990, pp 116-121.

24 Strikers set up the Sarmcol Workers' Cooperative (SAWCO) which in turn established a cultural group. SAWCO has continued to be creatively active notably through the production and performance of the play *Bambatha's Children*. On SAWCO see P Green, A Place to Work: Sarmcol workers' co-ops, *SALB* 11 (4), 1986, pp 17-23.

25 Sitas, The Flight of the Gwala-Gwala Bird, op cit, pp 7-16 (pp 10-11).

26 Sitas, The Flight of the Gwala-Gwala Bird, op cit, pp 17-37; also interview (with FOSATU Cultural Group), op cit, p 72. On uses of the notion of tradition in worker poetry see the following debate: A Sitas, A black mamba rising: An introduction to Mi S'Dumo Hlatshwayo's Poetry, *Transformation* 2, 1986, pp 50-61; A Spiegel, Transforming tradition or transforming society: Sitas, Hlatshwayo and performative literature, *Transformation* 6, 1988, pp 52-56; A Sitas, Response to Spiegel, *Transformation* 7, 1988, pp 87-90.

27 These arguments were gleaned from work done by Steve Kromberg on worker poetry or *izibongo*. They also apply, if in a slightly diluted form, to worker plays. Kromberg identifies four factors that have led to the emergence and recognition of worker

izibongo nearly all of which, he argues, centrally involve the audience. These factors are: the survival of *izibongo* conventions in many forms among the black working class; the formation of an interpretive community; the evolution from worker plays to worker poetry; and official authorisation. See S Kromberg, The Role of Audience in the Emergence of Durban Worker *Izibongo*. In E Sienaert, AN Bell and M Lewis (eds), *Oral Tradition and Innovation: New Wines in Old Bottles?*, for University of Natal Oral Documentation and Research Centre, Durban 1991, pp 180-202.

28 Von Kotze, Workshop Plays as Worker Education, op cit, p 92.

29 Sitas, Culture and Production (1), op cit, p 90.

30 On this and other arguments outlined below see Sitas, The Voice and Gesture, op cit.

31 Steadman has similarly argued that resistance theatre depends upon 'an interested audience that brings to theatrical performances a stock of experiences, keywords and ideas. The work's capacity to engage the audience depends on this reservoir of references'. See I Steadman, Theatre beyond Apartheid, *Research in African Literature* 22(3), Fall 1991, pp 77-90 (p 87).

32 In part this was because, as Sitas has noted, 'the theatre [narrowly defined] as an institution has a thin base in working class life in South Africa' (Culture and Production (1), op cit, p 90).

33 Sitas, Culture and Production (1), op cit, pp 103-4. This is one of nine 'contradictions' (see pp 93-104) that arise from the clash of moral orders between workers' attempts to express themselves and existing popular culture, and the fact that this struggle is conducted within and through the aesthetic hegemony of the current forms of culture. These 'contradictions' create the necessary tension to propel worker theatre to creativity.

34 The play *Bambatha's Children* created by SAWCO is given by Sitas (in The Voice and Gesture) as an example of successful innovation in the theatrical field. He lauds it as a 'new model, which now in its own right influences further work throughout Natal'.

35 B Peterson, Performing history off the stage: Notes of working-class theatre, *Radical History Review* 46(7), 1990, pp 321-9 (p 326).

36 See Tomaselli, From Laser to Candle, op cit; The Semiotics of Alternative Theatre, op cit. For a critique of some of Tomaselli's ideas see A Sitas, Culture and Production: The Contradictions of Working Class Theatre in South Africa (henceforth Culture and Production (2)), paper presented to the History Workshop, University of the Witwatersrand, 1984, pp 1-32 (pp 4-6).

37 The reasons for this are beyond the scope of this article, but surely include the more simple and direct performance dynamic of poetry and the survival of familiar *izibongo* conventions — 'rules and "tropes"', aesthetic models — on which poets and audiences could draw. Theatre lacked, as its central core, a similarly persuasive context of the familiar.

38 Sole, Black Literature and Performance, op cit, p 61.

39 MM Molepo, *Ilanga Le So Phonela Abasebenzi* (sic) (review), *SALB* 6(6), 1981, pp 49-51 (p 49).

40 See von Kotze, *Organise and Act*, op cit (Chapter 1, *The Dunlop Play*, pp 19-40); and Workshop Plays as Worker Education, op cit.

41 Von Kotze, *Organise and Act*, op cit, pp 102-6. For a different, five-fold classification of worker plays based on the following questions: a) For what occasion was the play made? b) Who are the central figures and in what context are they shown? c) What is the major conflict presented? see A von Kotze, Workers' theatre in South Africa, op cit (pp 89-90).

42 Rosanna Basso has written of transitory myths that flicker into brief and intense life during the course of collective events such as a battle, an uprising or a strike. In the heat of such an event a worldview is worked out which is strongly conditioned by the conflict being lived through. At the same time this new perception proves effective as a psychological means of identifying and directing the situation. Such a myth can offer a

way of controlling through fantasy the future that is wanted but cannot be conceived, and allows the natural to be challenged, the impossible to seem possible. See R Basso, Myths in Contemporary Oral Transmission: A Children's Strike. In R Samuel and P Thompson (eds), *The Myths We Live By*, London: Routledge, 1990, pp 61-9.

43 See note 34.

44 There has been considerable debate about the relationship between working class politics and culture and the non-class-specific anti-apartheid movements, and the need to encompass both specificity (in terms of class and the factory floor) and breadth of vision. See, for example, the following debate in the *SALB:* Sole, Black Literature and Performance, op cit; Naledi Writers Unit/Medu Art Ensemble, Debate: Working class culture and popular struggle, *SALB* 10(5), 1985, pp 21-30; K Sole, Politics and Working Class Culture: A Response, *SALB* 10(7), 1985, pp 43-56.

45 Ngoasheng, op cit, p 37, also p 35.

46 Difficulties faced in this regard are discussed throughout this article, but there are others that also need to be addressed. For example, the cultural movement is male dominated and female participation has been 'sporadic rather than regular and strong'. Among the reasons are: transport problems; the 'double-shift' worked by many women leaves little time or energy for cultural work; patriarchal attitudes (as a result most women who participate are young and/or single); and a socialised lack of self-confidence. See N Malange, Women workers and the struggle for cultural transformations, *Staffrider* 8(3 and 4), 1989, pp 76-80.

47 See Steadman, Theatre Beyond Apartheid, op cit, pp 79, 84, 89. M Fleischman, Workshop theatre as oppositional form, *South African Theatre Journal* 4(1), May 1990, pp 88-118 (pp 99, 103-4, 109-10). Fleischman also provides an interesting definition of workshop theatre (pp 88-9). With a worker constituency it has been identified as constructive in a number of ways. It enables participants to simultaneously learn and teach, subjects choices and opinions to broader evaluation, and fosters debate. New skills, such as role-play, are acquired that can be used in diverse contexts. Furthermore, it brings people together and to some extent overcomes alienation and isolation in the workplace; participants develop a renewed sense of self-confidence and self-worth; and actors gain an understanding of labour history, both in their company and nationally.

48 Kirkwood, op cit, p 666.

49 Von Kotze, *Organise and Act*, op cit, p 55.

50 Malange, op cit, pp 78-9. One of the apparent paradoxes of worker culture was that while preaching that everyone had a story to tell the story told was largely the same, it took on a kind of collective unity.

51 Obviously worker theatre has infused this model with a content in line with the political nature of its organising principle. However, at the level of structure this model is useful. At its most repetitive and formulaic worker theatre recorded an ideologically distilled public life of encounters between representative 'types' in archetypal situations. The battle lines were clearly drawn, 'the exploited' battled against 'the exploiters'. Infliction/defiance/consequence/assertion revolved around such issues as strikes and demands for union recognition. At the end of a play assertion often took the form of the singing of a unifying union song, proclamations of worker strength in unity or conversions to the cause.

52 Von Kotze, *Organise and Act*, op cit, p 23. Stated with reference to *The Dunlop Play* but probably intended to have general validity.

53 See Tomaselli, The Semiotics of Alternative Theatre, op cit, pp 17, 23-4, 28.

54 Von Kotze, *Organise and Act*, op cit, pp 27-9, 31 and Workshop Plays as Worker Education, op cit, pp 100-1, 103.

55 See Sitas, Culture and Production (1), op cit, pp 101-2. He refers to the segment of *The Dunlop Play* outlined above in rather different terms to von Kotze: 'a vast span of time was retold in very interesting ways but could not in any way be re-enacted the

way it was told. The strategy to solve this was to juxtapose a story teller with a "cranky" ... whereas the rest of the group acted out snatches of this unfolding history. In the process a lot of nuance was lost.'

56 Von Kotze, *Organise and Act,* op cit, pp 54, 82.

57 Von Kotze, Workers' Theatre in South Africa, op cit, pp 88-9; Interview (with Fosatu Cultural Group), op cit, p 74.

58 C Luther, South African Theatre: Aspects of the Collaborative Fringe, Doctoral Thesis, Leeds University, 1987.

59 Sole, Black Literature and Performance, op cit, p 71.

60 For example, Tomaselli has argued the need for 'empathy' (The Semiotics of Alternative Theatre, op cit, pp 20-1), while Kavanagh states that 'the criterion here is not membership of a racial/national group or class, but the actual function of the work produced' (R Kavanagh, *Theatre and Cultural Struggle in South Africa,* Zed Books, London, 1985, p 201).

61 For discussions of the role of worker cultural acitivists see Ngoasheng, op cit, who argues that the core of cultural activists have become, in Gramscian terms, the movement's 'organic intellectuals' in the cultural field; and D Bonnin, We Went to Arm Ourselves at the Field of Suffering: Traditions, Experiences and Grassroots Intellectuals, Natal Workshop, 1988, who discusses the idea of 'grassroots intellectuals'.

62 Von Kotze, *Organise and Act,* op cit, p 100; also see pp 70, 80, 81, 82, 84, 87, 89, 94.

63 Ari Sitas: The publication and reception of worker's literature (interview), *Staffrider* (8)(3 and 4), pp 61-8, (pp 63, 67-8).

64 See von Kotze, *Organise and Act,* op cit, p 97.

65 See L Passerini, Italian working class culture between the wars: Consensus to fascism and work ideology, *International Journal of Oral History* 1(1), 1980.

66 Sole, Politics and Working Class Culture: A Response, op cit, p 52.

67 Sitas, Culture and Production (1), op cit, pp 85, 104; also see Culture and Production (2), op cit, pp 3-4.

68 Sitas, Culture and Production (1), op cit, p 104.

69 New theatrical 'types' redrew the lines of engagement in black theatre. The 'new seriousness' of the worker moral order clashed with the moral order of much previous black theatre that assigned to vibrant, wayward 'types' — drunkards, *tsotsis,* shebeen queens — the task of creating dramatic excitement and engaging the audience. Worker theatre has struggled to find a politically acceptable yet equally engaging equivalent within their new pantheon of 'types'. Sitas notes the danger of 'middle men' becoming the strongest characters when counterposed against the faceless collectivity of the workers. Sitas, Culture and Production (1), op cit, pp 95-98.

70 As has already been mentioned, worker theatre has generally failed to situate its uniqueness politically and culturally. It has not, for example, adequately addressed the subtle interaction of continuities with and divergences from black and popular theatre, or, more generally, with past and present performance traditions.

71 Halton Cheadle, the lawyer who was instrumental in devising the play *Ilanga,* replied with disarming clarity when asked how he saw his role as a white intellectual within such worker theatre: 'I am not at all embarrassed about being intellectual and the workers are not embarrassed either. The form it takes would be our intervention. The substance is theirs. It is an on-going relationship. It is really hell of exciting' (as quoted from an interview in Tomaselli, The Semiotics of Alternative Theatre, op cit, pp 28-9).

72 Von Kotze, *Organise and Act,* op cit, pp 16, 99; Sole, Review of *Organise and Act,* op cit, p 120.

73 Interview (with FOSATU Cultural Group), op cit, p 73.

74 Doherty, op cit, p 100.

75 Sole, Politics and Working Class Culture: A Response, op cit, p 54; also see K Sole,

New Words Rising (Review of *Black Mamba Rising*). *SALB* 12(2), 1987, pp 107-115 (p 114).

76 Von Kotze, *Organise and Act,* op cit, p 23.
77 Ari Sitas: The Publication and Reception of Worker's Literature, op cit, p 67.
78 Orkin has noted the tendency of class-based analyses to privilege plays that deal with working class issues above others. The following is also of relevance: 'But contradictions seem to extend everywhere in theatre and theatre studies in South Africa. For instance, as intellectuals attached to the ruling classes, von Kotze and Sitas remain interventionists, confirming even in an overwhelmingly workerist constituency, an element of contradiction. Moreover, to date, what we know of such attempts at workers' theatre apart from the performances themselves, results mainly from their own mediation in reports, papers, published articles and a book ... Yet again, if, from another point of view, the involvement of intellectuals and sociologists in worker plays has been interrogated, these criticisms come ... from critics themselves not members of the working class — contradictions inevitably inform the positions of critics too!' (Orkin, op cit, p 196). I stand accused!
79 Kromberg, op cit, pp 197-8. On audience response to and evaluation of performance in worker gatherings also see Sitas, The Voice and the Gesture, op cit.
80 Sole, Black Literature and Performance, op cit, p 56.
81 A Sitas and D Bonnin, The Struggle over leisure: Durban workers, culture and education, *SALB* 15(2), August 1990, pp 61-4. They reach the rather spurious conclusion that 'involvement in cultural activities is significant, however low the percentage might be'.
82 S Smith, The autobiographical manifesto: Identities, temporalities and politics, *Prose Studies,* 1991, pp 186-212 (p 189).

Reflections on a Cultural Day of Artists and Workers on 16 April 1989

ALI KHANGELA HLONGWANE

This particular occasion on 16 April was seen as a day rededicating the people to the long wars of resistance when the colonists initially set foot on the shores of Azania on 6 April 1652. Such a merging of political and cultural activity is not new in our society, in fact it is becoming the norm. Certainly, since the early 70s artists and political activists have developed an awareness of the need for 'cultural activity and socio-political struggle (to) interact with each other'.[1] This stems from the realisation that artistic activity is one of 'the most potent forces rallying and uniting struggling peoples'.[2] At the present time this realisation shows itself in the continuous efforts to organise the arts — theatre, music, dance, oratory and fine arts at a mass-based level: arts education programmes have sprung up in different parts of the country; political organisations have their sports and culture secretariats which are far more active than in the past and trade unions are now initiating cultural units. In the 80s these activities took place against the background of a 'permanent' state of emergency: bannings, harassment of the press, and the ever-growing military presence in the townships as well as growing commercialisation and appropriation of the arts by the government controlled television.

This report reflects briefly on the works presented at the cultural day hosted by the Mafube Arts Commune at Lecton House in Johannesburg. It sees the event as a representative occasion of artistic activity which is mass-based. It also focuses on the interplay of 'popular', 'serious', traditional and new modes of expression in evidence in the works presented and touches on the ideological influences at play, the audience responses, and sets out for consideration the role of African languages in reaching the masses. Certainly the occasion showed the working of many expressive modes — there were slogans, in particular, 'Izwe lethu!' (Our land!), the singing of liberation songs, the recital of poetry, drama, all with a lot of mime, movement and drumming.

A feature of the day was that it drew together cultural activists from different operational bases. Well known writers like Ingoapele Madingoane, Maishe Maponya and Sipho Sepamla participated. Ingoapele Madingoane presented extracts from his poem 'Africa my beginning', as well as poems published in *Staffrider* Magazine and also recited from his as yet unpublished work, 'Africa must explain'. Maishe Maponya followed with poetical extracts from his plays *Gangsters* and *Busang Meropa*. Both of them recited and sang during their presentations. Sipho Sepamla, the director of the Fuba Academy read one of his poems, 'The Blues is You in Me'. He also read from his latest poetry anthology, *From Goré to Soweto*. But it was not only established artists who took part in the day's events. Community groups had their part to play as well. Pokela Cultural Group, made up of pupils coming predominantly from Selekele High School in Orlando East (re-named Sobukwe High by the militant school children) presented dramatised poetry fused with movement and with liberation songs. Then came a play, *Azania the Naked Truth*, presented by Busang Thakaneng from Sharpeville. This took the audience on a long journey to pre-colonial Afrika, showing them the coming of the settlers to the land and how they took it from the African people. The Africans resisted heroically but were finally defeated by the military might of the invading Europeans. As the play unfolded we were shown that colonial conquest was sparked by the Europeans' need for material resources for their own economic enrichment. For conquest to be effective, the play told us, the people had to be divided and mentally enslaved. Then later in the play the dispossessed masses rose and waged the just war of liberation. The play ended with 'free at last'.

Present during part of the day's proceedings was Ntate Zephaniah Mothopeng, President of the Pan African Congress. When he spoke briefly, he praised all the participating cultural groups and stressed the role of such groups in propagating the aspirations of the oppressed and the exploited. A performance which was a special tribute to 'Uncle Zeph' was put on by Mafube Theatre Unit. They adapted part of Ngugi wa Thiong'o and Micere Mugo's play, *The Trial of Dedan Kimathi*, and substituted the court scene in Nyeri where Kimathi is tried, with a scene from the trial known as 'The Bethal 18 Secret Trial'. In their adaptation, Ntate Mothopeng (like Kimathi) refuses to plead for mercy, turns his back on the colonial judge and addresses the Africans present in the court. The dramatic techniques of the Mafube group are aimed at showing their closeness with the audience. For instance, they do not wear costumes, instead they act in their everyday clothes. Nor do they tightly define their performance space. They mingle freely with the audience, involve them in singing, ululating and hand-clapping. As the play ended,

Ntate Mothopeng stood and called '*Izwe lethu*'; the audience responded with 'iAfrika', crying also, '*IBhubhesi*, uMothopeng, *iBhubhesi*!' (The Lion, Mothopeng, The Lion!). As he left, the youth of the audience followed him singing,

Mothopeng sikhokhele!	Mothopeng retaliate for us!
Mothopeng sikhokhele!	Mothopeng retaliate for us!
Siyongena eAzania!	We will gain Azania!

Workers' groups made their presence felt in the day's events as well. After Ntate Mothopeng's departure Media Workers Association of South Africa members from Perskor put on a poetry reading, and sang revolutionary songs accompanied by drums. The focus of their poetry was land dispossession and economic exploitation. For myself, the most memorable poem was one which highlighted the speaker's detestation of designations with racial connotations. Then came the turn of affiliates of the Commercial Catering and Allied Workers Union of South Africa. Their untitled play dealt with shop floor experiences and the home tribulations of a female worker. The central figure is dismissed from work after a long dispute between workers and management. On hearing about the dismissal of their colleague, the other workers take offence and down tools, pledging solidarity with their fellow worker. They shout the slogan, 'An injury to one is an injury to all! Long live worker control!' They also sing and chant '*toyi-toyi*' and this serves as a transition to the next scene which focuses on the problems of the man and wife relationship. It shows the abuse of female activists by ignorant men, who are apolitical. In one case we see a woman who is divorced by her husband because of her political involvement. So the play forces the audience to consider not only the exploitation of workers in general but the situation of women in particular. The play sets these themes within the broader struggle for national liberation. A professional actor sitting next to me remarked, 'Hmh! I thought these workers only complained about their wages!'

Taking the day as a whole, the audience responded remarkably to the different items presented. What struck me most was the absence of laughter in tragic incidents. This may seem a strange comment to make, but a number of performers have been grappling to understand why audiences among the oppressed tend to laugh at tragic scenes, as if, for some reason, they withdraw from total empathy at such moments. Somehow, on this occasion, performers and audience were as one, the painful scenes were clearly felt as such by the audience, and there was no laughter. Also, in many ways (and perhaps the absence of out-of-place laughter is somehow linked to this?) the total occasion was a reminder of how traditional African participatory theatre works: there was a great deal of singing and hand-clapping by the audience, a breaking down of any rigid performer-audience demarcation. At certain moments too, as in all theatre, the audience would alienate themselves from the presentation, obviously marvelling at the beauty, the craft and the artistry prevalent in some of the works. The entertainment aspect was also an inseparable aspect of the day.

Another overall feature which was very striking was that African languages tended to be the main medium of communication. Most of the works also juxtaposed English, Afrikaans and the different African languages and this is a trend which is generally on the increase. Also noticeable was the difference between these performances and those slavishly following the dictates of commercialism — the mixing of modes of expression which I have already mentioned, songs, poetry, dialogue, movement, mime and drumming and the way in which these were utilised was very different from what you find in commercially dominated shows.

To sum up, this surely was cultural action for social change. Everything was organised and performed for a grassroots majority, using accessible means of communication and styles, liberating art from the trappings of commercialism that holds hostage a number of so-called 'professional' artists. The work presented on the Cultural Day at Lecton House was free from the constraints imposed by venues that demand expensive sets, costumes and lights. This kind of activity was indeed conducted 'with due recognition of the political importance of cultural action'.[3]

1 *Free Azania*, 2, August 1988.
2 Pitso, *Journal for Azanian South Afrikan Arts and Culture*, Vol. 1, No. 1.
3 Robert Kavanagh, *Theatre and Cultural Struggle in South Africa* (London, 1985).

Marotholi Travelling Theatre: Towards an Alternative Perspective of Development

ZAKES MDA

My concern in this account is with theatre rather than drama, and I think it is important for us to clarify the distinction from the onset. 'Theatre' here refers to the production and communication of meaning in the performance itself, in other words a transaction or negotiation of meaning in a performer-spectator situation. 'Drama' on the other hand, refers to the literature on which performances are sometimes based, the mode of fiction designed along certain dramatic conventions for stage representation. The kind of theatre I am concerned with here is development theatre, in particular the Lesotho group known as the Marotholi Travelling Theatre.

The initial stage of any development activity is communication, and throughout the life of the activity communication continues. Without the essential social interaction through messages between 'development agents' and the people, the so-called beneficiaries of development actions, we cannot in any meaningful way talk of development.

When we examine various development projects in Lesotho we find that in many cases communication is top-down. In other words, planners from outside the community decide what is good for the community and impose projects without finding out from the 'beneficiaries' what their needs are. More often than not such projects fail to realise their objectives because people lack the motivation to participate in the projects of which they feel they are not part. In our tours of the villages we have in fact discovered that the general attitude is that the responsibility for failure or success of such projects rests with the 'government' (by which it is meant any development agency — be it government or non-governmental). People feel that things are being done for them, and it is up to the 'benefactors' to see to it that they succeed. They see themselves as mere recipients — an attitude which reinforces dependency.

For communication to be complete and effective it must be two-way instead of a top-down, one-way flow of information. However, for communication to be two-way it must take place among community members themselves. The need for a democratic vehicle to facilitate dialogue at community level gave birth to the use of theatre as an appropriate medium — a medium that can be used for both mass and interpersonal communication.

Marotholi Travelling Theatre

Marotholi Travelling Theatre is a theatre for development project of the National University of Lesotho. It was established in 1982 by a joint working party of the Department of English and the Institute of Extra-Mural Studies. The English Department initiated and got involved in this project because it had the skilled personnel in theatre. The Institute of Extra-Mural Studies became involved because of its expertise in rural development, non-formal education and adult education. The performers are students who have successfully completed a course on Practical Theatre, offered by the English Department.

Between 1982 and 1985, the theatre for development project produced a number of plays dealing with such themes as reforestation, co-operative societies and the rehabilitation of prisoners. From the beginning, the aim of the project was to use theatre as a medium of development communication, and secondly to use theatre for motivating communities into initiating and/or participating in development activities.

Agitprop Theatre

The first method used by the project was as follows: A group of students would go out to the villages and gather information on the problems of the target areas. The next step would be to analyse the information and prioritise it. It must be noted here that in most cases 'priority' would be from the point of view of the theatre group, and not the communities themselves. From these priorities a story would be improvised. The next stage would be rehearsal, and then the actual performances in the target areas. After every performance there would be discussion of the issues raised in the play among the community members, the cast, and the extension workers if they happened to be present. Finally there would be follow-up action by the Extra-Mural Department or another agency depending on the theme of the play. Follow-up action involves giving the people the actual practical advice on how to go about solving their problems. For example, if a community decides to establish a co-operative society for poultry farming, the Extra-Mural Department would provide the skills for them to establish and run such a co-operative themselves.

This is a method of theatre known as agitprop, and in our evaluation of previous performances[1] we discovered that, although it has a strong rallying force, it lacks real community participation since the play comes to the village as a pre-packaged message, and the spectators become mere consumers of a finished product. The level of critical awareness on specific themes is therefore not very high since it is raised outside the community.

We have now completely discarded this method for we feel that if the message is pre-packaged, the process does not differ much from the top-down communication that we are so much against. To us it seemed as though through our research in the villages people told us their problems, and through our theatre we 'solved' their problems by providing fully worked-out solutions. In other words this kind of theatre is geared towards persuasion — to influence people to do what we think is right for them, instead of trying to raise the level of their critical awareness so that they may examine and find ways of solving their problems themselves.

Indeed in using the agitprop approach there were post-performance discussions, but we discovered that in many cases such discussions led to individual action only on a short-term basis — a discovery which tallies with other experiences in various parts of the world where this method has been used as a medium of development communication.[2]

Development as Social Transformation

This led us to re-examine our own notion of what development really is. Initially all it meant to us was simply and vaguely: 'To bring about social change' and 'to improve the living standards of the people'. We discovered that development should indeed be a process of social transformation. However, many cases of social change in the developing world, and in the industrialised part of the world as well, do not lead to a better quality of life. Social change could also be anti-developmental. We therefore searched for an alternative perspective on development and settled for a definition which stressed that through development a society should achieve a greater control of its social, economic and political destiny. This, of course, means that the individual members of the community should have increased control of their institutions.

Now, this can be a dangerous perspective in many Third World countries, for it contends that development must imply liberation, a freeing from all forms of domination — of dependence and oppression. The ruling classes may not be amused by this perspective.

A related concept is critical awareness. For development to happen, people must have critical awareness, which should be brought about by a critical analysis of their situation. We found that although agitprop as used by the National University of Lesotho Theatre Project was able to arouse the emotions of the people, even sometimes to bring to their notice things they were not aware of, it fell short in that it was not able to be a vehicle for the people to examine their situation, critically analyse it, discuss among themselves, and if possible come up with solutions. Thus, after an initial period we felt that theatre for development should not instruct people on what to do, as our project had been doing, but should rather arouse the people's capacity to participate and decide things for themselves.

Participatory Theatre and Theatre for Conscientisation

Two methods that Marotholi now use in trying to overcome the shortcomings of agitprop are Participatory Theatre and Theatre for Conscientisation.

In Participatory Theatre community members themselves become performers. The Marotholi troupe become catalysts — outsiders with skills in theatre and in community development. This kind of theatre is able to raise community issues, to involve the people in discussing the issues, and finally to involve the people in making decisions. Since catalysts must get the people involved in presenting the dramatic programme, it was necessary for at least some theatre members to stay in the village for some time and to learn at first hand the peculiar problems of each village. This was in fact impossible for Marotholi members to carry out since the troupe had to travel throughout the country and could at most spend only one day in each village.

The most effective method therefore is now seen as Theatre for Conscientisation, which works as follows:

- Actors (catalysts) perform a short scene suggested by a local person.
- They halt the action at a crisis point.
- They then ask the audience to offer solutions.
- The actors become like puppets and perform the action strictly on the spectators' orders.
- The best solution is arrived at by trial, error, discussion and then audience participation.

• The final stage is follow-up action by the development agencies.

In this kind of theatre the action is not deterministic — everything is subject to criticism and rectification. Everything can be changed by any spectator at a moment's notice without censorship.

An even more effective variation of this is when the spectators themselves become actors. Participants tell a story with a social problem, then catalysts and community members together improvise, rehearse and present it to the group as a skit. The audience is asked if they agree with the solution. Any spectator is invited to replace any actor and lead the action in the direction that seems most appropriate to him or her. As before, the best solution is arrived at by trial, error, discussion, then audience consensus. The emphasis in this kind of theatre is self-education. Consciousness is raised from inside by group analysis of social reality and power relations.

Brief Case Studies

To illustrate the potency of Theatre for Conscientisation, I wish to cite in a summary form two cases where the method was used, and the community members were able to make resolutions to solve their problems. The first one involves migrant workers and their families in the Mohale's Hoek district, and the second, peasants in a village in the Mafeteng district.

In a village in the mountains of Mohale's Hoek we discovered that there were dissatisfactions among the women folk about the National Union of Mineworkers. They felt that their husbands go out to South Africa to work for their families, but when they get there they join such 'terrible movements' as the National Union of Mineworkers, whose main function is to call strikes. When strikes are called, their husbands are expelled from work, and their families suffer.

The catalysts performed a short scene suggested by a local housewife who was up in arms against the trade union movement. The scene depicted the irresponsibility of the men in the mines who forget about their families at home, and take part in the activities of trade unions. It also depicted the families that suffer at home as a result of these activities.

As usual, at a crisis point the action was halted, and the spectators were asked to offer solutions. This was a very controversial issue, and the community members participated enthusiastically. Some commented from the sidelines, while others came to the stage and took up roles in the play.

I shall briefly list some of the issues that emerged from the performance:

• A migrant worker indicated that he had been a member of the National Union of Mineworkers, but had resigned because the 'NUM is more concerned with South African politics, rather than with the problems of the workers. All we ever do is to sing political songs about South African political leaders, and about the evils of apartheid.'
• Another migrant felt that the National Union of Mineworkers is most active only when it comes to demanding increased wages from the employers. 'For instance, they now demand a 55% raise. This means that the owners of the mines will only get 45%. The mine owners will in fact get less than the workers. The workers want to own the mines!'
• A woman complained that she heard from her husband that the National Union of Mineworkers has always been quiet about white people who come to the mines and are trained by experienced blacks, only for these whites to become bosses over the blacks. The National Union of Mineworkers is useless on this issue because it is only interested in fighting for money.
• Yet another migrant indicated that the Union had called for strikes which were not agreed upon by the members. For instance in 1985, they went to negotiate with the Chamber of Mines, and when they came back they reported to the members that there was a deadlock, and if it was not resolved by the first of October, there would be a strike. They did not ask the members whether there should be a strike or not. Indeed, without any voting by the members, a strike was called on the first of October.
• Another migrant complained, 'I have passed Cambridge Overseas School Certificate, but I found at the mines the shop stewards are people with a Standard Six certificate. They mislead the miners'.

When emotive issues are raised, performances of this nature can easily get out of hand, and turn into shouting matches among the opposing sides. It therefore becomes necessary for some intervention, that is for the catalysts to be able to conduct the proceedings in an orderly and entertaining manner, so that every point of view is given a hearing. After many scenes of trial and error — in effect scenes of debate in a theatrical form within the world of the play, though constantly related to the world of the community — a consensus which showed some considerable shift in points of view was reached along the following lines:

• The structures that have created racial discrimination at the mines are political. That is why white people can be trained by blacks, only for them to become bosses. 'These are politics of apartheid,' a migrant said. 'For the union to be effective in fighting these issues, it must deal with the system that has created such discriminatory laws. An effective union cannot avoid politics.'

• The workers are not fighting to own the mines — which would not be a bad idea in any case — but for decent wages. The 55%–45% arithmetic of the other migrant was shown to be faulty. 'The union wanted our wages to be raised by 55%. This means 55% of your current wages.'

• On the issue that the union is only interested in 'fighting for money' the audience agreed with an old man — he had never been a miner but was a farmer — who said, 'You just complained that you do not get any recognition for the work you do. You complain that inexperienced whites are made your bosses. Again you complain that your union is only interested in demanding more wages. Is recognition not shown through money?'

• There was some disagreement among those who had been to the mines as to whether the National Union of Mineworkers ever called a strike that was not authorised by the members, and the catalysts did not have any information as to whether this was true or not. However, it was agreed that 'the union should not be the *boss* of the workers, for in that case the union would just be acting like the employers who always bully the workers. A union must be run by the workers according to their own wishes'.

• The complaint that shop stewards have little formal classroom education was dismissed with contempt and much ridicule. 'Is the union not a workers movement?' the women asked. 'Are the workers in the mines not our husbands who have not been to school? Who should run the movement if not the workers themselves?'

At the end of the performance the spectators-cum-performers took a resolution that migrant workers should join and participate in the activities of a trade union because trade unions benefit the workers. There was a minority which was adamant that Basotho miners had no business in South African affairs. They were 'like beggars in someone else's country', and should not participate in the politics of that country. They should rather realise that they went to the mines to earn money for Lesotho and for their families.

The second case I would like to cite concerns land. For many years Mafeteng was the foremost wheat-producing district in Lesotho.

However, of late very little wheat is produced in the district, and generally the standard of agriculture has deteriorated. In a village in the district the community members were keen on examining the causes of the poor wheat production in their village, and how this trend could be reversed. What started off as a harmless play with extension workers from some development agencies participating in the performance, and advising villagers on proper methods of agriculture, ended up exposing the corruption of the chief. Apparently for some years he had been encouraging the peasants to sell their fields as residential sites. He received a fat commission from such transactions. Although the sale of land is illegal in Lesotho, huge tracts of previously rich farmlands had been divided into small residential plots and people had already built their homes there.

The community members resolved that the sale of agricultural land should stop, and people should be allocated residential sites on the mountain slopes and rocky areas, in order to reserve arable land for wheat farming.

A lot of plays we do are not as controversial as the two cases cited. They deal with such issues as rural sanitation, immunisation of infants, and income generating activities for rural women.

Finally, it needs to be said that, depending on the level of consciousness of the catalysts and of their intentions, it is possible for popular theatre, particularly of the agitprop kind, to become an instrument of oppression — what has become known as 'theatre for domestication'. In the same way that Paulo Freire challenges us to make a distinction between education as an instrument of domination, and education as an instrument of liberation,[3] so is the distinction essential between theatre as an instrument of the domination of the peasants and urban slum dwellers through the ideology of the ruling classes, and theatre as an instrument of liberation.

1 Z. Mda, *Marotholi Travelling Theatre* (Roma, 1986), pp. 36–40.
2 Pru Lambert, Popular Theatre: One Road to Self Determined Action, *Community Development Journal*, 17, 3 (1982).
3 P. Freire, *Pedagogy of the Oppressed* (New York, 1970).

Theatre for Development in Zimbabwe: An Urban Project

R. MSHENGU KAVANAGH

In many parts of the underdeveloped world theatre is being used as a medium of education, problem-solving, dialogue and mobilization on development issues such as literacy, health, sanitation, agriculture self-help projects and co-operatives.[1] The following is an account of a theatre project in an urban area in Zimbabwe. Up to now most theatre for development work has been conducted in rural areas. The Matapi Hostels experience reveals the problems of such work in urban conditions and prompts certain doubts concerning the long-term validity of theatre for development itself.

Background

The hostels in Mbare, previously Harare location, were constructed by the colonial city council to house single labourers, the majority of whom were migrant. They consist of four-storied blocks of single rooms. During the liberation struggle in the 1970s families fled the rural areas and took refuge in town. They built shelters at Harare Musika (the market and main terminus for country buses). Many women with their children joined husbands and took up occupation in the hostels.

The Muzorewa regime, which immediately preceded independence, accommodated the influx into Harare in the hostels, among other places, as a temporary measure. At independence, when families could have been repatriated, they stayed on and were joined by yet others coming to Harare for jobs or to follow their husbands and relatives. What had been intended as single accommodation had now come to house whole families, many of them extended.

Mrs B.V. Matsvetu of the Zimbabwe Council for the Welfare of Children has been working in the Matapi Hostels for some years, mobilizing women, initiating hygiene and cleanliness campaigns and disseminating information on family planning. Much of her activity's funding is derived from an American foundation which lays stress on family planning as the answer to the problems in Matapi.

Mrs Matsvetu appealed to the Faculty of Arts Drama at the University of Zimbabwe to work with her in the hostels. Drama at the University of Zimbabwe consists of practical and theoretical courses in the B.A. General and Honours degrees in the English and African Languages Departments and extra-curricular activities. Between 1985 and 1988 there was an annual Faculty of Arts Major Production in which anyone either in or outside the University could participate. *Mavambo — First Steps*, a dramatization of Wilson Katiyo's novel, *A Son of the Soil* (published in University Playscripts in 1986), was the first, followed by an extremely popular and effective production of the Kenyan play, *I'll Marry When I Want* in Shona, *Kremlin Chimes* by Nikolai Pogodin, in which Lenin was played for the first time by a black actor, and *The Contest* by Mukotani Rugyendo.

In 1985 a political theatre group, Zambuko/Izibuko ('the river-crossing' in Shona and Ndebele), was founded, consisting of students, workers and unemployed youth. In addition to short agitprop pieces on special political occasions (*ngonjera*), Zambuko/Izibuko devised two full-length plays, *Katshaa!* on South Africa (published in University Playscripts, 1988) and *Samora Continua*, on Mozambique, and performed them in a wide variety of venues all over Zimbabwe.

A group of students were allocated to the project as part of a course begun in 1986 entitled Popular, Political and Community Theatre, in which students are expected to leave campus and involve themselves in practical drama work in the community. In previous years students had worked with the police, the army, convicts, nurses, women's clubs and the unemployed. In 1988, one group did a video on sexually-transmitted disease on the university campus, another followed up the previous year's work with the police and a third was detailed to work with Mrs Matsvetu.

The course was due to start in June and in the same month Zambuko/Izibuko performed its play, *Samora Continua*, in the Matapi Hostels in order to stimulate an interest in drama before work in the hostels began. As a result of discussions with Mrs Matsvetu, it was decided that the Matapi students should be divided, one group to work with the adults on a play on living conditions in the hostels and another with the youth in order to help establish a drama group which would provide an occupation and a source of income. In addition, in collaboration with the University Centre for Educational Technology a video record of the project would be made.

The Process

The process began with a briefing session at the University, at which Mr C. Chisvo, Senior Youth Development Officer in the Department of Housing and Community Services in the Harare City Council, Mr Gweshe, in charge of the hostels themselves, and Mrs Matsvetu would brief the students on the hostels. As it happened only Mrs Matsvetu turned up and she introduced the students to her organization and to the living conditions in Matapi. The students had meanwhile discussed their project beforehand and agreed on ways to approach and work with the community. Their course included discussion of the methodology of theatre for development and various case studies, including the uses of theatre in the Great October Socialist Revolution, socialist, workers and 'alternative' theatre in Britain, Kamiriithu (Kenya), Laedza Batanani (Botswana), Zambia, Malawi and the Murewa workshop in Zimbabwe (1983).[2]

During the first visit to the hostels, in one of the vast public dining halls, which was bare except for its concrete tables and benches, introductions took the form of some words of explanation, dancing and singing. As one of the student participants explained it:

We introduced ourselves to the women. We had to make much more personal introductions so as to create personal relationship with the community. At the end we realised that some of the community members really knew our families, like myself. I met people from my village. This really inspired the community.[3]

In addition, the women acted a play they had worked on as a result of seeing *Samora Continua*. The plot depicted a girl who is made pregnant. The father, a young boy of her own age, refuses to accept responsibility. She is about to abort then she is told of the Zimbabwe Council for the Welfare of Children, where she receives help. The session ended with the parents who were to work on the Matapi play, and the youth who were to establish a drama group, meeting separately and planning their next meeting. It was agreed that the women would take the students around the hostels to see the conditions for themselves.

When this was duly done, a report back took place at the University to enumerate the problems the students had witnessed, namely overcrowding, unemployment, prostitution, fighting, drunkenness, especially caused by drinking *kachasu* (an illegal home-made gin), theft, noise, breakdown of the family, shortage and inadequacy of ablution, toilet and recreation facilities and police harassment.

The cold shorthand of this list obscures scenes of wretchedness and inhuman squalor which deeply affected all those who were involved in the project. The following is one student's record of what she saw:

> There was one bathing room for all women in the block and two for men. This inconvenienced a lot of working people and school children who were to bath in time in the morning. There was also one place for washing plates and this caused a lot of stealing. The places where plates were washed were adjacent to the toilets . . . There were so many children running around, some sitting idly or lying about, most of them very dirty with wounds and they appeared to be victims of malnutrition. The three rooms that I personally visited were overcrowded. One woman told me that she had nine children and a lodger because she could not afford the rent as she lived on selling vegetables.[4]

It was decided that this list now be taken to the women in Matapi and discussed and analysed together with them. A storyline would then be devised. Discussion revealed that the burning issues were low wages and unemployment, high rents for inadequate rooms and facilities, no repair of breakages and men's dereliction of family responsibilities. The following scenario was collectively agreed on:

- Two men, A and B, returning home from work on a Friday. Pay-day. A goes to the bar, B goes home.
- The bar. A squandering his pay on girlfriends and drink. A young boy selling matches in the bar is forced to smoke and drink. Prostitution, drunkenness, fighting and noise characterize the bar, which is actually situated in one of the hostel buildings.
- A's wife and family in their room in the hostel. A arrives drunk, demanding food and falling all over the children who are trying to sleep on the floor. He beats his wife when she fails to produce satisfactory food. There is a fight. A's daughter is trying to study but she is forced out into the corridor by the noise.
- The corridor. She is reading. A man suggests she come to his room, which is quieter. Ultimately she agrees. Later we hear she is pregnant.
- B's room in the hostel. Also over-crowded. He hands over his pay-packet. His wife attempts to work out how it will be used to cover their expenses. It is insufficient. The wife suggests they use some of the money to buy vegetables in order to sell and make some extra money.

• Women, including B's wife, selling vegetables by the roadside near the hostels. They are discussing their problems, e.g. one sink to wash body, plates, nappies and food in; broken windows left unrepaired, a child fell through a broken window to her death; no doors on bathrooms so that as women they are seen naked when washing; lack of privacy in the rooms, lack of ceilings so that 'what's happening in one room, can be heard in the other'.[5]

It had now become clear what the aim of the performance was to be. It was agreed that the women would present their play to an audience made up of people from the community and people in authority so as to initiate a dialogue between them aimed at improving conditions in the hostels. In order to do this it was important that the play should not be a performance but a facilitator of dialogue. The students therefore began introducing the women to the idea of incorporating discussion of issues raised by the play itself, that is, between the actors in character and the audience. This had been done extremely successfully by Chris Kamlongera of Chancellor College in rural development work in Malawi and students had seen a video of this.[6]

The students and the women then began rehearsing the play, including one abortive attempt to rehearse outside the hostels so as to open up the rehearsal process to the community. A first performance was agreed on, to be held in the same indoor area where *Samora Continua* had been successfully performed. This area was on the ground floor of one of the hostels and contained a row of kiosks, pin-ball machines and table soccer.

The performers, that is, women and students, marched down the main road past the hostels singing and informing the people of the performance. They gathered a vast army of small children and entered the performance venue. A small number of adults gathered as well and the play began. It was not long before the children were making too much noise for much to be heard of the play and efforts to initiate discussion during the performance proved abortive. The video camera began to dominate and towards the end performers and audience were speaking straight into the camera lens. Coincidentally, Mr C. Ngorima, Director of Housing in the City Council, who happened to be passing by, dropped in to see what was going on and students engaged him privately in debate after the performance. He was very concerned that the students' intentions might be hostile to his administration.

The next meeting took place at the University to evaluate the first performance. A second performance was planned and measures taken to avoid the blunders of the first. A film show was arranged for the children by Mrs Matsvetu and it was suggested that students playing parts like that of a policeman should play them sincerely rather than make it obvious that they considered them to be the villains of the piece. A new venue was chosen, namely the dining hall where the first meeting had taken place, and Mrs Matsvetu agreed to invite local City Council and party officials to attend in order for there to be dialogue between the community and the authorities. The programme was to consist of a play by the women alone, the combined women-student play and then a performance by the youth of a play they had rehearsed with the other group of students entitled *Imwe Chanzi Ichabvepi?* by William Chigidi.[7]

The second performance took place on 15 October. In addition to members of the Matapi community, present were the MP for the area, Mrs I. Mashonganyuika, Director of the Department of Housing in the City Council, Mr C. Ngorima, and other councillors and party officials. The programme proceeded as planned. The in-character discussion with the audience was greatly improved and the MP and councillors participated enthusiastically as did Matapi residents. The children had abandoned the film show in favour of the drama so the bulk of the audience was again children and noise levels were still high. More men were attracted into the audience on this occasion and one spoke out passionately against *kachasu*. There was to have been a discussion at the end of the entire programme but in reality it rather took the form of speeches by the dignitaries present.

As a mechanism for achieving dialogue the drama did achieve certain limited objectives: 'The leaders learnt the people's problems while the people in the community were made aware that there were some problems they could solve by themselves'.[8] The authorities expressed shock at some of the issues raised. Mr Ngorima, for instance, claimed that the Council was not aware of the scale of the overcrowding in Matapi and said that if it was true then 'action should have been taken yesterday and not tomorrow'. He expressed concern over the lack of doors and, noting that the audience was seated on the floor, promised to furnish the dining rooms. He also undertook to have broken windows and blocked sewage pipes repaired but called for the formation of hall committees to prevent vandalism. He also appealed to residents to turn off water taps after use and promised to install neon lights in the hostels to curb theft of bulbs. At the same time the visitors strongly warned the students not to incite the people against the government and to keep the process of dialogue away from the media.

The Situation in the Matapi Hostels and Participatory Theatre for Development

Matapi was the result of colonial labour policies, which in certain sectors relied on single, migrant workers earning a wage adequate only for themselves and not their families. These were expected to feed themselves on the produce of their land in the rural areas. Even before the war the system was under strain as the black population of Rhodesia had been restricted to areas of poor soil and erratic rainfall. Over-population, overgrazing and overcropping in these areas had already made it increasingly difficult for families to subsist and they depended on the worker's wage for crucial inputs and basic commodities, not to mention taxes, schooling and medication.

The war led to total breakdown in many parts of the countryside. Rhodesian forces, in retaliation for peasant support for the guerillas, destroyed homesteads and swept up whole populations into 'keeps' or fortified villages. The rural leg of the colonial labour system could no longer stand and families converged on the cities. After independence the repressive machinery was no longer in place to enforce the colonial labour system in all its aspects. Families who had remained in the countryside were now free to join their husbands and relatives in town. Despite a number of hikes in the minimum wage, which were effectively eroded by price rises, the colonial wage system remained substantially unreformed. The combination of massive expansion of the education system, influx to the towns, low wages and a stagnant economy led to a drastic rise in unemployment and increased urban poverty. The situation in Matapi is a dramatic and extreme manifestation of what in other areas is there but less visible.

Solutions to the problems of Matapi encountered by the students in their work were resettlement, self-help in various forms and birth control. The students did not carry an analysis of the situation in Matapi to the residents and at no time suggested solutions. They did raise the question of resettlement and the women made it clear that they refused to be dumped in rural poverty away from their men, who, they said, would only philander in town and fail to send home money to their families. They preferred to remain close to the cash source in order to divert some of the money at least to the uses of the family. No satisfactory answer was received from the unemployed as to why they rejected going to the resettlement areas except for statements along the lines of: 'Let us rather be poor and enjoy electricity than be poor in the dark'. Despite unemployment and poverty the city does provide facilities the country cannot rival — water, electricity, education, health and the hope of employment.

The women did dutifully refer to birth control and, working under the Zimbabwe Council for the Welfare of Children, they did make a play advocating it but in discussions and rehearsals with the students the women never raised the issue. Clearly the fundamental problems in Matapi are unemployment, low wages and accommodation. These result in promiscuity, high birth rate, drunkenness, theft and vandalism. It became clear that calling for birth control until the fundamental problems have been solved is ineffective. The Matapi hostel-dwellers need jobs, a living wage and accommodation.

This raises some fundamental questions concerning theatre for development work. Development problems present themselves as causes and effects. To take the case of Matapi, promiscuity, drunkenness, theft, vandalism, high birth rate, baby-dumping, fights, breakdown of the family, lack of hygiene, are all effects. The causes of these behaviour patterns are economic, the material conditions of the hostel-dwellers lives i.e. unemployment, inadequate wages and no accommodation. It is apparently easier for theatre for development workers to tackle the effects. This results in reformism. How does one tackle the causes, the material base? Revolution? Is theatre for development a substitute for theatre for revolution? What development can be meaningful if it is not revolutionary development?

In early 1988 students at the University of Zimbabwe closed the University down. They were protesting on a number of issues — failure to raise the student grant as promised, transport, accommodation, library facilities and so on. Since independence the University has expanded from 800 students to 8 000. Students are no longer a small protected élite. They now have to contend with at least some of the problems that face the Zimbabwean urban masses, transportation and accommodation being the most obvious.

The demonstration culminated in an invasion of the campus by police, involving beatings and tear-gas. Students increasingly came to perceive the cause of their problems as 'the corrupt system'. Before starting work in Matapi such views were expressed by the students' discussion. However to have gone into Matapi with such an analysis and attempted to work with the residents on the basis of such rhetoric would have been for a number of obvious reasons counterproductive.

It was decided that the main function of the students was to listen to the residents, facilitate their own articulation of their situation and bring about a dialogue between them and those in authority with a responsibility for living conditions in Matapi. In other words neither a theatre of reform nor a theatre of revolution but instead a process of participatory theatre encouraging articulation of problems and leading to dialogue. However, the process, without any imposition of an analysis, still led to the conclusion that the basic causes of Matapi's problems are a system, a system that creates unemployment, pays low wages and does not accommodate its people.

In October 1988, a week or so before the second Matapi performance, the students demonstrated again. This time they targeted their protests at what they alleged was corruption in the leadership of the party and government. Demonstrating simultaneously with their fellows at the Harare Polytechnic, the students attempted to leave the campus but were opposed by the police, who sealed off all exits and another round of invasion, beatings and tear-gas followed, worse than the first. In the wake of the 'anti-corruption' demo, a Marxist lecturer, a Kenyan exile in the Law Faculty, was deported on a 48-hour order. Four other lecturers and a dozen students were charged in court. The President and a number of ministers strongly condemned the demonstrations on television and at rallies all over the country.

This accounts for the strong warnings issued by the MP and The City Councillor at the second performance that the students should not incite the people against the government. Thus they expressed their appreciation that the students were concerning themselves with the problems of the people and participating in their development, but feared that they might try and do this out of the context of party and government programmes and policies.

The students were obviously treading a tightrope. And what, if anything had been achieved? This brings us to the question of follow-up. Among the students who helped establish a theatre group with the youth, one who lives in Mbare continued to liaise with them during the holidays. At the same time it was decided that the students would attempt to interest the Mbare Project — a World University Service project organised at the University of Zimbabwe to do outreach work in Mbare — to take the group on and give it initial backing in the form of funds, transport and publicity until it established itself independently. Unfortunately, the Mbare Project collapsed soon afterwards.

As far as the women's group was concerned, some repairs were undertaken in the hostels. But this in turn introduced fresh problems. For example as soon as taps were installed they were stolen. How could the community and the authorities work together to ensure that any improvements would be sustained? This became the basis for the next round of work with the women.

Theatre for Development: Town and Country

It was mentioned earlier that Dr Chris Kamlongera's work in Malawi had been influential in the students' approach at Matapi, particularly the technique of discussion with the audience in character during the performance. Other examples studied included the Murewa and Chindinduma workshops in Zimbabwe, Chikwakwa Theatre (Zambia), Laedza Batanani (Botswana), Nhlangano workshop (Swaziland), Malya, Msogo and Bagamoyo (Tanzania), Maska, Samaru and Bomo (Nigeria).[9] Kamiriithu is not included in this list because it was a frankly political, in fact, revolutionary cultural campaign, involving a direct challenge to a patently tyrannical neo-colonial regime. All the examples of theatre for development in Africa available to the students were rural projects. Their work in Matapi however was urban. It was discovered that there are significant differences and a number of intractable problems to be encounterd in working in poor, urban neighbourhoods as opposed to rural villages, mostly relating to rehearsal and performance.

The problems encountered in Matapi were also different from those encountered in the theatre for development work of the previous two years — at the King George VI Barracks and the Central Prison, for instance, and the rigidly hierarchical bureaucracy that made work difficult. By way of illustration, it was necessary to have a signed order from above to move a table and chairs outside for rehearsals. In the Central Prison it was the suspicion and inhumanity of an archaic, colonial attitude to imprisonment that reduced the effectiveness of the work. It took the students months of patient slogging to get permission to work with the convicts in the first place — and then only with those attending the adult education class. It was stated that it was against prison regulations that convicts mix with the public and so the students were forbidden to do warm-ups or act with the convicts. Ultimately, the play was acted by the adult education students to others in their class. No performance was permitted to the other convicts in the prison. The army, the prison, the police and Parirenyatwa Hospital all presented problems of suspicion or lack of imagination or understanding on the part of a rigid hierarchical bureaucracy. In Matapi this did not exist at all. The difficulties were of quite another order.

In participatory theatre for development it is essential that the people be involved in every phase of the process. It is always the aim to expand as much as possible the input (or participation) of the community beyond that of those who are actively working on the play. Open rehearsals are an effective way of doing this. The making of *I'll Marry When I Want* at Kamiriithu was a notable and successful example of this. Members of the community, who were free to attend all rehearsals, contributed with dialogue, characterization, songs, dance, language and at times actually joined the cast as a result of contributing in this way.[10] The students working in Matapi likewise wished to open up the process of rehearsal to the community and a rehearsal was conducted outside one of the hostels.

Unfortunately the experiment had to be abandoned as the environs of the hostel are extremely dusty and littered with trash. It was impossible to sit on the ground and all scenes had to be acted standing up. The area is also extremely noisy with small children playing all over the place and large trucks and buses moving past. Whereas traditional meeting places in the rural context are outdoors, in the urban context they are indoors — for the same reasons that make outdoor rehearsals at Matapi impossible. Yet to rehearse indoors was to remove the activity from the sight of residents and passers-by so that it became a secluded event.

The ubiquity of small children proved to be a problem not encounterd by those working in the villages. Traditionally discussion of problems of development are not considered fit for the participation of small children. In fact, in some societies even adult women might be excluded from such discussions. At Matapi both efforts to discuss such problems, that is, through performance, attracted large numbers of small children. High birth rate, no recreational facilities and inadequate daycare have combined to produce large numbers of unsupervised children. At performances they soon began to make noise despite the efforts of adults to restrain them, made dialogue between performers and audience difficult and inhibited the attendance of adults.

Though it had been decided that they would be excluded from the second performance, the attempt to attract them to a film failed. Yet there was no doubt that their presence almost destroyed the process of dialogue. This is not to say that they were in actual fact badly behaved. Simply that it was too much to expect them to remain silent while such topics were discussed in performance. In addition some of the material of the play was not appropriate for children, for example, seduction. Children in Matapi are exposed from birth to the sexual activity of adults as a result of over-crowding and many of them mimic what they see and hear at an early age. However to legitimate this by exposing them to such topics in a performance is clearly not desirable. This is a problem which many contemporary community theatre groups in Zimbabwe need to pay attention to as a high proportion of audiences at theatre performances in working class venues are young children and so far there are few signs of either keeping them out or ensuring that the content of the plays is suitable.[11]

In the rural community there is also a strong tradition of contributing to a discussion in a disciplined way, with each speaker being given a chance to speak in turn without interruption until he or she finishes.[12] In Matapi, especially in the presence of children, this did not exist and efforts to promote dialogue between performers and audience often collapsed into questions being answered by an undifferentiated chorus of shouts.

The key obviously to future work of this kind in the Matapi Hostel is the exclusion of the children. These should and need to be catered for by their inclusion in the audience at performances of plays, like the *Samora Continua* staging which they attended and did not substantially disrupt. *Samora Continua*, being as it is a historical analysis of Mozambique's struggle for socialism, was obviously not really appropriate. There is therefore a strong need for children's theatre in order to involve them both as actors and as audience.

In a more disciplined environment restricted to adults, the technique of in-character discussion with the audience could prove more successful — as indeed it did when another group of students undertook a similar project with the Zimbabwe Republic Police.[13] This is what future work in Matapi will have to strive to achieve.

A Postscript

Work continued the following year in, among other communities, Mbare. Students worked again with the women and the youth theatre group. The women were keen to present another play dramatizing the current situation and illustrating what had and had not been done since they last performed to the authorites. They aimed to invite them back again for another round of dialogue, thus illustrating that in theatre for development work the process does not culminate in a definitive 'performance' but is a continuing process of dialogue and problem-solving. Students working with the youth assisted the theatre group by re-rehearsing their play, understudying parts played by erratic members, helping to organize performances and videoing their play. Meanwhile students in the Theatre in Society course reworked the women's original scenario into a piece of theatre realism entitled *Chero Tiro MuHarare*, which simply means 'It doesn't matter as long as we are in Harare'. Their intention was to give the material an effective artistic treatment and to bring the conditions prevailing in Matapi to the attention of a wider audience, placing them too in the wider context of the general struggle in Zimbabwe to eradicate such poverty and suffering.[14]

1 For a comprehensive bibliography of theatre of this kind see R. Kidd, *The Popular Performing Arts, Non-Formal Education and social Change in the Third World: a Bibliography and Review Essay* (The Hague, 1982).

2 See D. Bradby and J. McCormick, *People's Theatre* (London, 1978); C. Itzyn, *Stages in the Revolution* (London, 1980); M. Etherton, *The Development of African Drama* (London, 1982), ch.8; Ngugi wa Thiong'o, The Language of African Theatre in *Decolonising the Mind* (London, 1986) pp.34-62; R. Kidd, The Repression of Popular Culture in Kenya, *Third World Popular Theatre Newsletter* (Caribbean Edition), 3 (1983); Popular Theatre Committee, Laedza Batanani, Institute of Adult Education, Gaborone, n.d.; C. Kamlongera, Theatre for Development: the Case of Malawi, *Theatre Research International*, 7, 3 (1982); and R. Kidd, *From People's Theatre for Revolution to Popular Theatre for Reconstruction: Diary of a Zimbabwean Workshop*, Centre for the Study of Education in Developing Countries (The Hague, 1982).

3 B. Mazaiwana, Report on Matapi Hostel Project, Faculty of Arts Drama, University of Zimbabwe, 1988, ms. p.2.

4 S. Ndlovu, Report on Matapi Hostel Project, Faculty of Arts Drama, University of Zimbabwe, ms. pp. 2-3.

5 Mazaiwana, Report, p. 5.

6 For an early description of Kamlongera's work in Malawi see his article in *Theatre Research International* referred to in the previous note. He has subsequently developed the programme and produced both conference papers and unpublished reports. A video record of work at Mwima has been made and in addition students of Chancellor College have done undergraduate papers on the work. It is therefore relatively well documented but unfortunately little is published as yet.

7 W. Chigidi, *Imwe Chanzi Ichabvepi* (Where Will Another Chance Come From?) (Gweru, 1986).

8 Mazaiwana, Report, p. 8

9 The students had the following record available for study: A. Boeren, Theatre in Swaziland, *Third World Popular Theatre Newsletter* (Caribbean Edition), 3 (1983); *The Report of the Workshop on Theatre for Integrated Development* (held at Nhlango Farmer Training Centre, October 1981), published by the Department of Extra Mural Services, University College of Swaziland; D. Kerr, Mchira wa Buluzi: The Process of Creating a Popular Vernacular Play, Malawi, unpublished; J. Mschenye, The Development of Popular Theatre for Development, Zambia, unpublished; the complete text of P. Muhando (Mlama)'s national entry on Tanzania which appeared in abbreviated and edited form in M. Banham (ed.), *The Cambridge Guide to World Theatre* (Cambridge, 1988); in addition to sources already quoted above and numerous other materials on, among others, Nicaragua, Jamaica, Bangladesh, and the Philippines.

10 Cf. Ngugi wa Thiong'o, *Detained*, pp 34-62.

11 Until a few years after independence, theatre in Zimbabwe was dominated by settler minority theatre. The present situation is that grassroots theatre groups have come into existence all over the country, including many that are full-time, prominent examples being: Batsiranayi, Zvido/Izifiso, Theatrical Manoeuvres and Zimbabwe Theatre Works. These groups now tour extensively all the provinces of Zimbabwe, performing plays on social and political themes in schools, mines and working class suburbs and holding discussions and workshops.

12 For a description of traditional forms of public discussion, e.g. *Lekgotla* (Tswana), *pitso* (Sotho), *inkundla* (Nguni) and *dare* (Shona) see I. Schapera, *The Bantu speaking Tribes of South Africa* (London, 1937), Political Institutions.

13 The group of students working with the Zimbabwe Republic Police had a particularly tough assignment, given the relationship between police and students in the aftermath of the first student demonstration. The project was almost scuppered by the outbreak of further hostilities between police and students a matter of days before the final

performance. As it was, the performance did take place before a combined student-police audience. It was highly dramatic as the play depicted the confrontation of police and students in a re-enactment of recent events on campus in which the police played police and students students. It came to a climax when one of the students who was *acting* throwing stones at the police received a real message from police headquarters that he was urgently required to go and face charges for throwing stones at the police in the recent demo. Despite the tensions, the scene-by-scene discussions of police-student relations, though frank and at times passionate, were disciplined and productive.

14 By way of acknowledgement, most of the organization, time, creativity and energy that brought this first Matapi project to a successful conclusion was contributed by the students themselves, who put into it very much more than the requirements of the course. For example, transport from the university to Matapi repeatedly failed to arrive and often students were forced to get there by emergency taxis. In addition the above account relied considerably on the written reports of the students, in particular those of A. Dzinotyiwei and B. Mazaiwana.

Mental Colonisation or Catharsis? Theatre, Democracy and Cultural Struggle from Rhodesia to Zimbabwe

PREBEN KAARSHOLM

Introduction

Drama is arguably the most dynamic and social of cultural forms. Where there are areas of conflict in world view, and tensions between the forces of dominance, acceptance and revolt, theatre often serves to illuminate self-understanding and to articulate precise needs and aspirations. Working through the medium of language and physical expression it reworks mythologies, formulates utopias and represents either a symbolic reconciliation between the individual and the social or the tragic impossibility of such endeavours. By presenting and arousing 'pity and terror', as Aristotle has it, theatre effects 'the proper purgation of these feelings'[1]. Or to quote a modern theoretician, theatre:

> drives human beings to see themselves as they are, lets them drop their masks, exposes the lie, the spinelessness, the baseness, the sanctimoniousness; it shakes the suffocating inertia of a materialism, which attacks even the clearest assertion of the senses; and by placing collective groups of human beings face to face with their dark powers, their secret strength, it invites them to assume a heroic and aloof attitude towards the fate which they would never have attained without theatre.[2]

The pre-eminence of drama is striking in the short, but intense cultural history of Rhodesia and Zimbabwe from 1890 to the present day. Firstly, because white-dominated Rhodesia as a conquest society from the outset was in dire need of legitimisation of its very existence and values — both in order to consolidate and harmonise the white community internally and to put on a show of civilisation *vis-à-vis* the world of black Africans which was being expropriated or excluded as primitive and non-cultural. This historical drama expressed and interpreted itself in a wealth of historical romance, travelogue and novelistic fiction,[3] but also and emphatically in theatrical performances.

Secondly, in a later phase, Rhodesia was decolonised in the course of a violent and traumatic war that gave rise to its own genres of cultural expression, and in which drama again played a prominent part — to fortify bastions of white pride and supremacy on the one side and to mobilise black African people and promote mental decolonisation on the other.

Finally, drama has fulfilled a special function in the cultural and political development of Zimbabwe since 1980. In a situation in which, until recently, political debate was restricted and dominated by an increasingly anachronistic nationalist rhetoric, and where other cultural manifestations have been characterised by a surprising reticence and self-censorship,[4] popular theatre has provided an outlet for frustration and a possible forum for the articulation of criticisms that would otherwise have been kept quiet or exploded as unarticulated violence.

Township theatre groups have focused on the politics of everyday life and have insisted that the personal and the social belong to same world, and that political and moral conflicts stem from one set of roots. I shall attempt to show that Zimbabwean grassroots theatre has been directly influential in changing the agenda for political discussions within society as a whole, in placing anti-corruption and democracy issues at the centre of debates and in bringing about the spectacular reorientation in the cultural and political climate towards more genuine areas of contestation that have occurred since 1988.

Theatre and the Cultural Hegemony of Rhodesia

Theatre was an integral part of Rhodesian settler society from the earliest days of conquest in July 1890, when the 'pioneers of progress' entered the 'emptiness' of the African interior beyond the Limpopo. As a colonial historian recalled, the area at the time:

> contained not more than half a million Bantu, many of whose forebears had arrived there only 50 years before, and the life they lived was primitive, both in its working methods and in the nature of its infrequent amusements. The pioneers, by contrast, came for the most part from environments which had all the sophistications of the nineteenth century, environments which for their relaxation, required entertainment of the standard civilised type — theatre, music, variety.[5]

Certainly, early settler society in Salisbury, Bulawayo and even Fort Victoria and Umtali, was enthusiastic in putting on amateur drama. There was a steady fare of plays such as *The Turned Head* and *Black Justice*, or operas like Luscombe Searelle's *The Wreck of the Pinafore, Estrella* and *Isadora*. Before World War One, undoubtedly the most popular single play was *Charlie's Aunt*, and British music hall was a favourite genre — in 1892, a variety show by the famous Madame Blanche so inspired a family in the process of settling between Salisbury and Marandellas that they decided to call their three farms 'Tarara', 'Boom' and 'Deay'. Such early dramatic performances established a pattern which continued to dominate Rhodesian cultural history up to 1980 and even characterises much of white theatrical sub-culture after independence.

The pattern was one of almost surrealistic European-ness, of an acute keenness to imitate or reproduce the latest or at least recent fashion in London West End theatre and thereby to reinforce in audiences a conviction, not perhaps that they were not in Africa, but that Africa was a continent of ultimate emptiness and extreme primitivity into which colonial civilisation had to be introduced.[6]

In this respect there was a certain structural difference between Rhodesian culture as it manifested itself in the performance of drama and in the writing of fiction, inasmuch as local novels from the early twentieth century on were struggling to construct a Rhodesian national identity which was different from the British equivalent and which was more authentic and belonged more naturally in Africa than black African non-culture.[7] But even here the construction of identity takes place against a background of African emptiness — Gertrude Page, for instance, goes into rhapsodies about Rhodesia as a land of loveliness 'never seen by human eye' and lets a male character dream sadistically about clearing the landscape of polluting Africans — 'I should like to see the whole of the black race made into a huge bonfire, and stand by to help with the stoking ... I believe ninety per cent of the white men all over the world would be ready to do the same. As a matter of fact, burning is too good for them'.[8]

The officially-sponsored Rhodesia Literature Bureau encouraged the creation of an African language written literature which extolled the virtues of 'traditional' life or bemoaned the tragedies of its disintegration. At a workshop organised by the Bureau in 1964, 'stars' of the white cultural scene like Wilbur Smith and Adrian Stanley tried to impart to black colleagues a sense of the professional skills required for the production of novels and drama, while 'veteran' African writers like Paul Chidyausiku gave advice on suitable topics to write about — in an atmosphere of stark unreality.

Wilbur Smith made his point by comparing the writing of a story to the serving of 'an eight course meal to fifty assorted guests, some of whom have ulcers and others have diabetes. You have to balance everything off. The hors d'oeuvres to sharpen the appetite, the soup not to fill them too much, the fish, the white wines to go with it — everything has to be right'.

Chidyausiku recommended existential and apolitical themes as subjects for literature — the conflict between tradition and modernity as experienced by 'the educated African', the conflicts and joys of childhood, youth, family life and old age. Bishop Chakaipa thought that 'it is only by writing in the vernacular that African culture can be enriched and preserved' and Adrian Stanley lamented that 'there is no tradition of theatre in the European sense, as we know it, in Africa,' but it was badly needed:

> We have a few local plays based, supposedly, on the political situation, which I think have been very inept, because they have over-simplified our problems completely, by using extremes. You get the African extremist, you get the white settler extremist, and these are over-simplifications and, I think, a bit tiresome. The country badly needs a comedy, a local comedy. I think it's time we laughed at ourselves a bit. We have got quite enough to worry about ... I think that the famous Greek tragedy, Oedipus Rex, would translate very well into an African setting.[9]

Rather than dismantling differences, this parody of dialogue served to consolidate the gulf which existed and was being deepened between the cultural worlds and possibilities of white and black Rhodesians.

The engulfment in a segregated world was felt particularly strongly in the case of white theatre in Rhodesia. Not only was the repertoire exclusively European, but membership of theatre organisations and the right to attend performances was also restricted. One of the most prominent institutions, the Salisbury Repertoire Players (or Reps Theatre) debated the question of accepting 'non-European' members in 1954, but decided against it, and only gradually and without enthusiasm, was membership at least theoretically made available to non-whites.[10] It was hardly any wonder if extremely few black or 'Asiatic' members of society decided to take advantage of an entry into the cultural world of whites that was granted so reluctantly.

Yet white Rhodesian theatre was also in many ways a genuinely popular cultural movement and fired by a special energy and commitment because of its basis in amateur mobilisation. Audiences were never big enough to allow for the development of professional institutions and performances, government support was not available, and drama associations had to rely on their members' resources as far as funds, actors and directors were concerned. Yet hardly any plays were written locally. A few dramatisations of Gertrude Page novels were shown in Salisbury and Bulawayo in the 1920s, but only after they had been produced in London.[11] Being involved in theatre was synonymous with maintaining a close link with the culture of the British motherland, and visits from British performers were major events in what might often be experienced as the provincial backwaters of Rhodesia.

Only very exceptionally a play or script emerged that in both genre and contents challenged the very structure of the ruling hegemony. One rare instance was Judith Todd's satirical farce *A Guide to the Thoughts of Ian Smith and his Friends* circulated anonymously in 1971.[12] The play consists almost entirely of cut-up and rearranged quotations from parliamentary debates and speeches by the Prime Minister and other white culture heroes like Pieter Kenyon Fleming, Voltelyn van der Byl and Desmond Lardner-Burke — Ministers of Information, Justice and Law and Order respectively in the Rhodesian Front government. It was never performed, but was passed around and read out clandestinely to hilarious effect. In spite of its sub-cultural status it managed to gain a certain influence. After independence Todd's play helped one of the more successful pieces of drama of the new Zimbabwe, as we shall see below.

Theatre and African Nationalist Counterculture

In the face of attempted marginalisation and manipulation of black African culture within the ruling hegemony, it is not surprising that a uniform response of African nationalist organisations, regardless of political differences, was to dedicate themselves to the promotion of an original, self-reliant and 'authentic' African culture. The need for the reconstruction of a proud, precolonial cultural tradition, whose institutions, genres and self-confidence had been suppressed or expropriated by settler domination would feature prominently on their programmatic agendas.

The promotion of African cultural tradition was to serve the purpose of 'mental decolonisation' and a break away from 'cultural imperialism' — the recreation of the confident sense of African selfhood that Frantz Fanon expounded in a famous speech 'On National Culture' in 1959. African culture would take on 'substance', gain new vigour and experience a renaissance away from mere folklore through being incorporated into the people's struggle for freedom.[13]

The necessity for formulating a cultural programme became increasingly urgent as the battle between the Rhodesian regime and the African nationalists for the hearts and minds of the people became an outright war from the early 1970s. As camps and schools for refugees and for the training of guerillas were set up in Zambia and Mozambique, and armed nationalist forces began to penetrate the countryside, questions of socialisation, propaganda, motivation and cultural interaction became matters of strategic importance.

In an article in ZANU's *Zimbabwe News* in April 1978, Nathan Shamuyarira described the basic struggle as one against an imperialism which has 'plunged our people into a morass of emotional and spiritual confusion' in a 'mental process that has taken years of intense cultural aggression, and which has resulted in the loss of our cultural heritage ... Our country will need mental decolonisation just as much as it needs political and economic independence.'[14] Parallel with this, PR-ZAPU before the independence elections in 1980 campaigned for a policy of 'preserving' cultural values.[15]

There can be no doubt that during the struggle for independence, appeals to 'traditional' culture were often made in an opportunistic fashion, and the progressiveness of such appeals met with serious criticism within both the two major nationalist organisations.[16] On the other hand, it is also clear that the appropriation of 'traditional culture' could help to transfer energy from earlier and more clandestine forms of anti-colonial cultural resistance to the modern political organisations and assist in unifying their nationalist aspirations.

Thus a parallel discussion was going on in the nationalist camps between 'traditionalists' and 'modernists' about the usefulness and progressiveness of appeals to traditional religion and culture in mobilising the civilian population inside Rhodesia and in the educational and socialising work that was taking place in the refugee and guerilla camps. Was the building of nationalist socialism to take the form of a continuation of traditional cultural forms, or did these — and traditional religion in particular — represent modes of mystification that had to be combated and done away with just as radically as, for instance, the repressive cultural influence of Christianity?

Over the more secular forms of dance, song, choir performances and enactment of dramatic tableaux there was less controversy, and these could be encouraged in the camps both as forms of entertainment and as stimulants of cultural nationalism. In the ZAPU camps for instance, members were encouraged to develop a proficiency in all three major languages (Ndebele, Shona and English), and cultural performances from different regions and linguistic areas of Rhodesia were researched and promoted in an effort to bring about 'unity' — to incorporate different groups into the liberation movement, emphasise the coherence of their endeavours and develop a new sense of nationality.[17]

Performances would also be encouraged to evoke a sense of 'life at home' and keep up the spirits of camp members who were often children and young people who had lost their families or left them behind in Rhodesia. A wide-ranging repertoire of 'classical' song and dance genres was investigated and kept intact — dancing and singing for rains and harvests, hunting and war occasions, to appease spirits or welcome homecoming family members, for funerals, to celebrate the installation of a new chief or for social occasions like weddings and beer parties.

Also in the ZAPU camps in Zambia, traditional songs and dances in praise of Mzilikazi or Lobengula would be performed by school children in intricate attire, exploiting the ambiguity of praise poetry through which admiration can be combined with utterances of criticism of authoritarianism; they can also combine eulogy with the humour and ambiguous statements now being levelled at unpopular teachers and camp leaders, or perhaps even, in 1978-79, at Joshua Nkomo whose image as 'Father Zimbabwe' was being promoted at the time.[18]

Similarly, the popular urban tradition of *Mbube* choir singing would be carried on through cultivation of an old repertoire of songs as well as through the production of new songs often with a political message. Players would also develop the sketch-like qualities of the performance in which the lead singer/dancer alternates with the rest of the group.[19]

There was, though, a radically 'modernist' stand present in the cultural debates of the camps which would request that tradition be exposed to criticism or suppressed along with other forms of 'feudal' or 'bourgeois' mystification and replaced by a properly socialist and scientific ideology. Attwell Mabhena, who played a major part in organising educational work in the ZAPU camps in Zambia, remembers how Joshua Nkomo and party leaders would try to act as moderators and reconcile tradition and socialism, for example as regards the relationships between men and women in the camps and the setting up of separate schools for boys and girls, while younger camp members 'moved ahead' and developed attitudes that would eventually make it difficult for them to adapt when they returned to Zimbabwe.

The theatrical equivalent of the 'modernist' or Marxist-Leninist position on cultural policy would be a type of propaganda play based on slogans, often taking the form of a series of consecutive educational tableaux, interspersed with *chimurenga* or *impi yenkululeko* songs. Capitalism was seen as a sickness requiring therapy and medicine in the form of correct ideology, and in ZANU camps a Maoist influence contributed towards making formulation of the corrective ideology sometimes extra-schematic.[20]

ZANU's *Zimbabwe News* of July-August 1978 has a description in photos and text of the play *The People Are Invincible* which, like the choir performances referred to above, works with an altercation between soliloquy and chorus intervention:

A 'peasant' (with scarf) denounces the 'internal settlement' and is particularly infuriated by Chirau with whom he 'herded cattle ... heartless brute he was! Fond of pinning innocent lizards to trees with his arrows. Became a sergeant in the fascist Rhodesian police force ...'

ZANLA: We must not be fooled by these stooges. Muzorewa, Sithole and Chirau. They are not for genuine independence. We have the sacred task of intensifying the armed struggle and liberating Zimbabwe.

And the play ends with the chorus singing a revolutionary song — 'From the Zambezi to the Limpopo, the people of Zimbabwe are suffering'.[21] A different ZANU play, which is perhaps more in harmony with cultural nationalism and a conciliatory attitude towards tradition is described by Sr Janice McLaughlin in a paper from 1981:

The play called 'Black is Beautiful' was written and performed in the camps. It depicts an African youth who is so alienated from his culture that he pretends he is 'coloured' and is drafted into the settler army. He is eventually captured by the freedom fighters who take him back to his village where he is reunited with his people. The play ends with the freedom fighters telling him to be proud of his people and culture.[22]

In ZAPU camps, there were varieties of drama. Since the schools for refugee children were often dependent on old textbooks from Rhodesia, and students were still meant to prepare for Cambridge Certificate examinations, plays like *Macbeth* and *Julius Caesar* would be performed, and a teacher from the schools would introduce the play and relate it to the political situation and to everyday life in the camps. Other plays were produced by the teachers themselves or by students, and a third category was made up by propaganda pieces to illustrate the positions of the Party.

Within both nationalist movements there were forces trying to come to terms with different understandings of culture and searching for a cultural programme that was at once socialist and democratic. Some of the contradictions come out in a paper produced by ZANU's Education and

Culture Department for a teachers' course at Matenje Camp in Mozambique in September 1979, which states on the one hand that '*Culture is universal*. All people have and therefore share a common humanity,' and on the other that 'there are no identical cultures and hence *culture is incomparable*'. At the same level of contradiction, the document claims that '*Culture is organised*' and constitutes a 'coherence and structure among the patterns of human behaviour and meaning,' but also 'rarely intrudes into conscious thought' and represents 'certain norms of *unconscious reaction* to varied situations of every aspect of life'.[23]

What is at stake here is a confrontation between a dogmatic view of culture as something that can be rejected or preserved, and another view according to which culture is created through articulation, critical discourse and interaction between conscious and self-reliant human beings. The latter, more democratic understanding of culture was developed further in the new pedagogic principles that were tried out in the teaching of refugee children in Zambia and Mozambique as experiments with a new, socialist organisation of education. Among the principles were: integration of manual and mental work, dialogic teaching methods, collective organisation and administration, co-operation instead of competition, promotion of culture and equality of women.[24] Students, it was put in a lecture to teachers in Mozambique, had to learn to work together as well as to be critical and anti-authoritarian individuals, and teaching should be conducted in an atmosphere of 'mutual and comradely criticism'.[25]

The new philosophy was presented systematically in a long article by ZANU's Secretary for Education and Culture, Dzingayi Mutumbuka in *Zimbabwe News* in November 1978, in which he compared the passivity induced by the colonial system with the new principles of dialogue and criticism which would characterise the new revolutionary education, culture and mentality of independent Zimbabwe.[26]

One channel for expressing the new initiative, self-reliance and critical capability of young Zimbabweans who were students in the ZANU and ZAPU camps was through the production of drama. A play called *The People Are Invincible* was produced by Form 4 youth, and Attwell Mabhena remembers how students at the J Z Moyo school in Zambia would produce political plays without scripts:

> Plays were written by the students themselves ... these things were just written on pieces of paper ... I don't remember seeing anything like full scripts ... they would think of a situation, a war situation in Zimbabwe they were fighting, and make it in such a way that our forces are on top of the situation

and so on, and how the Rhodesian forces are murdering our parents at home and so on.

But another kind of theatre would also be tried out, dealing with the everyday problems and politics of the camps — an early variety of community-based drama:

We used to have a big kitchen, so they would dramatise and show how they were going to get the food and so on, the problems they were facing, how the teachers were treating them, going to the food. Those unkind teachers who would be displayed, they would be very cruel, the kind ones, very kind. This was all done by the students themselves ... Some of the [teachers] were not pleased about it, but that was the fact of life.

The fact was that the students in the refugee schools were extremely difficult to handle, and that some of the democratic pedagogic principles of group and project work and dialogic teaching were the results of necessity as much as anything else. Most pupils had left their families behind or had been orphaned in the war, and some of the 'schoolchildren' would be young men and women in their twenties. So often students tended to be 'wild' and anti-authoritarian and impatient to put the ideals of the new social order into practice in the everyday life of the camps. ZAPU's Schools Co-ordinator, Paulos Matjaka, remembers that a certain type of 'bastard culture' would be characteristic of students:

At the same time as the old African culture was being revived, a new type of culture was developing because of the circumstances, and this was reflected in entertainments and performances in the camps. Some were plays about the older people — the Chaka type of person, the Nehanda type of person, the Lobengula type of person — but most of them were written by the teachers or the students themselves ... What they used to do would be to dramatise something anti, to express thoughts they had to play down, and they did it, spontaneously.[27]

Dramatisation became a way of expressing your needs and getting what you wanted. In this way, a tradition of discussion theatre, of drama dealing with and directly articulating the political grievances of everyday life, developed in the camps alongside the tradionalist revival of cultural nationalism and the ideologically orientated propaganda tableaux organised by Marxist-Leninist commissars. In all likelihood, this was the most innovative form of cultural manifestation to emerge within the nationalist counter-culture — a venture that radically challenged deep-seated colonial habits of self-obliteration and authoritarian behaviour.

While inside Rhodesia the repressive measures of the white regime prevented any open or underground development of an African nationalist or aggressively democratic theatre — 'in the townships there were police and informers everywhere, and people were too scared to experiment with anything like that'[28] — the experience of the youngsters of the refugee camps of being uprooted and on the move led to new genres of dramatic activism which came to represent the most potent agents of decolonisation and renewal in Zimbabwe after independence. Politics and the future were not just things to be told about — they were matters to be discussed and acted out in practice.

Zimbabwean Drama since Independence

After independence, theatre in Zimbabwe continued to be characterised by the high level of dedication that had surrounded it before 1980. Indeed, drama may be said to be the form of cultural expression which has experienced the most spectacular flourishing during a period that has been remarkably quiet as far as literary and artistic development is concerned. Whereas in literature and pictorial arts the country has not yet seen the great outburst of articulation and creativity that might have been expected to follow the demolition of colonial cultural repression, theatre has provided an outlet for a variety of needs for expression.

There are at present more than a hundred dramatic groups active in Zimbabwe at different levels of ambition and organisation — nearly thirty of these performing regularly in and around Bulawayo, where — because of the special circumstances that existed until the Unity agreement between ZANU(PF) and PF-ZAPU in December 1987 — drama has developed a special importance as a forum for debate of issues that it was difficult for a long time to discuss more directly and politically.[29] Fundamentally, theatre in Zimbabwe has retained the amateur nature and level of personal motivation it had in Rhodesia. Without substantial amounts of public funding, there is no basis within the foreseeable future for the establishment of fully professional dramatic institutions.[30] But the balance of strength and influence between the types of drama within the country has shifted. They now occupy different situations in the changing hegemony, and their messages and impact have been transformed accordingly.

From representing the epitome of civilisation within the dominating white culture of Rhodesia, white European theatre in Zimbabwe has been transformed to a nostalgic, but still very confident sub-culture. As if nothing had happened, Harare's Reps Theatre stages Agatha Christie thrillers and performances of the ballet *Giselle*, standards of the London repertoire or anachronisms like *Golden Music Hall* with Queen Victoria on the stage and boisterous singing of 'Ta-ra-ra-boom-deay' just as in the earliest days of settlement. But the institutions in the white professional theatrical world have changed and the National Theatre Organisation — the former Southern Rhodesia Drama Association — has succesfully broadened its scope, redefined its main objective as 'To unite Zimbabweans through the Medium of Theatre and Drama',[31] made its fund-raising, library and workshop facilities available to a wide variety of drama initiatives, and turned its Annual National Theatre Festival and Play of the Year Competition into major stimulants and forums for dramatic productivity. In relation to the contents of individual plays and the frameworks of genres, there have been important and succesful attempts to break down old boundaries and fuse creatively a variety of influences. Thus some of the contents, formulations and devices that used to belong exclusively within the realm of European or 'western' modernism have been appropriated and mixed with African background influences to produce powerful results in plays by Dambudzo Marechera and Andrew Whaley. Their plays seem to represent a radically new departure in post-independence Zimbabwean theatre. Whereas in the 'traditional' Rhodesian white drama that continues to exist in Zimbabwe, Western European genres are introduced and performed in a manner emphasising their alienness from and superiority to African culture, Marechera and Whaley attempt to 'naturalise' modern international aesthetic discourses and techniques by fusing them with local realities and idioms, to create theatre which is at once modern and Zimbabwean.

Marechera's dramatic writings are only sketches or fragments and have never reached the performance stage, but they nevertheless represent an important effort to make the achievements of an international modernist style available for Zimbabwean culture. The desperation, outspokenness and absurdity of the three small plays contained in *Skin of Time: Plays by Buddy* — The Coup, The Gap and Blitzkrieg — probably captured central characteristics in the world view and experience of young urban Zimbabweans in the early 1980s better than most other writing, and it is hardly any wonder that the publication in which they were printed has become a cult book in Zimbabwe — especially since the author's death. Marechera's revolutionary anarchism in approaching dramatic convention seemed to signal the possibility of a new freedom of artistic creation.[32]

A similarly successful application of international modernist discourse can be seen in Andrew Whaley's *Platform Five*, which won the first prize at the Annual National Theatre Festival in 1987 and became internationally known when it was later performed at the Edinburgh Festival. The play was written for the group Zimbabwe Arts Production, which had in it some of Zimbabwe's strongest actors (Ben Sibenke, Friday Mbirimi, Dominic Kanaventi and Walter Muparutsa), and it very convincingly fuses an absurdist world of tramp life and dialogue, of games over meaningless power among the down-and-out and powerless, which could have come from Samuel Beckett, with an articulation of life experiences that are immediately recognisable as realistically Zimbabwean.

The play at one point salutes the figure of Marechera — a man with dreadlocks 'that sprout just now like vegetables' who lives and writes in the town parks like a tramp himself[33] — but the characters of Whaley's play are less aggressive and more gently drawn than Marechera's. It is a play driven forward by an eloquent dialogue which gets the most out of the misunderstandings that arise out of an English language that is spoken with unequal competence by different characters and becomes an instrument of power itself.

Equally dynamic and original in its fusing of international styles and local traditions — both white Rhodesian and African — is a second play by Andrew Whaley called *The Nyoka Tree* — a comedy produced by Meridian Theatre which won a trophy as the best, new, locally written play at the 1988 Annual National Theatre Festival.[34] The play is steeped in intertextuality — most centrally by parodying the pastoral genre that was prominent in white Rhodesian literature and self-understanding before independence, but also more specifically as when Nyoka's 'Prologue' mimics the metre of Milton's *Paradise Lost*.[35] There are repeated direct and indirect quotes from the Bible, from Chairman Mao and not least from Ian Smith, whose voice and phrasings come through in the television announcements from 'Himself' — the ruler of Paradesia. In this manner, the play takes up the tradition of satirical sophistication initiated by Judith Todd's *A Guide to the Secret Thoughts of Ian Smith and his Friends*, which was constructed entirely out of quotations. Further, *The Nyoka Tree* brings into play nationalist songs of resistance — songs in Shona as well as Ndebele panegyrics of Mzlikazi and Lobengula.

Another shift from the pre-independence pattern of drama is that performance genres that show continuity with the pre-conquest past are now prominent rather than marginalised. A policy of setting up 'culture houses' has been introduced by the Ministry of Youth, Sport and Culture to encourage local cultural initiatives, though so far only a single institution of this kind has been established at Murewa. Similarly, a series of attempts have been made to rework traditional performance genres, explode their conservative folklore character and incorporate them into more modern theatrical institutions and forms of expression. At the Second National Music, Dance and Drama Festival organised by the Ministry of Youth, Sport and Culture in August 1987, traditional dance clubs and choirs were performing alongside township theatre groups and political community-based theatres and took part in the same discussion workshops to share 'information experiences, techniques and skills' and 'to demonstrate the importance of performing arts as a tool for national development, cultural identity, the preservation of cultural values and the promotion of socialist culture'.[36]

Individual plays have also experimented with the incorporation of elements of traditional singing and dancing, as well as with a modelling of plots over themes and characters originating in a black African narrative and dramatic heritage. So far this has often taken a form that is not very different from the moralistic comedies which dominated African drama in the 1970s. Ben Sibenke's *My Uncle Grey Bonzo*, which was the first African play to be performed at the National Theatre Festival in 1981, is a didactic fable about the confrontation in a high-density suburb between two brothers — Grey Bonzo, who is a successful and selfishly individualistic businessman, and Gwenzi, who represents traditional values of family and community solidarity.

Another play, Karl Dorn's *Murume Murume* written in 1984, secularises tradition by putting ancestral spirits directly on the stage, but is otherwise a moral fable in the old mould about a rich man who 'smells very much of selfishness and greed' and has forgotten culture and tradition.[37]

While plays like these to a large extent carry on the moral focus and domestic didactism of pre-independence African theatre and avoid pointing to political solutions, a different type of agitation drama has since emerged in Zimbabwe which endeavours directly to carry on and develop the traditions of dramatic propaganda that were established in the nationalist camps in exile during the war. The small drama unit set up within the Faculty of Arts at the University of Zimbabwe has played a special part in promoting this field of theatre with the support of the Ministry of Youth, Sport and Culture, and the drama lecturer Robert McLaren, who was appointed in 1985 together with Thompson Tsodzo as 'staff development fellow', has been strongly influential in elaborating its theory and producing some of the most spectacular shows.[38]

One of the first performances that was put on by the University's Faculty of Arts Drama group was a dramatisation of Wilson Katiyo's 1976 novel, *A Son of This Soil* called *Mavambo, First Steps*. It is an interesting play in many ways which, according to Stephen Chifunyise, until recently the Director of Arts and Crafts at the Ministry of Youth, Sport and Culture, 'sets a stage where visual presentation of the history, aspirations, struggles, successes, failures and revolutionary zeal of the people of Zimbabwe becomes the priority concern of Zimbabwean theatre' and creates 'a uniquely Zimbabwean dramatic idiom'.[39]

The idiom is created through the incorporation of mbira music and traditional singing and dancing as well as through the use of bilingualism — *Mavambo* incorporates both English and Shona. Like Katiyo's novel, the play operates on two levels in time. Its introduction, through a flashback representing the narrative of the old Sekuru, presents typical episodes during the colonisation of Rhodesia from the point of view of ordinary African people: 'History is not made by heroes alone'.[40] The resistance of the local community, led by Chief Chuma, is broken — first in military confrontation with a brutal gang of settlers who are after diamonds, land and cheap labour, secondly through the disintegrative influence of a Christian missionary, who is welcomed into the village to set up school and a church. The 'traditional ways' are lost, and the villagers turned into 'slaves' and 'beggars'.

The second part of the play deals with the 1960s. Young Alexio moves from his village to Highfield township outside Salisbury and with his cousin Rudo experiences the early confrontation between nationalist mobilisation and police repression. He is framed, arrested and tortured, but at the end of the action he manages to escape and make his way into the mountains, where preparations for a renewed 'battle of Nehanda' are under way. The continuity with the resistance tradition of the past is re-established, and the play concludes in a tableau with guerillas coming on stage and the whole cast singing 'Nyika yedu yeZimbabwe' — 'Our country, Zimbabwe'.[41]

Mavambo is characterised throughout by a heavy didacticism which is not unlike the moralistic and educative tone in the colonial African theatre of Rhodesia. The action is continually interrupted to let the actors address and lecture the audience, and the 'bad' characters in particular are drawn so crudely in order to provide a lesson that they come close to being caricatures. The message of *Mavambo* is not meant to be argued with — the audience is expected to join in a celebration of the righteousness of the struggle against evil.

A similar tendency makes itself felt in the play *Katshaa! The Sound of the AK* which was produced by the Faculty of Arts Drama and performed by the group Zambuko/Izibuko in 1986.[42] The theme is one in which the issue of good and bad is even more clear-cut — the struggle against apartheid in South Africa — and the idea behind it as to the intended mobilisation of audiences is perhaps best described in Stephen Chifunyise's introduction:

> *Katshaa!* is a sample of theatre which is ideologically clear and one which illustrates the role and function of theatre artists in the political and cultural struggle in Southern Africa. It is an example of a performing art where artistic zeal is properly couched in indefatigable ideological commitment to socialist revolution and the victory of the majority of South Africa ... the [play's] technique ... is effectively used to enable the audience to identify immediately and consistently with a clear ideological analysis.[43]

The purpose of the performance is clearly not to produce an argument, but to make the audience identify spontaneously with a correct ideological standpoint. As drama, *Katshaa!* suffers from being far too much an illustration of points — it is based on an International Defence and Aid Fund pamphlet, *This is Apartheid*, which is reproduced in its entirety in the printed edition. To a much higher degree than *Mavambo*, the play falls apart in a series of semi-allegorical tableaux that demonstrate different ways in which apartheid is an evil system of government. As in Zimbabwe it is a part of official policy towards apartheid, and the play's audiences are generally well aware of the South African system's brutally repressive and racist nature, the effect of *Katshaa!* becomes not so much critical as celebrationist: the play confirms rather than tests attitudes that may be taken for granted.

The celebrationist aspect is also conspicuous in the examples of Zambuko/Izibuko ngonjeras that are published as an appendix to *Katshaa!* Ngonjera is a Tanzanian term for a short theatrical performance to be organised 'on political occasions'.[44] Thus one of these dramatic happenings, 'Ngonjera for Mandela and Nyerere' was prepared 'on the occasion of the conferment of Honorary Degrees by the University of Zimbabwe on Cde Nelson Mandela and Mwalimu Julius Nyerere' and another 'Ngonjera for NAM', for the Cultural Gala for Heads of States at the Non-Aligned Movement Summit in Harare in 1986.[45] The main point of these brief manifestations is an expression of unquestioning faith in their political leaders on the part of a group of loyal subjects — with no sign of the ironies and ambiguities which were referred to above as characteristic of traditional praise performances.

The Faculty of Arts Drama group continued its work in 1987 and 1988 with productions of two plays called *Samora Continua!* and *Samora Continua! Two* which expressed grief at the death of the Mozambican President, Samora Machel, in an air crash in 1986 and a determination to continue the struggle against the South African regime which is suspected of having monitored the disaster. More interesting, however, was a large-scale and popular Faculty of Arts Drama production in late 1987 of a classic of 1940s Soviet 'socialist realist' theatre Nikolai Pogodin's *Kremlin Chimes*. The play is part of a monumental trilogy dealing with the life of Lenin, and the occasion of the performance in Harare was the 70th anniversary of 'the Great October Revolution', but it endeavoured to make Pogodin's message relevant to the political conditions of a recently independent African state. Thus Lenin's struggle against negative criticism concerning the impracticability of socialism and electrification in backward Russia was presented as an allegory to prove the need for a similar optimism for present-day Zimbabwe.

The political message of the play, however, does not only stress the need for optimism, but also for an iron discipline and a necessary ruthlessness in dealing with counter-revolutionaries in a way that betrays the script's Stalinist origins. In one of the final scenes of the play the idea of a democratic socialism is ridiculed through being propagated by a pretentious, British upper-class caricature of H G Wells — impersonated with great gusto by Robert McLaren in the Harare performance — and rebuked by Lenin as follows:

> You have made up a nitty-pretty Christmas-tree socialism. I stand for the dictatorship of the proletariat, for without the dictatorship of the proletariat nothing will be done. Dictatorship is a harsh word — bloody and appalling. Not a word to use idly, but without it there will be no dreaming of electrification, or of communism, or of socialism! Time, the march of history, will show which of us is right![46]

What constituted the greatest appeal, however, of the quite lavish production of *Kremlin Chimes*, which made use of the extensive costume collections of the Reps Theatre, were the humorous episodes that arose out of the mixing of Soviet history with modern Zimbabwean reality. As for example in the scene where two peasant girls find themselves under a big photograph of (the historical) Lenin and are spoken to by a fellow black actor (the excellent Todd Winini), who insists HE is Lenin:

> *Natasha*: Shoot it! You are not Lenin, just a stranger, a peasant come to visit us. You are not at all like Lenin — look at his picture, and you'll see.
> *Lenin*: This stuffy looking gentleman, is it a bit like Lenin?
> *Natasha*: And you are, I suppose?

In episodes like this, the programmatic moralism of *Kremlin Chimes* was undercut by farce to the obvious delight of both actors and spectators.[47]

An important trend in post-independence drama has been the development of so-called 'community-based theatre'. The idea of this form of theatre is to get local urban or rural communities together in order to discuss their problems, conflicts and grievances and to dramatise the arguments and points of view they want to express. The basic political concept behind community-based theatre is therefore in a sense the opposite of that of the propaganda theatre discussed above — the purpose of performing is not to make an audience identify with a specific ideology or political line, but to promote grassroots articulation and popular participation in the definition of political and developmental goals.

The Zimbabwe Foundation for Education with Production (ZIMFEP) — a private organisation that operates with the support of the Zimbabwean government — has played an active part in the promotion of community-based theatre. One of the objectives of ZIMFEP has been to run schools for the refugee children who returned to Zimbabwe after the war and to continue the experiments with radical educational reforms that were conducted in the camps in Zambia and Mozambique in the late 1970s. It has therefore been an obvious move for the organisation to adopt the idea of community-based theatre to develop further the use of drama to democratise education and also to extend the principle into projects for local participation in communities outside its own schools.

In 1983, a workshop involving about 100 participants from a variety of African countries was organised at Murewa to debate and experiment with 'theatre for concientisation and mobilisation'. Shortly after that ZIMFEP employed the Kenyan lecturer and playwright, Ngugi wa Mirii, who had come to Zimbabwe as an exile after the suppression of the Kamiriithu Community Education and Cultural Centre in 1982.[48] Through his experience Zimbabwean theatre has been able to learn from the experiments with democratic resistance drama in Kenya, and since 1983 Ngugi wa Mirii has organised several workshops in different parts of Zimbabwe to teach people theatre skills and encourage them to form drama groups and cultivate their local dramatic traditions. He has also, with the support of the Ministry of Youth, Sport and Culture, played a leading role in the formation of the Zimbabwe Association of Community Theatre (ZACT) which was set up in 1986-7.

Another influence has been the notion of 'theatre for development' which has been important in Malawi and Zambia, and which may be defined as drama for local audiences with a specific didactic theme and purpose and a low political profile.[49] Examples of the genre can be found in the short pieces educating audiences on water pollution and safety in the workplace that were produced by Iluba Elimnyama in Bulawayo in 1987, (See Globerman p. 75), or in the plays of Stephen Chifunyise. These deal with conservative attitudes and institutions — belief in love potions, male chauvinism and the plight of rape victims, generation conflict over the payment of roora or bride price — presenting them as factors which constrain development in everyday life.[50]

But the attempt to introduce grassroots theatre from above and with government support has not been without problems and paradoxes. Community-based theatre is supposed to further the articulation of local grievances, but not surprisingly people in power positions have reacted to criticism with anger, and Ngugi wa Mirii has had drama workshops closed down at schools, for example, when female students started dramatising sexual harassment by teachers. A more basic contradiction lies in the fact that community-based theatre is supposed to be at once democratic and to offer a platform of expression to people who would otherwise have difficulty making themselves heard, yet must also base itself on 'authentic' national cultural traditions and a correct ideology. In 1987, Stephen Chifunyise defined community-based theatre in the following manner:

> The concept as we are using it here in Zimbabwe simply means theatre being produced by individuals within their community, and that theatre addressing issues or cultural interests or aspects of that particular community predominantly and then also being performed in that particular community predominantly ... Community-based theatre should contribute to the political orientation of our people, to the fight against cultural imperialism as well as to the fight against elitist cultural attitudes, so you could say that it has a lot to do with the politicisation of the masses.[51]

To some extent the programme for expressing local grievances through community-based theatre has been restricted by the demand that it should be self-critical and informed by a correct ideology and a 'true' consciousness. Further, the objective of placing the community-based theatre movement prominently in a struggle against 'cultural imperialism' has meant in practical terms that a somewhat unproductive 'cold war' exists between the Zimbabwe Association of Community Theatre and the National Theatre Organisation.[52]

In spite of organisational difficulties, restrictions and disagreements about how to define the scope of popular theatre, a tradition of political 'discussion theatre' has been emerging in Zimbabwe since the mid-1980s which has managed to build a strong local base for itself and to produce highly original plays with a strong impact. This development, which has been spearheaded by the group Amakhosi Theatre Productions in Bulawayo, has been able to base itself partly on the achievements of the community-based theatre movement and partly on the experiments with a more satirical kind of political drama that were carried out in earlier plays by T K Tsodzo and Habakuk Musengezi. Tsodzo's 1983 work *Shanduko*, for example, attacks the immorality and hypocrisy of certain members of the elite in independent Zimbabwe — people who 'preach vigilance, hard and honest work on one hand while on the other they practise graft, shirk duty, cheat and exploit the very public they profess to serve'.[53]

Musengezi's *The Honourable M.P.*, written in 1984, is less cautious in its portrayal of Shakespeare Pfende — a member of the Zimbabwean parliament — and his wife Immaculate.[54] Pfende is a great womaniser, his greed for imported goods, money and farms is gargantuan, he is a powerful speaker who knows how to manipulate his audiences at political meetings, and at the same time he is as meek as a lamb, whenever Immaculate shows up to assume control. The self-indulgence of the politician is contrasted with the poverty and misery of the members of his constituency, and at the end of the play it is not the state that intervenes like a deus ex machina to correct his evil ways, but the local peasants who have had enough of a representative who does not concern himself with their needs and has even helped to have them evicted from an area that has been designated a game reserve.

A similar outspokenness is characteristic of the plays written and performed by Cont Mhlanga and Amakhosi Theatre Production from around 1985. The group was started as a karate club in 1978 in Makokoba Township — one of the oldest of Bulawayo's 'western suburbs'. The club offered classes in karate to children and young people three times a week at Stanley Hall, one of the few facilities besides beer gardens and churches available in the township for cultural activities, and the aim was both to give training in self-defence in a community which had a high crime rate and to give youngsters self-respect through the semi-religious discipline of karate.[55]

After participating in NTO workshops at Stanley Hall and in Harare in 1980 and 1981, the group started experimenting with the production of plays and with a mixture of karate and drama. In 1982 Mhlanga began writing his own plays. The first, *Children, Children*, was performed in 1983 followed by *The Book of Lies*, and in 1984 Amakhosi performed *Diamond Warriors*. Like the karate club, the drama activities were meant to be an integral part of township life:

The intention was to make the group known in Makokoba, make it a local institution. People should know who Amakhosi were and where they could find us, no matter when. We wanted what we did to be of significance to a local audience, and they should be able to recognise themselves in what we were doing. So the lines in the plays were to a large extent based on what I heard people saying and the way they talked, in the workplace, in bars and so on ... We were building an audience at the same time as we were learning how to write plays — if they didn't like what we did, they would get up and leave.[56]

Gradually, drama became more prominent than karate in the performances of the group, though karate training continued to contribute to the physical fitness and body control of the actors, and elaborate fighting scenes based on karate remained major attractions of the shows. Amakhosi had their breakthrough in 1985 with *Nansi lendoda* — a play dealing with youth unemployment, nepotism, and sexual humiliation of women. As with all Amakhosi productions it was (and is) performed in three versions — in Ndebele, in English and in 'Ndenglish' to make it possible to communicate with different audiences in town and in the countryside.

The play looks at the world from the point of view of the underdog, in this case a highly qualified young person who is unable to find a job. Judgement is passed, but not as a final solution to the conflicts of the plot, rather as something to be thought about and debated.

Nansi lendoda made Amakhosi known outside Makokoba, in the Bulawayo area and around Matebeleland, where the play was performed at schools and community halls. The next year, in 1986, the group produced *Workshop Negative* in the hopes of relating to a local audience as well as of producing 'discussion theatre' that would be of interest on a national level and in the other SADCC countries.

Workshop Negative tells the story of a tool-making workshop in post-independence Zimbabwe. The owner of the shop is Mkhize, an ex-guerilla, and among his workers is Ray Graham, a member of the former white élite and of the Rhodesian Defence Force (played by the very competent white actor and karate fighter Chris Hurst). Another recently employed worker is Zulubou, also a former freedom fighter who was engaged in direct fighting with Ray's regiment during the war. At the beginning of the play the main conflict exists between Zulu and Ray. But the oppositions soon become more complex. Mkhize, like 'the leaders of this nation', wants 'reconciliation ... and it must start right here in this workshop', and at the same time he himself is emerging as a profit-maker and an exploiter of workers who is not essentially different from the people who used to call the tune in pre-independence times — only he wants to be addressed as 'Comrade' instead of 'Sir'.[57]

Performances of *Workshop Negative* brought about a liveliness of discussion and controversy over culture and politics in Zimbabwe that had not been experienced before. The reason for this was partly the popularity of the play and its unusual efficiency and outspokenness, but also the fact that the authorities responded to it rather obstructively by refusing to sanction a tour to Botswana and Zambia.

Workshop Negative was also attacked for its lack of realism and representation of 'untypical' events. In February 1987, a panel discussion at the University of Zimbabwe about the play drew a large and committed audience, some of whom reacted with boos and laughter, others with applause, when Stephen Chifunyise, representing the Ministry, claimed that the play — in spite of its artistic qualities — misrepresented the history of Zimbabwe.

The controversy over *Workshop Negative* was further fuelled when the group wanted to take the play abroad and present African nations with this apparently wrong-headed and unrealistic portrayal of Zimbabwean society. Though the play was never censored and Amakhosi were not forbidden to take it abroad — they were only denied 'the Government's blessing' — the controversy still produced uneasiness among writers and theatre people in Zimbabwe. The Writers' Union of Zimbabwe saw the case as one involving the rights of freedom of speech and artistic expression, and drama groups were worried about the official discouragement of statements encouraging critical discussion. 'There was a definite intake of breath,' as Susan Hains from the National Theatre Organisation put it:

> a lot of theatre groups became very frightened, certainly from the play-writing point of view ... there was a fear about writing, not just plays, but possibly novels, poems. People were nervous about writing anything that could be construed in any way as being critical in any way or talking about sensitive issues.[58]

Amakhosi Theatre Productions, though, has carried on producing discussion theatre in line with *Nansi lendoda* and *Workshop Negative*. In 1987, the group did two plays — *Children on Fire* and *Cry Isililo!* — and in 1989, *Citizen Mind*. And the development in the overall political situation of Zimbabwe has meant that democracy and a promotion of channels for articulating frustration and criticism now figure much more prominently on the political agenda than at any time since independence.

The Unity agreement between ZANU(PF) and PF-ZAPU in December 1987, the amnesty offered to the 'dissidents' of Matabeleland in May 1988, the student demonstrations in Harare in September-October 1988, and the Bulawayo *Chronicle*'s and later the Sandura Commission's public exposure of corruption and nepotism in high political circles have provided the basis for a new type of realistic rather than rhetorical debate over social and political issues.

There can hardly be any doubt that the tradition of a grassroots-based democratic theatre of discussion going back to the liberation war, and the activities of Zimbabwean drama groups have helped considerably to bring about the new political climate. Not only were the issues of corruption and nepotism that were at the centre of the campaigns by students and the press in 1988 first articulated openly by drama,[59] but the confrontation between drama groups like Amakhosi and the authorities in early 1987 helped to clarify and increase understanding of the impact of different political philosophies of culture. And most importantly, the day-to-day work of the drama groups in the communities has stimulated discussion, self-respect and a culture of participation among the 'little people' — the workers, peasants and unemployed men and women of the country.

The correction and the change in the situation was underlined symbolically when on the evening of 30 September 1988, at the height of the student's demonstrations and battles with the police, Amakhosi performed *Workshop Negative* at the University in Harare — this time with a new ending celebrating the Unity agreement in December 1987. And the following day, the Bulawayo group performed the play once more at Kwanzura Stadium in Highfield township at a unity rally organised by ZANU(PF) youth organisations. By furthering articulation, theatre may bring about necessary confrontations, but at the same time it helps to heal conflict by exposing wounds to the fresh air, bringing the repressed out into the open and making it available for transformation through discussion and communication.

The argument presented in the article was developed through earlier presentations in a programme on Radio Denmark produced together with Jesper Bergmann in April 1988 and at seminars at St Antony's College, Oxford, in December 1988, the Center for Research in the Humanities in Copenhagen in March 1989 and the Institute for Commonwealth Studies in London in November 1989.

---

1 Aristotle. Poetics. In W Jackson Bate, *Criticism: The Major Texts*. New York, 1952, p 22.

2 Antonin Artaud, Le Théâtre et La Peste. In *Le Théâtre et Son Double* (1933), *Oeuvres Complètes*. Paris, 1978, p 31.
3 Cf AJ Chennells. Settler Myths and the Southern Rhodesian Novel. Doctoral Thesis, University of Zimbabwe, 1982.
4 Cf P Kaarsholm. Quiet after the storm. Continuity and change in the cultural and political development of Zimbabwe': *African Languages and Cultures*, II, 2, 1989, pp 175-202.
5 CTC Taylor. *The History of Rhodesian Entertainment*, 1890-1930. Salisbury, 1968, p 13.
6 Cf the interpretation of a similar pattern in South African pictorial art and poetry in JM Coetzee. *White Writing. On the Culture of Letters in South Africa*, New Haven, 1988, pp 36-62.
7 Cf Chennells, Settler Myths, p 186 and P Kaarsholm, From Decadence to Authenticity and Beyond. Fantasies and Mythologies of War in Rhodesia and Zimbabwe, 1965-1985. Paper presented to conference on Culture and Development in Southern Africa. Copenhagen, 1988, p 4.
8 Gertrude Page, *Love in the Wilderness, The Story of Another African Farm*. London, 1907, pp 94, 52.
9 Wilbur Smith, The Writer. Paul Chidyausiku, Sources of Material for Creative Writing, Patrick Chakaipa, Vernacular Literature Now and in the Future and Adrian Stanley, Play-Writing. In EW Krog (ed), *African Literature in Rhodesia*. Gwelo, 1966, pp 17, 44-48, 52, 89. Cf EW Krog, The Progress of Shona and Ndebele Literature, *NADA*, the Annual of the Ministry of Home Affairs, xii, 1, 1979, pp 67-71. As far as making European classics available in 'an African setting' is concerned, the Literature Bureau never got as far as *Oedipus Rex*, but did bring out, in 1975, a shortened Shona version of *King Solomon's Mines*.
10 Robert Cary, *The Story of Reps, The History of Salisbury Repertoire Players, 1931 to 1975*. Salisbury, 1975, pp 110, 149.
11 Taylor, *A History of Rhodesian Entertainment*, p 115. Similarly, despite all the energy dedicated to symphonic music, Rhodesian compositions were extremely rare, exceptions being a few pieces by Hugh Fenn or Robert Sibson's *Rhodesian Fantasy* written for the colony's 50th anniversary in 1940. Cf John Wylcotes, The Development of Symphonic Music in Bulawayo, *Arts Rhodesia*, 1, 1978, pp 37-40.
12 Anon, *A Guide to the Thoughts of Ian Smith and his Friends*, n p or d.
13 Cf Frantz Fanon, *The Wretched of the Earth*, Harmondsworth, 1967, p 189.
14 Nathan Shamuyarira, Education as an instrument for social transformation in Zimbabwe, *Zimbabwe News* (Maputo edition), X, 2, March, April 1978, p 61.
15 Cf *The Patriotic Front in Government. Election Manifesto*, n p, 1980.
16 In an interview in February 1987, ZANU's Deputy Political Commissar, Joshua Tungamirai, told Sr Janice McLaughlin that using African religion and spirit mediums in the process of mobilisation 'was a way of luring people. We lured them by what they believed in'. Quoted in J McLaughlin, 'We Did It for Love'. Refugees and Religion in the Camps in Mozambique and Zambia during Zimbabwe's Liberation Struggle. In CF Hallencreuz and Ambrose Moyo (eds), *Church and State in Zimbabwe*, Gweru, 1988, p 139. A similar view was expressed by Saul Ndlovu, who edited ZAPU's *Zimbabwe Review* during the war, in an interview with me in Bulawayo on 20 September 1988. Acknowledging the success of ZANU appeals to traditional culture, he regretted that ZAPU had not used them more, but that such a policy would have alienated the organisation's strong representation of 'young, urban, literate people'.
17 Interview with Valo Mabi, 15 September 1988; interview with Attwell Mabhena, co-founder of the ZAPU Victory Camp and JZ Moyo schools in Zambia during the liberation war, Nyamandhlovu, 12, September 1988.
18 Cf Leroy Vail and Landeg White, The Art of Being Ruled. Ndebele Praise Poetry, 1835-1971. In Landeg White and Tim Couzens (eds), *Literature and Society in South*

Africa, London, 1984, pp 41-59. This type of drama is still being performed on festive occasions at ZIMFEP's JZ Moyo Secondary School in West Nicholson, which was founded to carry on the tradition of revolutionary education from the wartime schools in Zambia.

19 The genre has its background in the *ingoma ebusuku* or 'night music' that was developed by Zulu and Swazi 'bombing' choirs in the townships of South Africa. *Imbube* ('lion') was the title of a particularly popular 'night music' song that was recorded by Solomon Linda's Original Evening Birds in the early 1940s. It became known worldwide through a subsequent recording by Peter Seeger and the Weavers under the title 'Wimoweh' or 'The Lion Sleeps Tonight'. David B Coplan, *In Township Tonight! South Africa's Black City Music and Theatre*, London, 1985, p 154ff. Since independence in Zimbabwe, and more particularly since the recent rise to world-fame of *Ladysmith Black Mambazo*, the popularity of imbube choirs has experienced a renaissance, particularly in Matebeleland, and they have become something of a speciality among the extremely competent cultural groups at the ZIMFEP secondary schools in Nyamandhlovu and West Nicholson. Zimbabwe's best-known *mbube* group at present is the *Black Umfolozi* which consists of former students from the TG Silundika School in Nyamandhlovu.

20 Cf 'Political Re-Education in ZANU. Interview with a Police deserter', *Zimbabwe News* (Maputo edition), X, 2, March-April 1978, p 8: 'ZANU believes that capitalism is a contagious disease which poisons human minds, pollutes the bodies and stunts human potentialities for healthy development. A capitalist society eventually produces sick and poisoned people in dire need of therapy. Any Liberation Movement such as ZANU, inspired by Marxist-Leninist-Mao-Tsetung Theory, believes that political and ideological education is the indispensable medicine to recovery and health.'

21 ZANU-Day Play: The People Are Invincible, *Zimbabwe News* (Maputo Edition), X, 4, July-August 1978, p 8ff.

22 Sr Janice MacLaughlin, Creating a New Mentality. In *Education Zimbabwe: Past, Present and Future*, Harare, 1986, p 31.

23 ZANU(PF) Education and Culture Department, Culture for National Liberation. Reprinted in *Learn and Work*, I, 2, June-July 1986, p 8.

24 Sr Janice MacLaughlin, Creating a New Mentality, p 27ff.

25 The Teacher is a Guide. Reprinted in *Learn and Work*, II, 1, April-May, 1987, p 27ff.

26 Dzingayi Mutumbuka, Foundation of a New Mentality, *Zimbabwe News* (Maputo Edition), X, 6, p 55ff and p 58. Cf Paulo Freire, *Pedagogy of the Oppressed*, New York, 1970, *Education for Critical Consciousness*, 1968, New York, 1973 and *Education, the Practice of Freedom*, 1968; London, 1976.

27 Interview with Paulos Matjaka, Madjoda, 21 September 1988. Mr Matjaka has described other aspects of life among Zimbabwean exiles in Zambia in an unpublished novel, *Khanya — What a Mess! Or, Marriage in Exile*, 1977.

28 Interview with Cont Mhlanga, Copenhagen, 9 September 1989.

29 Interview with Norman Takawira and Nhlanhla Sibanda, chairman and secretary of the Bulawayo Association of Drama Groups, Bulawayo, 9 September 1988; information from Evie Globerman, consultant to the group Iluba Elimnyama, 22 May 1989. Other groups are Strong Wave Drama Group, Art Roots Co-Op Society, Drama Force, Progress Youth Collectives, Bazooka Performing Arts, Amakhosi Theatre Productions, Young Warriors, Tose Sonke, Amaswazi, Tropical Age Theatre, Kuwirirana Drama Club, Amasiko Drama Theatre, Core Force, Vulture Drama Club, Inhlamwu Zika Mthwakazi Drama Group, Vukanani Comedy Theatre Club and Bulawayo Western and Eastern Writers and Actors.

30 The Repertory Players, *Golden Music Hall*, devised and directed by Noel McDonald, Reps Theatre, Harare, 17 September to 3 October 1987.

31 Aims and Objectives of the National Theatre Organisation, Harare, 1988.

32 Dambudzo Marechera, *Mindblast, or The Definitive Buddy*, Harare, 1984.

33 Andrew Whaley, *Platform Five*, Harare, 1987, ms, p 26ff.

34 Andrew Whaley, *The Nyoka Tree*, Harare, 1988, ms, pi.

35 For Rhodesian pastoral, cf Chennells, Settler Myths, chapter 3, The Search for Place: Pastoral Elements. Nyoka's prologue was apparently left out of *The Nyoka Tree* after the first performances. This may be an indication that appreciation of Milton in Zimbabwe is not what it used to be.

36 Objectives of the Festival. In *Programme, 2nd National Music, Dance & Drama Festival*, Harare, 27-30 August 1987.

37 Karl Dorn, *Murume Murume*, Harare, 1984, ms, p 2.

38 Robert McLaren is an exiled South African, who taught drama in Ethiopia before coming to Zimbabwe. His theoretical views on the development of a theatre which gives voice to the aspirations of the masses are put forward in the book *Theatre and Cultural Struggle in South Africa*, which he published under the name Robert Mshengu Kavanagh (London, 1985).

39 SJ Chifunyise, Introduction. In Faculty of Arts Drama, University of Zimbabwe, *Mavambo, First Steps*, Harare, 1986, p i. In 1989 'Youth' was moved to a new ministry of Political Affairs and the Ministry renamed the Ministry of Sport and Culture. There seems to be a good chance that 'Culture' will in the near future be reintegrated into the Ministry of Education, where it belonged just after independence.

40 Ibid, p 1.

41 Ibid, p 34.

42 Zambuko/Izimbuko, University of Zimbabwe, *Katshaa! The Sound of the AK. A play in solidarity with the heroic struggle of the South African masses*, Harare, 1988.

43 Ibid, p i-ii.

44 Ibid, p v.

45 Ibid, pp 33-7 and pp 43-50.

46 Quoted from tape recording of the performance at Beit Hall, University of Zimbabwe, 3 October 1987.

47 Ibid.

48 The story of the Kamiriithu Centre and Theatre is told in Ngugi wa Thiong'o, *Decolonising the Mind*, London, 1986, pp 34, 64. Ngugi wa Mirii was the co-ordinating director of the Kamiriithu Centre and the co-author with Ngugi wa Thiong'o of one of the most famous productions, *Ngaahika Ndeenda (I will marry when I want)*, in 1977. Cf also Penina Muhando Mlama, *Culture and Development: The Popular Theatre Approach in Africa*, Uppsala, 1990.

49 The idea of 'theatre for development' and its historical background in colonial extension and literacy programmes is described in Mlama, *Culture and Development*, p 94ff.

50 Interview with Memory Kombota and Patrick Mabhena from Iluba Elimnyama, Mzilikazi, 28 October 1987; Stephen Chifunyise, *Medicine for Love and Other Plays*, Gweru, 1984.

51 Interview with Stephen Chifunyise, Harare, 13 November 1987.

52 Dwindling Funds Endangers Theatre's Welfare, Record Festival Entries — but Theatre Remains Deeply Divided, *Parade*, August 1989, pp 48-9.

53 Zinyemba, *Zimbabwean Drama*, p 82.

54 H G Musengezi, *The Honourable M.P.*, Gweru, 1984. The original title of the play was *I Will Become a Socialist When I Want* — a line spoken by Pfende — and echoed the title of a play written by Ngugi wa Thiong'o for the Kamiriithu Theatre, *I'll Marry When I Want*. Cf Zinyemba, *Zimbabwean Drama*, p 93ff.

55 Interview with Cont Mhlanga, Makokoba, 30 October 1987.

56 Interview with Cont Mhlanga, Copenhagen, 8 September 1989.

57 Cont Mhlanga, *Workshop Negative, A Play*, Mzilikazi, 1989, ms, p 8 and p 5.

58 Interview with Susan Hains, Harare, 3 November 1987.

59 Cf, for example, the student demonstrators' Anti-Corruption Document of 29

September 1988; Geof Nyarota's editorials and articles on corruption in *The Chronicle* in November and December 1988; Stanley Nyamfukudza's article Zimbabwe's Political Culture Today. In *MOTO*, 71, November 1988; and Report of the Commission of Inquiry into the Distribution of Motor Vehicles. Under the Chairmanship of Mr Justice WR Sandura, Harare, March 1989.

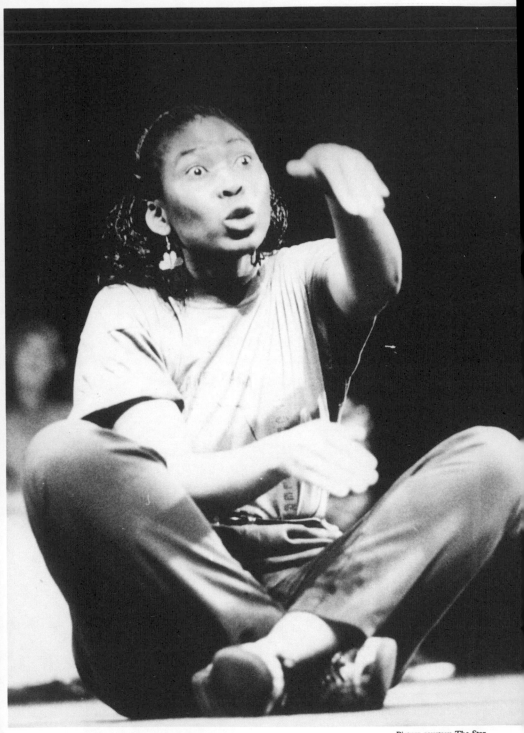

Gcina Mhlophe dramatically tells the mystical tale of *The Impala* in a performance at Johannesburg's Market Theatre in October 1993 (see Interview with Gcina Mhlophe)

Patronage, the State and Ideology in Zambian Theatre

STEWART CREHAN

In this examination of the relations between Zambian theatre and the state, I shall argue that the early promise of benevolent, enlightened patronage has not been fulfilled, and that the development of Zambian theatre has been hampered by a prevailing attitude of patient reliance on state patronage, part of a larger problem of identifying the nature and role of the Zambian state itself, which lies beyond the scope of this study. The attitude nevertheless reveals certain unresolved contradictions, some of which I have tried to deal with elsewhere[1], and needs to be objectively analysed when discussing the attempt to create an articulated Zambian identity. Although the Zambian state has been liberal compared to most African states, and does not practise open censorship of plays and productions, the habit of self-censorship on the part of playwrights and theatre practitioners has made its task easier.

The ideological and formal limits of Zambian drama, with its cautious stance towards experimentation, and apparent contentedness with a loose mixture of realism, comedy, didacticism and melodrama, have subtle links with this same attitude of reliance on state authority to which I have referred. The praise song, in which a chief or king is eulogised, and the traditional moral tale, in which a clear message is defined through a straightforward linear narrative, may be of relevance here, while the fantastic, non-realist elements found in traditional oral narratives have, for the most part, been restricted in Zambian drama to a preoccupation with ghosts and witchcraft. Popular theatre in its various forms and modes thrives in Zambia. However, a revolutionary synthesis of traditional and modern, popular and elitist forms has not yet occurred, for reasons possibly traceable to Zambia's own history, and to the nature of its ruling Party, UNIP. As the representation of fictional events, drama is a refraction of social change both in the way its content and form refract other ideologies (political, religious, social, moral and aesthetic), and in the way it is constituted as a social institution. Hence in looking at its economic mode of existence (in this case, patronage) we shall also be looking at the development of Zambian theatre and drama as art and as a vehicle of ideas.

The Colonial Legacy

Between 1953 and 1958, at the height of the copper boom, the government of Northern Rhodesia, the mining companies and the municipalities made a significant investment in white settler culture. Seven little theatres were built along the line of rail, one in Lusaka, the rest in the mining towns of Broken Hill (Kabwe), Kitwe, Ndola, Luanshya, Mufulira and Chingola. Until independence the proscenium stages of these solidly-constructed establishments were tramped exclusively by the feet of white thespians performing their anodyne amateur theatricals before settler audiences. Even up to the early eighties, expatriate productions still tended to predominate in most of the little theatres. According to Stephen Chifunyise: 'these drama clubs grew to become the strongest colonial establishment for the propagation of white culture and the enforcement of racial segregational laws in the colony'.[2]

The policy was really one of exclusion and subordination rather than cultural assimilation. Only when theatre was in danger of being turned into a political weapon in the late fifties did the colonialists seriously try to incorporate Zambian artists into their 'white culture'. Moses Kwali writes:

> They did not allow us to take part, except for very special reasons. No one is blind to their colonial policy, a policy full of hypocritical contradictions, of separate development based on Native Authority enactments. It then becomes obvious that they taught us to appreciate their drama so that we could only be an observing mass to be exploited as a market where they sold their drama.[3]

In equating settler culture with 'white culture', however, cultural nationalism often mistakes the dummy for the man. Settler culture, unlike the creative theatre work in Zambia of progressive whites such as David Wallace and Michael Etherton, was always a parasitic phenomenon, incapable of creative innovation. A sterile dependence on the metropole gives settler theatre its special character. Invariably middlebrow, sentimental and escapist, it is locked in a genteel past which perhaps only a little theatre in Africa can preserve intact. Settler drama repeats the same flat theatrical landscape that constituted the bulk of English drama up to the thirties, nostalgically keeping alive the a-political suburban drama typified by the well-made play. And yet the little theatres were completed in Northern Rhodesia precisely at a time when English theatre was going through a historic renaissance with the drama of Osborne, Pinter, Wesker and Arden. Mistaken for the real thing, amateur settler theatre helped to drive a wedge between emergent Zambian drama and radical developments in Europe, masking a dynamic cultural reality behind the smiling falsehood of a tailor's dummy. That the dummy has been taken for the man has done nothing to advance Zambian theatre.

As Dickson Mwansa has said, 'the road to professionalising performing arts in Africa is slow and hazardous'.[4] Zambia's own slow development in this area has its origins in the colonial past: in racial segregation and the colonial education system. Segregation created social structures, institutions and mental habits which, twenty-five years after Independence, still exist, albeit perpetuated in ways other than the purely racial. Between the élite club, such as the Lusaka Playhouse or Kitwe Little Theatre, and the tavern or bar where the male-dominated beerhall atmosphere is less pompous, there is an abyss almost as great as that which exists between the rural and the urban areas. Formerly segregated institutions have acquired a more purely class character that makes them easier to demystify; yet the legacy of a colonial education system that bred intellectual mediocrity and cultural inferiority as a matter of policy should not be forgotten.[5] Up to 1946 only one secondary school existed in Northern Rhodesia. At independence in 1964, Zambia had only a hundred graduates. The nature of the Zambian élite thus militated against the kind of conscious cultural reaction that occurred in the Francophone countries, while the serious manpower shortage at independence meant a continued reliance on expatriate personnel up to the eighties (hence the continued strength of the white-dominated Theatre Association of Zambia, TAZ), and an educational expansion that had to supply deficiencies in the vocational, technical and managerial fields before the liberal arts and higher professions could be Zambianised. These factors help to explain what some have seen as the Philistine mediocrity of the Zambian ruling élite and its inability to formulate a 'cultural policy'. They also help to explain the ideological faith in state intervention and bureaucratic measures as solutions to the development of theatre in Zambia.

Where the membership and committees of the little theatre clubs have become Zambianised — a process that is now largely complete — the initial, and in some cases lingering picture has not been one of cultural resurgence and theatrical innovation, but rather an influx of 'drinking members'[6] such as the 'state agents'[7] (Special Branch officers), UNIP

Party chairmen, ward officials, police officers, parastatal executives, civil servants and clerks who regularly patronise the Lusaka Playhouse. Most of these members prefer to stay in the bar during a theatrical performance, thus revealing their complete lack of interest in theatre.[8] Similar situations have been reported in the little theatres of Kabwe, Ndola and Mufulira, while at Kitwe Little Theatre the entire executive (members of the local élite) was dismissed in January 1987 for its failure to produce plays, its inept administration, and failure to keep account of finances.[9]

Kaunda and State Patronage

Above this sea of philistinism, corruption and 'falling standards'[10] the Head of State enjoys a unique status as the nation's most enlightened patron of the arts. Quoting from a 1983 Presidential speech ('We need playhouses and theatres in our cities, towns and villages. Let us organise ourselves to provide these. Let us build.'), Mwansa and Banda affirm: 'He is one person who has interest in the development of the arts'.[11] In 1977 Kaunda urged Tikwiza Theatre to take the message of Masautso Phiri's elegiac solidarity play *Soweto* 'to all corners of the world'[12]; in 1979 he praised Dickson Mwansa's controversial play about prison life, *The Cell* — which some members of the government wanted to ban — as 'an eye opener'[13], and in 1984 he honoured Graig Lungu, author of *Song of the Shanties*, a play about corruption and workers' rights, with an award. Such 'radical' gestures have helped to legitimate Kaunda's role as a supporter of socially critical drama while at the same time confirming his paradoxical image as an omnipotent patriarch sadly hamstrung by an entourage of unimaginative mediocrities.

In October 1967 the recently-formed Department of Cultural Services organised a huge festival to coincide with the third anniversary of Zambian Independence. President Kaunda conveyed the following message:

> I am pleased to announce that the festival will be an annual event that will climax Zambia's cultural expression ... I am still confident that my Government will, before very long, be able to build an Arts Centre that will incorporate a National Arts Gallery and a National Theatre here in Lusaka.[14]

Twenty-two years later there is still no functioning arts centre and no national theatre; not one new theatre house has been added to the seven that were completed over thirty years ago, and until 1974 the only annual drama festival in Zambia apart from schools drama was that held by the

Theatre Association of Zambia, which represented the little theatres.

A few Zambian theatre artists have observed that despite some support, the state has done relatively little to encourage the development of theatre in Zambia.[15] The majority nevertheless continue to hang on to every word the Head of State happens to drop on the subject of theatre. In April 1988 he 'gave theatre artistes marching orders to support methods of improving theatre'.[16] This was immediately picked up as a major policy statement, and top-level meetings went ahead to discuss a 'National Cultural Complex'.

A rapprochement between the state and Zambian artists, with its hint of increasing direction of the arts from above, is in no way resented by the artists themselves. On the contrary; even if only for economic reasons — leaving aside the battle for a Zambian cultural identity — Zambian artists and performers eagerly look to the state for recognition and support, for protection and guidance, regardless of whether the personnel who make up the leadership have the qualifications or the resources to satisfy such demands. Far from fearing Zhdanovism and censorship, most Zambian artists continue to believe in the liberal benevolence of a state headed by a man who is himself an artist.[17] The fear is not of being smothered, but of being abandoned. In 1984 the chairman of the Zambian Union of Musicians, for example, complained that 95 per cent of entertainment premises were 'occupied by foreign musicians'[18] and that the government was doing nothing about this situation which, he said, 'makes an artist feel like a motherless child with no shoulder to cry on'.[19]

In this context, Baylies and Szeftel point out that the Zambian petty-bourgeoisie is 'more dependent on the state and state assistance than the more successful members of the bourgeoisie and therefore more in sympathy with its policies'.[20] This is certainly true of many Zambian theatre artists, young writers and musicians. Their populist orientation and occasionally xenophobic outbursts evince their embattled situation. As Moses Kwali, author of a series of radio plays sponsored by the Anti-Corruption Committee, puts it:

[Whosoever] is actively engaged [in the story of play writing in Zambia] is by the connivance of events immersed in his own rich experiences which, for better or worse, blot out the objective viewpoint and turn him into a debater projecting his side of the motion. To try to convince him to be objective is like asking a rat to consider and agree that the cat needs a rat for its meal. For the bystanders, perhaps it is easy from the sidelines to be objective.[21]

One consequence of this embattled subjectivity is to view the state —

against all evidence to the contrary — as a saviour; a view which has deep historical and ideological causes.

The interaction of various theatre groupings charts the struggles against, and compromises with, state patronage. In 1983-4, radicals in the Zambia National Theatre Arts Association, founded in 1974, advocated firm action against the Theatre Association of Zambia (branded as a bastion of reactionary 'enclave theatre' blocking the development of indigenous Zambian theatre) and called on the state to nationalise the little theatres, giving the Zambia National Theatre Arts Association hegemony. But since the President had condemned the Zambia National Theatre Arts Association–Theatre Association of Zambia rivalry as divisive, both associations were dissolved and in 1986 the National Theatre Association of Zambia was formed. The Zambia National Theatre Arts Association, having made a bid for power in defiance of the President's call for unity, was seen as an undisciplined and rebellious child by the press. Yet the rebel quietly succumbed. One historical reason for this was that its formation in 1974, although in some ways a continuation of the work of the university group, Chikwakwa:

> involved lobbying for support in the cabinet and the Central Committee. The founding leaders exercised top secrecy so as not to alarm T[heatre] A[ssociation] of Z[ambia] amongst whose leaders were some men of high influence even in the high echelons of state power. At the same time they were aware of the strained relationship between the State and the University which had resulted in the closure of the University, so they were cautious not to make the government link the creation of the new association with the rising tide of student 'radicalism'.[22]

The K5,000 annual government grant that had been given to the Theatre Association of Zambia since 1971 was transferred to the Zambia National Theatre Arts Association soon after the latter was formed. A second reason for the Zambia National Theatre Arts Association's acquiescence in the unification with the Theatre Association of Zambia was the expectation (more or less fulfilled) that the National Theatre Association of Zambia would be little different from the Zambia National Theatre Arts Association in terms of plays, personnel and orientation. Segregationist habits remain deeply ingrained in Zambia, and while a Zambian or two may be involved in a white production and *vice versa*, blacks and whites involved in the theatre still tend to operate separately. A third reason was the as yet unassailable ideological and political authority of Kaunda himself. Apart from his reputation as a champion of liberation in Southern Africa, the other 'radical' side that made him generally acceptable in Zambian theatre circles was cultural nationalism, strongly articulated in his Watershed speech in 1975, delivered two years after the declaration of a one-party state:

> The whole issue, therefore, becomes one of identity in terms of culture. It becomes one of deliberately developing those cultural values which we recognise as good in our own past. It becomes one of rejecting and indeed fighting those cultural activities from other lands which may destroy our cultural values, thereby not only dehumanising us, but also making us faint carbon copies of themselves.[23]

Chifunyise has said that Kaunda's Watershed speech supported 'the ideological line' of Chikwakwa Theatre, which in turn owed much to Unzadrams, the University Drama Society founded in 1966.[24] It is true that the aim of Chikwakwa was to develop 'a truly Zambian theatre for the people'[25], portraying the Zambian way of life in vernacular languages and using Zambian songs and dances. However, whereas the main emphasis in the Watershed speech was on nationalist resistance to the 'invasion of our cultural values by those of the West'[26], Chikwakwa emphasised the need for a mass, popular theatre geared to the 'unfolding social revolution'[27], an emphasis which later became more explicitly revolutionary:

> It is socially committed drama. The participants are aware of the need for a revolutionary theatre to present the problems of economic and social development in the on-going Zambian revolution. The plays present such problems as the new role of women in modern society, the conflicts between upper and lower classes, the need for self-reliance and organisation of the people in the agrarian revolution ...[28]

The official representatives of the national bourgeoisie, unlike Chikwakwa's founders, were less concerned with mobilising the rural masses in 'the on-going Zambian revolution' than in legitimating their own status as leaders. This fundamental intention, namely, to legitimate the state and party machine, could be seen in the conspicuous visibility of 'senior Party and Government officials', in the front row at a Tikwiza Theatre Club gala performance. After the performance a few speeches would be made, as they are by any national leader at a tribal ceremony, and the similarities of purpose at both kinds of gathering are obvious.[29]

Drama, I shall argue, is useful to the Zambian ruling élite not because of any inherent value it might have as dramatic art, but because it provides a platform, can be instrumental to various causes, and has an important ideological function. (It can also, of course, be dangerous for these same reasons.) Like the airport dancers, whose rhythmically clapping female chorus sings appropriate songs of praise in the presence of a leader, or like the talented school choirs, whose patriotic songs about UNIP and Kaunda are sung on suitable occasions such as the President's birthday, drama's usefulness as a tool of the state has long been recognised. In February 1987 the theatre critic of *The Sunday Times* even asked: 'Why not use drama to woo shy voters?' Noting 'the low momentum of the just ended registration exercise for the Party elections', the writer suggested that 'district councils could have used drama to help publicise the election campaign'.[30]

In fact Kaunda's speeches and writings, and the various comments he has made at performances, suggest a somewhat old-fashioned, mission-school approach to art and culture rather than a radically enlightened stance. Christian hymns with plenty of spiritual uplift; moralistic plots whose messages are always 'loud and clear'; commonsense values that adhere to a righteous sense of duty ('Don't worry too much about setting the whole universe to rights, just try to make sense of that little patch in which God has placed you and do *something* with it.'[31]) — this homely mix, if it has not set the tone for a good deal of Zambian writing and drama, has undoubtedly helped to set the ideological and formal limits responsible for a widespread habit of self-censorship that is one of the most crippling aspects of literary and theatrical expression in Zambia. (It is one of the reasons why there has been so little need for overt censorship.) Radical innovations in theatrical form and style initiated by Chikwakwa and later by Tikwiza; sharp deviations from empirical realism and the linear plot; attempts to demystify the ideological mechanisms of patriarchy and power[32], and any critique of religion[33], are rare. The prevailing everyday ethos of learning how to put up with a multitude of sins in the name of some Christian-humanist sentiment has proved insidiously pervasive, despite a rapidly declining economy.

Zambian Theatre: Servant or Critic?

If there is one theatre club in Zambia that has played the role of the Head of State's praise-singers, echoing his stance on issues such as South Africa, it is Tikwiza Theatre. From the advantage of hindsight, Tikwiza's 'revolutionism,' demonstrated in such disciplined, high-energy productions as *Uhuru wa Ndonoo* (1976), *Soweto* (1976), *The Trial of Dedan Kimathi* (1980) and *Che Guevara* (1982), was both a validation of Zambia's Front-Line support for freedom struggles and a diversion from domestic issues. In 1982 Tikwiza's rare production of a Zambian play, *The Cell*, received a warning phone call from a senior Party official: if certain changes were not made, he said, the production would be terminated. (No changes were made, and nothing happened.) Tikwiza has received considerable moral and financial support from the state and various parastatals, to the extent that, as Mwansa points out, other groups felt that the club was being unduly fostered with its 'extra-territorial messages'.[34] Masautso Phiri, the club's leading creative force, was Senior Editor at Neczam, the national publishing company, when it published *Soweto: Flowers Will Grow* in 1979. Mumba Kapumpa, later chairman of the club, is a state attorney. Other members have included accountants, an economist, a quantity surveyor, a broadcaster, a statistician, clerks and secretaries in various parastatals.

When the multimillion kwacha, Chinese-built Freedom House complex that will house the UNIP Party headquarters was still in its design stage, leaders of Tikwiza Theatre put pressure on the government (unsuccessfully, as it turned out) to include the long-awaited national theatre in the architect's plans. (Tikwiza, an amateur club with professional attitudes and ambitions, seems to have harboured hopes of its own members forming the nucleus of a national theatre company.) Six years later, during early discussions concerning the 'National Cultural Complex', Tikwiza presented a 'Working Paper' proposing a Zambia Cultural Commission, 'a fully fledged parastatal with a board of directors'[35] that would 'implement cultural policy', train playwrights and directors, 'register and license all workers in theatre' and 'grade (sic) all artists including actors, directors and playwrights'.[36] Happily, this somewhat desperate-sounding bureaucratic fantasy was not endorsed. Between 1983 and 1986 the club appeared to have folded, but in late 1986 it came back to life. Phiri, now a protocol adviser at the American Embassy, made a come-back in 1988 with his *Waiting for Sanctions*, a somewhat lukewarm plea for sanctions against South Africa which, said the programme note, should be applied 'as sanctions are a lesser evil compared to apartheid'.

The play relies heavily on documentary material and actual utterances by Reagan, Thatcher, Botha, Mandela, Tambo, Mugabe and Kaunda, delivered with at times statuesque monotony by the actors. The opening night was attended by the President himself, and a unique event occurred in Zambian theatre as Kaunda watched himself talking and crying on stage in a piece of masterly mimicry by Edmond Ngula. Yet politically the play is ambiguous. The first-night audience was noticeably confused when the South African Garment Workers' Union entered with clenched fists *denouncing* sanctions, and one actress's speech brought hearty applause in agreement until some members of the audience realised that it was Margaret Thatcher who was speaking. The confusion was perhaps symptomatic: Zambia had been accused of sanctions-busting when Zambia Airways introduced its DC10 flight to New York (now regularly used by white South Africans) with a connecting flight from and to Johannesburg, after the United States Congress had deprived South African Airways of its landing rights. *Waiting for Sanctions* had not been sponsored or helped by the ANC, whose headquarters are in Lusaka; nevertheless, after the gala performance Kaunda donated K20,000 to Tikwiza Theatre, and the production went to the Party National Council before touring the country. (Later, and somewhat ironically, Tikwiza performed the play to raise K10,000 for the Party Headquarters, a building that would not look out of place in Bucharest.)

One notable thorn in the side of the Zambian ruling party and its government has been the University of Zambia. Chikwakwa, Unzadrams and the Department of English (now Literature and Languages) drama courses made the University a vital radiating point of new theatrical ideas, talented theatre artists, original productions, and dedicated Zambian teachers who went on to create the school drama clubs that would later compete in the Zambia National Theatre Arts Association festivals. Despite the deportation of Etherton and Horn, Chikwakwa continued as an active force until 1980 due to the presence of Fay Chung, Stephen Chifunyise and David Kerr. In 1982 a student protest against the opening of an Institute of Human Relations aroused the wrath of the Party leadership: the students alleged that the Institute was merely an attempt to foist the Party's 'bankrupt' petty-bourgeois philosophy of Humanism on the University community in order to provide a foothold for UNIP, castigated in a leaflet as 'a byword for capitalist corruption'. The ensuing strike and closure led to suspensions and expulsions that netted some Unzadrams leaders, and the deportation of more expatriates. A student production of Kabwe Kasoma's *Black Mamba*, a play about the independence struggle that features Kaunda's rival Simon Kapwepwe, was banned. Thereafter, the University became more of an instrument of state policy with little real autonomy, and since the students (most of whom the Party was unable to recruit) had no union, all students activities were severely curtailed. Censorship was introduced by the University administration, and Unzadrams became a shadow of its former self. By 1983-4 the drama courses had collapsed, so that all hopes were now pinned on the new Centre for the Performing Arts, which had been mooted in 1973 by Professor Kashoki. At the time of writing the Centre has no students, one member of staff, and some dancers.

Another challenge was presented by the Zambia National Theatre Arts Association. The rapid expansion of the Association after 1979, the radicalism of some of its plays, and its leaders' call for its recognition as the sole theatre organisation in the country, reduced its grant to K1,000 in a period of rising inflation. The mushrooming of affiliated independent adult theatre groups along the line of rail and in provincial towns such as Chipata signalled a major renaissance in Zambian theatre. The thematic evolution of the plays themselves, progressing from tales of culture conflict, back-to-the-land homilies and domestic melodramas to critiques of witchcraft, gerontocracy, urban poverty, corruption, dictatorship and employer-worker relations reflected the Association's growing independence — financial, artistic and ideological — from the state. The Presidential directive to form a unitary association was thus the chance to bring the Zambia National Theatre Arts Association, which was frequently attacked in the press, back into the fold.

The distinction between loyal criticism and oppositional criticism in Zambian drama is often a fine one: even a praise singer has the licence to criticise through oblique reference, circumlocution, and significant choices or omissions within the eulogistic repertoire. Toleration is, of course, to some extent a measure of self-censorship and fear of reprisal as much as it is of the state's own liberal attitude: I have never seen a play that featured miners on strike, for example, or homosexuality, or students on a boycott being beaten by paramilitary police. Apart from one or two instances where a sensitive social issue aroused the wrath of the state, such as one particular play that showed a child dying in a stampede for mealie meal, social criticism has been tolerated, and even encouraged. Veiled criticism of the leadership or of 'the system' tries to strike deeper than the tragi-comic critiques of social conditions, though it does not always make for better drama. This type of play works through allusion, or through allegory, like Zhaninge Theatre's *Make That Broom Sweep* where the oppressed office sweeper muses, in a manner reminiscent of Armah's *The Beautiful Ones Are Not Yet Born*, on the ingrained dirt beneath the surface polish. Whenever the audience see an office desk on stage, they can expect another attack on The Boss, and hence, by implication, on the bureaucracy; when sofa and two chairs, they can reasonably expect another unmasking of The Bad Husband or The Tyrannical Father (a well-plotted, lively example being Ikafa's *Parents*). Yet it is remarkable how many plays at the Zambia National Theatre Arts Association and the National Theatre Association of Zambia festivals have portrayed corrupt bureaucrats, dictatorial chiefs and selfish, hypocritical fathers, while no one involved in the festivals will ever utter one word of criticism in public against the actual leadership.

One of the most pointed critiques of the Zambian *status quo* is Graig Lungu's *Horses on the Rider*, a play which has mysteriously faded from the repertoire. (Its author, a lieutenant in the Zambia National Service, was sent for training as a 'political facilitator' after the play was performed.) The riders are a lazy, corrupt, drunken parastatal boss and his luxury-loving, pretentious, servant-berating termagant of a wife. The idealised horses are two virtuous and long-suffering servants, male and female, who keep their master's house in order. The play's kick, and that of its maltreated horses, is in the ending: the bankrupt, improvident master and mistress are made to leave the house by the industrious, thrifty servants, who take over. The lesson — that Zambia's leaders have proved to be bad housekeepers and should be ousted by the masses — hardly needs spelling out. Eviction and punishment of bad leaders and bad fathers may refer, in traditional moralistic fashion, to bad eggs and rotten apples or, more obliquely and allegorically, to the élite in general. In a recent play by another author, the director of a 'Human Resource Centre' is told by one of his colleagues at a crisis meeting: 'You have led a double-faced life; the life of a hardened dictator in our midst and that of a sensible, knowledgeable leader outside the circles of our company ... So, we demand your resignation'. Few Zambian audiences would miss that kind of political allusion, or fail to realise that patient submission had now given way to the final, angry warning.

The political and social criticism in some Zambian plays, however, is so muted as to be almost negligible. An interesting ideological shift was noticeable in Kabwe YMCA Theatre's new production of *The Tramp's Whistle* at the 1988 adult festival in Kabwe, where a measure of self-censorship was apparent in the doctored script. The tramp Santana (played as before with confident skill though less verve by Mike Tembo) was no longer a keen source of satiric irony directed at the hypocritical rich who uphold Zambia's national myths; instead he had become a lazy charlatan and an exploiter who deserved our condemnation. Ifilundu's award-winning production of Julius Chongo's *Kings Are Born*, a well-constructed play about traditional African politics, contained certain anachronisms: 'We are in a State of Emergency', 'The situation is political. It does not require military intervention', and 'You never get power on a silver plate. There are tactics in the corridors of power'. The play invited (and at the same time frustrated) allegorical readings; yet what was notable in the production was the repeated intrusion of an anachronistic register that hinted at the cynicism of Zambian power politics while implicitly endorsing the conservatism of the slogan: 'Vote KK No Change'. (The play was subsequently performed at State House in April 1989 on the occasion of Kaunda's 65th birthday.) In other plays that try to be critical, a moralistic didacticism prevails. Plots that resolve contradictions for the audience instead of confronting audiences with the need to resolve these contradictions themselves, imply the existence of a benevolent force at work in the world, thereby endorsing a fundamentally religious attitude of passive dependence. This is the same attitude which, as I have already argued, looks to State and President as a beneficent, almost parental force guiding the nation. An intended political or social critique may thus be short-circuited.

In the present context, an ironic contradiction manifests itself. Zambian theatre artists have repeatedly called for intervention by President, State and Party. In the early post-independence period, during Zambianisation, this was undoubtedly progressive. But at a certain point, when the Zambian ruling class had consolidated itself and could no longer blame the Zimbabwean war for domestic problems (i.e. after 1980) intervention promised to be repressive rather than supportive. At this point, Zambian theatre becomes aggressively critical and self-confident, and Tikwiza goes into a decline. When the Zambia National Theatre Arts Association has been tamed, Tikwiza revives and calls for state control. Given Zambia's present economic decline, greater state control is understandable, for the ideological sphere is crucial in legitimating policies that must bring suffering. A small yet significant result of that suffering could be the further bureaucratisation and censorship Zambian theatre will have to undergo in order to gain a professional national theatre that has been so long in coming.

Popular Theatre and its Patrons

During the fifties, with the rise of African nationalism, a dance such as Fwemba arose to become a vehicle of protest and a symbol of revolutionary discipline; M'ganda parodied and at the same time celebrated formal military discipline, while the Nyau dance, part of a traditional ceremony, developed new satirical characters such as 'sajeni', the colonial policeman. Dance forms, songs and paradramatic forms that were connected with the liberation struggle were soon seen by the colonialists as a threat. The colonial government had no ideological objection to African culture *per se*. What it feared were cultural forms that served as vehicles for political agitation. From 1958 onwards, moves were made to incorporate more Zambians into white-controlled theatre through community centre youth groups, schools, colleges and drama festivals, moves that varied from the paternalistic to the radical. Independent activity by Zambian theatre artists who supported UNIP bore fruit with the independent, UNIP-sponsored Zambia Arts Trust (1964-9). The Arts Trust had a Department of Traditional Arts directed by Gideon Lumpa and a Department of Theatre and Drama directed by Kenneth Nkhata, thus bringing together dance and drama. Dance drama, an original African form, was an important weapon in the nationalist movement, employing traditional and modern forms and techniques in its satirical, anti-colonial sketches. Since independence, its focus has been mainly on developmental issues, though as a form it has much unexploited potential. In 1967 the Arts Trust mounted a lavish production called *The King Must Die*, a shortened version of *The Oresteia* involving sixty dancers and ten drummers, and combined 'classical Greek dance-drama with Zambian traditional music and dancing'.[37]

The combination of dance-drama and revolutionary politics that began with Fwemba and other dances could have been the most dynamic and explosive contribution Zambia has made to theatre if a further original synthesis in terms of *form* had been created. As it was, dance and drama were brought together in the theatre without fully cross-fertilising, even in the early Chikwakwa plays.[38] The gulf that continues to exist between popular and élitist forms could, I suggest, have something to do with the way in which Zambian independence was achieved and consolidated. Revolutionary forms answer revolutionary needs. It might therefore be argued that a revolutionary synthesis of popular and élitist forms in Zambian theatre could only have occurred if the class alliance between the nationalist petty-bourgeoisie and the masses had been based on a struggle for social transformation rather than just flag independence and 'Zambianisation'. This is merely a hypothesis, but the gulf is especially striking at a Zambian drama festival where one may see an electrifying performance of a Fwemba dance on stage, full of great energy, concentration and split-second timing, and then, later, a sloppy performance of a scripted play in English in which, perhaps, some of the same artists take part, performing like grounded albatrosses with slow entries, badly-timed cues, unconvincing gestures and curtain changes that last several minutes. At such moments it seems that dance and drama inhabit different aesthetic universes.

Other aspects of the dichotomy between traditional and modern, popular and élitist might be mentioned. There still exists, for example, an almost schizophrenic attitude towards language. The highly figurative language of Bemba, with its metaphors, similes and hyperboles, may occupy one part of the mind of a certain kind of playwright who, for cultural and ideological reasons, and not for reasons of linguistic competence, is simply unable to translate that figurative richness into English. It is as if English were restricted, according to his way of thinking, to certain élitist and bureaucratic registers, functions and contexts that precluded such a transfer. Yet another problem is the attitude to scripted plays. If the 'embattled subjectivity' we noted above as typical of some Zambian playwrights can be linked to an atomised dependence on the state, it also goes with the delivery to drama groups starved of Zambian material of hastily-written, frequently 'half-baked' playscripts which their authors have neither the time nor the inclination to revise, expand or polish. One reason for this, I suggest, is an ambivalence towards the written playscript. If it is written, it will always be in English. The playscript is thus indirectly associated with 'white culture,' western forms of drama, and hence with the little theatres. Those Zambian playwrights whose basic sympathy is with popular drama (associated with the unscripted vernacular performance improvisation and collective authorship) frequently display an indifference, possibly even a latent sense of guilt towards their own written scripts as finished products. Their interest is in the *performance*, not in the play as something to be read, studied, or appreciated as literature, for this may remind the playwright (especially if he is in his middle or late thirties) of expatriate teachers, Shakespeare, and the colonial syllabus. This shamefaced attitude towards the conventional stage play and the written script may therefore be related to broader attitudes engendered by racial segregation and a colonial education policy.

There have been, though, attempts to produce a scripted Zambian theatre tradition which was innovative in its dual emphasis on an oral-based performance aesthetic and on experimental Western theatre techniques. With its specially-constructed open-air theatre and student travelling theatre, Chikwakwa Theatre attempted to fuse what was most vital in Zambian popular culture with the most progressive tendencies then current in European theatre: theatre-in-the-round, experimental use of different stage levels, audience participation, 'taking theatre to the people' (as in the popular and street-theatre movement of the late sixties), the fluid, open-ended action of Brechtian epic theatre (as in the production of Andrea Masiye's *Kazembe and the Portugese*), and a deliberate avoidance of the smooth progressions and clichés of the well-made play. All were part of what Michael Etherton called the 'new aesthetic'.

Chikwakwa's influence was considerable, yet it was not until after the

Chalimbana Workshop in 1979 that the theatre for development concept, which had been applied by Laedza Batanani in Botswana and the Kamiriithu community project in Kenya, began to take root in Zambia. An important distinction here lies between what can be called 'campaign theatre', where ready-made or pre-rehearsed plays and sketches (usually unscripted) are taken to the compounds and rural areas and are performed in the appropriate language by outsiders, and a process in which a play arises out of participatory research and collective discussion, between the animateurs and the local people, of the problems and issues which the people themselves find most relevant. The specific target population are involved at every stage, including the final performance, the aim being to raise consciousness through drama so that, ideally, it is the people themselves who learn to overcome problems whose solution the play has demonstrated. Interestingly enough, Tikwiza Theatre carried out their own theatre for development exercise, of a kind, when, after having discussions with pupils at Namwala Secondary School long-standing problems and grievances at the school were uncovered which the resulting play helped to solve. What also happens fairly frequently in Zambia, particularly with the professional travelling theatre groups, is that once a play has been developed with the help of some theatre for development techniques, or more thoroughly as part of an aided project, the play solidifies as an addition to the group's repertoire and is then taken to other communities and performed in other languages as a 'campaign' play.

The spread of Zambian popular theatre, now largely identified with theatre for development projects and educational campaigns, has been sponsored mainly by aid agencies and NGOs. The International Theatre Institute Theatre for Development Workshop held in Mongu in 1983 was sponsored by Oxfam, CUSO and the Frederick Naumann Foundation. The Kanyama Theatre Production Unit, a well-established professional travelling theatre group sponsored by DANIDA, performed in Denmark in 1988. Mwananga Theatre, based in Chipata, are sponsored by the Wildlife Conservation Society of Zambia. Their Nyanja 'campaign' play, *The Problem*, which combines dance drama and dialogue, deals with the economics of poaching, the involvement of foreigners (such as Senegalese), and the need for a greater environmental awareness among villagers. In *The Solution to the Problem* a district secretary explains the solution to the villagers while the local ward Party chairman, well oiled, repeatedly stands up to shout, 'One Zambia!' while the rest are compelled to answer: 'One Nation!'

The Pamodzi Travelling Theatre, another professional group formed in

1979, has been sponsored by the Ministry of Health, the Frederick Naumann Foundation, UNICEF, the ANC, the British Council and Luanshya District Council. An original unscripted play in the group's repertoire (performed both in English and in Nyanja, depending on the audience) is *Two Clever Fools* by Lukah Mukuka. In the play two sacked employees in Lusaka, after duping each other with fake commodities, come to appreciate each other's cleverness and go to Katete in the Eastern Province where one of them pretends to be the son and heir of a friend's dead father. When, providentially, they return to collect the dead man's death certificate and registration card the villagers see through the deception. The two tricksters are tried and sentenced by a village court. With effective use of humour and an economy of means, the play succeeds in raising topics such as unemployment, the shortage of essential commodities and black marketeering, inviting discussion by urban audiences; yet it also shows village audiences how, for once, they can thwart the exploitative intentions of 'clever' townspeople, thus indirectly alluding to the robbery of natural resources such as ivory and emeralds.

The emergence of AIDS in Zambia has had profound cultural as well as social consequences. The linking of the syndrome with homosexuality and prostitution made the state at first reluctant to publicise its presence. As late as 14 June 1987 the editor-in-chief of the government-owned *Zambia Daily Mail,* Komani Kachinga, used space in his newspaper to assert: 'Zambia for example has not got a big problem of prostitutes. The few girls who work for money in the few bars and hotels are a strange part of Zambian society,' adding: 'One has to be a crank to be a homosexual in Zambia'. Both statements were no doubt inspired more by the government's concern with Zambia's image than with the facts. AIDS nevertheless provided an opportunity for sponsored theatre groups to assist the government's AIDS education campaign that had already begun. In October 1988 Fwebena Afrika's *AIDS Bulepaya* (AIDS Kills) was performed in shanty townships, schools and colleges in Kitwe, sponsored by NORAD as part of the Copperbelt health education project. Kanyama Theatre mounted their own AIDS play, sponsored by WHO and the Ministry of Health's Education Unit, as did Tikondane Theatre and the University Teaching Hospital's drama group in Lusaka.

The best-known AIDS play in Zambia, however, has been Dickson Mwansa's *Father Kalo and the Virus,* directed by Masautso Phiri. Sponsored by the World Health Organisation and the Ministry of Health, the play introduces the abortion issue as well as AIDS to develop a three-sided debate between the Catholic priest Father Kalo, a doctor and a traditional healer. Without playing down the sense of tragedy (a Catholic couple who both have AIDS are advised by their doctor that the wife, who is pregnant, should abort), Father Kalo symbolically preserves the existing social order in the face of a human catastrophe by balancing the claims of all three institutions: the traditional healer's medicines are not dismissed as the tricks of a charlatan, and we do not find out if the wife defies her priest or her doctor.

The most controversial part of the production is when the doctor throws condoms into the audience as AIDS leaflets are being distributed — something that would have been wholly inconceivable a few years ago. Such plays have helped to break down traditional taboos. Yet in none of them is homosexuality discussed, while in Tikondane's *AIDS Campaign*, the professional street prostitute is eschewed in favour of the more familiar bar girl. As in other AIDS plays, the focus is on a man who contracts the disease from a girl who is promiscuous rather than the other way round.

Another recent development in Zambia is 'institutional theatre'. Fewer community theatre groups are now sponsored by city councils: in Kitwe, Bakanda Theatre, once on a par with Tikwiza, have seen their community hall being allowed to fall into neglect by the council. Instead, parastatal institutions such as the Zambia National Commercial Bank, the Bank of Zambia, the National Provident Fund and Zambia State Insurance are sponsoring theatre groups formed by their own employees, following the example of Zambia National Service, Zambia Air Force, and Zambia Medical Stores. The sponsored drama group, like the sponsored football team or darts team, forms part of the employer's welfare programme.

This contrasts with the arrangement whereby an institution sponsors an independent group. Independent groups such as Zhaninge and Bwananyina in Kitwe and Tapeza in Ndola have had stormy relationships with their patrons, Bwananyina having to compete in Zambia Consolidated Copper Mines' Social Club with drinkers and discos before being evicted. The institutional arrangement privileges those in employment. Whereas popular theatre groups and independent community theatre groups often have school drop-outs and unemployed as members, the institutional group has a more acceptable, even petty-bourgeois image, especially since banking etiquette dictates that the employee is expected to wear a suit and tie at all times when at work.

It could be argued that the patrons of institutional theatre are a subtle extension of or substitute for state patronage, a means of curbing the radical, independent community theatre groups that infused the Zambia National Theatre Arts Association with such energy between 1980 and 1985. If so, the patronage of popular theatre groups by aid agencies and NGOs may impose another kind of limitation in that technical and practical issues are emphasised at the expense of 'consciousness-raising', binding groups to the parameters and objectives of particular projects.

I have not dealt here with radio drama, though the weekly Bemba programme *Ifyabukaya* (Local Lore), sponsored by a pharmaceutical company, is extremely popular, managing to be entertaining, critical and topical without offending Party or government, from which it takes some of its cues for themes and topics. Like the weekly television programme 'Players' Circle', which is in English, *Ifyabukaya* has an air of improvisation and naturalness, excelling in the tragi-comic ironies of domestic situations. The importance of drama in Zambia, both live and in the media, is unquestionable. Thousands of school children participate in plays every year, and the spirit of competition in the various festivals (in 1987 the UNIP Youth League staged its own performing arts festival) is keen. The potential Zambian audience for drama and live theatre, at least in the main urban centres, is growing.[39]

Benevolent state patronage has repressed rather than encouraged diversity, yet in spite of this, what is emerging is a confident variety of forms within Zambian theatre. These articulate a range of urban and rural consciousness and use forms both scripted and unscripted, élitist and popular. This vital range gives contemporary Zambian theatre culture a dynamic quality which, in the eyes of some, will only survive and flourish if it is guided by a generous hand rather than by one that merely slaps.

1 See Fathers and Sons: Politics and Myth in Recent Zambian Drama, *New Theatre Quarterly*, 3, 9 (February 1987).
2 *An Analysis of the Development of Theatre in Zambia, 1950–1975*, MA Thesis, University of Californiaa, 1977, p. 40.
3 Moses Kwali, Zambian Playwrights, in Dickson Mwans (ed.). *Zambian Performing Arts: Currents, Issues, Policies and Direction.* (Lusaka, 1974), p. 80.
4 The Theatre Situation in Africa, in Dickson Mwansa (ed.), *Zambian Performing Arts*, p. 194.
5 See P.D. Snelson, *Educational Development in Northern Rhodesia 1883–1945* (Lusaka, 1974), pp. v, 164, 210, 246 and 238.
6 An attempt to rule that the theatre bar be closed during performances failed at the Lusaka Playhouse in 1985.
7 Dickson Mwansa and Franciso Banda, The Zambia National Theatre Arts Association (ZANTAA) in Mwansa (ed.), *Zambia Performing Arts*, p. 39.
8 Theo Samuheha, commenting on the fact that club members stayed in the bar during a performance of John Kibwana's *The Grand Race* at the Lusaka Playhouse, wrote: It is so maddeningly irritating that something really needs to be done, and done as soon as possible before the place becomes just another noisy bar, *Sunday Times of Zambia*, 8 February 1987.
9 See Victoria Findlay, Zambian Theatre and the Direction it has taken since Independence, M.A. Thesis, University of Zambia, 1987, p. 82; *Sunday Times of Zambia*, 26 April 1987; *Zambia Daily Mail*, 11 March 1988, and *Sunday Times of Zambia*, 25 January 1987.

10 Nedson Sichula refers to 'a sea of falling standards' in the *Zambia Daily Mail*, May 27, 1988.

11 Mwansa and Banda, The Zambia National Theatre Arts Association, p. 38.

12 The play subsequently went to FESTAC in Lagos in 1977, then to Cuba, Botswana, Kenya and Zimbabwe.

13 This was after the play was performed in the The Zambia National Theatre Arts Association festival at Munali Secondary School, Lusaka.

14 Message from his Excellency the President of the Republic of Zambia, *Zambia Arts Festival Handbook*, 1967, 3.

15 See Mwansa and Banda, The Zambia National Theatre Arts Association, p. 37, and Dickson Mwansa, Zambian Theatre: Politics and Art, *Ngoma*, 3, 1 (1989), p. 55.

16 *Zambia Daily Mail*, 6 May 1988.

17 President Kaunda has written poetry and also sings, accompanying himself on the guitar.

18 Agudu Chimenya, The Zambia Union of Musicians: A Quest for Identity, in Mwansa (ed.), *Zambian Performing Arts*, p. 72.

19 Ibid., p. 74.

20 The Rise of a Zambian Capitalist Class in the 1970s, *Journal of Southern African Studies*, 8, 2 (April 1982), p. 210.

21 Moses Kwali, Zambian Playwrights, p. 82.

22 Mwansa and Banda, The Zambia National Theatre Arts Association, p. 34.

23 Kenneth Kaunda, *'Watershed' Speech, 30 June 1975*, Zambia Information Services, Lusaka, 1975, p. 28.

24 See Stephen Chifunyise, Chikwakwa Theatre and Its Offshoots, in *Zambian Performing Arts*, pp. 5–9.

25 Youngson Simukoko, Chikwakwa Theatre, *Chikwakwa Review* 1971, p. 2.

26 *'Watershed' Speech*, p. 28.

27 Youngson Simukoko, Chikwakwa Theatre, p. 2.

28 Chikwakwa flier, Luapula Province, 1977.

29 At the Mutomboko Ceremony at Kazembe in 1986, during the visiting Party dignitary's address, I heard complaints that this address had nothing to do with Lunda tradition.

30 Hicks Sikazwe, *Sunday Times of Zambia*, 22 Feburary 1987.

31 Kenneth Kaunda, *Letter to my Children* (Lusaka and London, 1977), pp. 138–9.

32 See my analysis of *The Witchfinder* in Crehan, Fathers and Sons.

33 In Moses Kwali's *Brotherman*, a musical play about Garden Compound, a shanty compound next to the council sewage works overlooked by Parliament Hill (used symbolically in the play), there is a song about how the Church hoodwinks the poor. When I produced the play at Lusaka Playhouse in July 1983 it was for a members' evening only; a public performance was felt to be asking for trouble.

34 Mwansa and Banda, The Zambia National Theatre Arts Association, p. 43.

35 Working Paper, 25 June 1988, p. 9

36 Ibid., p. 8.

37 *The King Must Die*, programme, 1967

38 Cf. Etherton's comment on the contrastive use of M'ganda with 'old songs from the Western Province' in *Kazembe and the Portuguese*, that 'the musical argument was too intellectualised and obscure for this stage of development in an integrated music and dance theatre for Zambia', *Chikwakwa Review* (1971), p. 11.

39 Despite its 'beerhall atmosphere', Lusaka Playhouse attracted full houses over a period of weeks in 1987 and 1988 to adaptations of two West African novels: *The Chief Minister's Daughter* and *The Old Man and the Medal*. Other plays such as Ngugi's *I Will Marry When I Want* have also attracted large audiences, refuting the belief of former white members that African plays can never make money. The success of these productions has shown that a paying Zambian theatre audience in the capital now exists.

Interview With Gcina Mhlophe

TYRONE AUGUST

1989

Q: *Can we start off by talking about the question of language as it is central to what you are trying to do in the theatre? Why do you write in English when you grew up speaking another language?*

A: I wrote for the very first time in Xhosa, because I was doing Xhosa at school, and it was a language I admired. In the process of learning it, I discovered the richness of the language. So I wrote poetry in Xhosa, and songs and short stories. I think it was only in 1979 that I started writing in English. I don't even think it was a conscious decision. I just found myself writing in English. Now I write in both languages. It depends on what is needed at that time. At times I write out of inspiration, something that I feel I should express. Other times I'm asked to write something. For example, I was asked to write a poem for Miriam Makeba in 1985 when (singer) Thembi Mtshali did a tribute to her. There was no way I could write it in English and say properly what I wanted to say, so I had to do it in Xhosa.

Q: *Do you think there is a tendency in local theatre to use English when addressing serious issues and to switch over to the vernacular when addressing less serious issues?*

A: Language should be something that should be respected. I know we have a problem — when some people want to swear in a play, they put it in Zulu or in Sotho so that only a certain section of the audience understands. And then they switch over to English when they want to speak about the serious things. I don't know what the purpose of that is. It sort of makes our languages less important and that needs to be corrected. But sometimes when people tell jokes for instance, they just don't know how to put them in English. It's a problem. We find ourselves forced to write in English because it's the most accessible language, especially in Johannesburg. And in showbiz you are on stage to be understood ... But, because English is our second language, you jump at any word you can get hold of. If it was your language, you would use the best word, but because you're using your second language, you find you're just grabbing at any word. The fact that I've worked for *Learn and Teach* (a monthly literacy magazine) helped me a lot. Having to break down what I'm saying all the time means that I now have a better understanding of the English language, and that has helped me to be able to switch to children's writing. I have a sense of those different levels, and that is an advantage which I should learn to develop even more.

Q: *Why did you choose to write* Have You Seen Zandile? *mainly in English?*

A: It's a very universal story. It could have happened to anybody in any part of the world. Using English was so that it could be seen by most audiences. If I had chosen to write it in Zulu, for instance, how many people would have understood it?

Q: *You say a lot of people wouldn't have understood it. That is linked to the kind of audience you envisaged for the play. How then, did you define that audience?*

A: In Johannesburg people speak Xhosa, Zulu, Shangaan, Venda, Tswana, Sotho. So if it was performed in the townships, different people would understand different things. The first half of *Zandile* has sections in Xhosa, and the second half things that are in Zulu. That's all. But only people who understand those languages would have understood the play if I had decided to do it completely in those languages. The rest of the audience would not have been able to — even if they were not white or English-speaking.

Q: *Would the same considerations apply to your folk tale* The Snake with Seven Heads?

A: I think I'm going to have to do a lot of work on that. The book is going to be translated into all the (local) African languages. That is definite. Secondly when I do the stage version, I would also like to do it in African languages in rural areas so that it can be accessible.

Q: *So you still see English as a starting-point?*

A: Yes, yes. I'm still going to use a lot of English. I'm writing in English now because there's a need for that. If I was living in Durban or the Transkei, where my mother is from, I wouldn't be writing in English today. There wouldn't be a need. But I don't speak all the different African languages spoken in Johannesburg. And I want to be accessible to people. I want people to understand what I'm saying.

Q: *Why do you think folk tales like* The Snake *are important in local literature?*

A: There was a time in African culture when the setting of the sun announced that it was time for story-telling. It was natural for grandfathers and grandmothers — they were more patient and more experienced — to tell stories. That time is gone now. Now everybody in the family works. When the children come from school, they roam the streets. Even if they are given things to do — homework and housework — there's no guarantee that they'll do it. So there's all kinds of break-downs in normal African culture because of the kind of lifestyle we lead, in the cities especially. The television and the radio and the disco are taking over. And that's something which should not be allowed to happen. There's wisdom in folk tales. Folk tales are educational. They have lessons to be learnt — whether it's to do with people telling lies, being untrustworthy or being selfish. Another thing: with television today you don't use your imagination. If they talk about a dinosaur, they show you a dinosaur. That kills something of the child's imagination. And it's probably the only time we have free imaginations — without any prejudices or confines of society. And there's the aspect of human contact. Story-telling should not conform to theatre rules. People should be able to sit in a circle and participate in the chants, in the songs. We're working towards that. For me, it's just the beginning, working from what I know best — the theatre. And some of the things we talk about in folk tales. They are not just out of the blue; they happened and people chose to tell stories about them. So these stories are very realistic. They don't always have to end 'happily ever after'. There are stories that end sadly. There's a Xhosa expression that says a wheel goes round and round in everybody's life. And sometimes the wheel turns on the wrong side.

Q: *In story telling, you can assume the role of various characters ...*

A: The fact that you have to be all those different characters in one, and not use any sound effects or musical instruments, is a very important skill in story-telling. That's what makes *you* a story-teller. It comes from inside; it's not something that people are appointed to do. As an individual, you are very mobile. You can tell stories virtually anywhere. It's inexpensive entertainment. It's one of the natural advantages of story-telling. All you need is one person and people's imaginations, but now that we live in the kind of times we do, we should really work towards putting them on paper. Because we just don't have enough people who are into this. We should put the stories on video if we can. It's important to do that so they don't die. They belong to a certain culture; they are worth retaining. Not only the story of Noddy or Pinocchio or Snow White. Those stories have lived for ever. Our stories are being repressed because they are supposedly from a barbaric culture. This generation should make sure — with all the skills and facilities we have — to tape them, to record them. Why can't we do that? And our stories are fresh because they've been suppressed for so long.

Q: *To shift away from folk tales. The aspect of being a woman. Have you consciously tried to use that in your work?*

A: I got involved in show business at a good time in my life. That was an advantage. If I had started younger, maybe I would have been confused on that aspect. But I started after I had fallen in love with myself. I had accepted myself. I had accepted the kind of person I am. So I see things whatever way I see them, and I don't feel: Am I female? Am I male? Am I black? If I see them, and come out as a black person, that's a natural process. It's not a conscious thing that I work on. And if things sound like it's a woman talking it's only natural. When I told people I was writing a new play called *Somdaka,* they said: How come? You're a woman. But if a man fascinates me, then I write about a man. If a woman fascinates me, then I write about a woman. I write what comes into my mind and impresses me. And if it comes out as a woman looking at a man, then that's fine as well. Why not?

Q: *In general, the theatre is dominated by men in South Africa. How can that be addressed?*

A: I'm aware that there are few women writers in theatre. It's pathetic. But I don't think I should force myself to write about women only. I'm conscious that I should hold up the point of view of women, but if something comes at a certain time to me, I allow that inspiration. I don't push things.

Q: *Let's take a work like* You strike the Women, You Strike the Rock *(directed by Phyllis Klotz). Do you think it's part of the attempt to redress the balance?*

A: It definitely is, because women want to tell it their way. They look at certain events from their point of view. Let's take (the Battle of) Blood River, for instance. How many women have you heard mentioned there? Did those men have no sisters, no mothers who helped them? Our history is very unbalanced. There's so much to do for a women's writer. The rivers won't dry for a very long time.

A: You Strike the Rock *was overtly political, because it was based on a real event, whereas* Zandile *was more of a personal story. Do you feel it's more important to focus on the personal?*

A: I think both are equally important. The choice is with the writer. But certain times call for things to be ... When you're in debating society, for instance, you don't put yourself first. You think of your group, your school. So the fact that overtly political plays dominate, it's because people put *themselves* back and think of what is important to say about what is happening in this country. Also, that has partly been sparked by white people speaking for us. Now black people are wanting to speak for themselves, wanting to say it their way. Expressing the anger, the joy that goes through them. Because you can't say those things in the streets, you say them in whatever art form you can. I think it's also possible for women to do that, to say: Okay, the men have spoken too much; let's speak. So we'll end up — say 10 years from today — with women dominating theatre and maybe using too much rhetoric. It always depends. And me giving priority to myself sometimes; it's just that I think of myself as important, as well as national issues. Also, I have the belief that I'm not a unique person. There's got to be somebody who's gone through it before and that gives it another point of view altogether. And because people go through the same kinds of things for different reasons, I think they've got something to share in my life. I think we need to think of it — the personal and the political — as equal all the way. Politics changes every day, but the fundamental things that are important to human beings last a long, long time.

Q: *We've talked about the distinction between the personal and the political. What do you think should be the relationship between politics and art or culture?*

A: 'Politics' is just a word that describes life. You don't decide to be in a politically explosive part of the world. You're born there and you're governed by what happens — whether the sun shines or it rains for months. These things affect people in different ways. Some people would find cause to celebrate, others to mourn. In art or culture, we portray what we see around us. People sing about love every day, because that is what they long for. Politics, for me, is just another part of life; it's another way of looking at life. So when you decide to portray things that are political, you're looking at a certain aspect of life. So art and politics should mix, by all means.

Q: *In your own work, do you intend concentrating on one more than the other?*

A: I let my course just run. The more well-known you become (for something), the more you find your choices being defined. You can choose to follow those choices defined by your audience, or you can choose to say: I am capable of *this* as well. So it depends on how strong you are in your views. I don't want to do anything that is not good. If I do something, it has to be worth everybody's time. So my work has to come from inside. I have to be truthful. I hope that comes across in what I do.

Q: *You use the words 'showbiz' and 'enjoyment' when you talk about your work. How do you regard your work? Primarily as show-business?*

A: I've been very choosy in the things that I do. I can't do any old play, maybe because if I don't enjoy myself I don't think the audience will enjoy themselves. You talk with your face. Even my friends, I can't bluff them and say I'm happy with something when I'm not. People are able to see inside me, through my face.

Q: *You don't have any intention of saying certain things in the theatre?*

A: Yes, there can be a message. But I don't sit down and write: the message is *this*. I just write it as it happens and then a message is found there. If something is important enough to force me to wake up, to write it, then there must be some value there!

Q: *To move to another issue. Your play* Zandile *was by its very nature a universal story, so it was accessible to overseas audiences. But there does seem to be theatre being created specifically for export. What are your views on that?*

A: When plays go overseas it's wonderful. It's important to share. But for me, I choose to give priority to the people of my country. Black artists don't go to university to learn skills, they learn from the people around them. They should plant back. We owe our community the right to share what we've achieved. We shouldn't create specifically to go overseas. The overseas interest in our art started very innocently, but it has escalated and reached the stage where people won't audition for a play if it's not going overseas. We have to give value to performing in our own country, if for no other reason than that we draw from our community.

Q: *If you look at local theatre, what gaps would you say there are? What should be done that isn't being done?*

A: I feel there's very little that people plan to do in terms of writing scripts, proper scripts. Closing the door, being alone, letting your characters live on paper, hearing their voices, seeing them get dressed, that's lacking in our theatre. Also, if we want to have audiences which are receptive, we should start with children. They either watch television or adult theatre. Yes, they *can* learn from adult theatre, but there should be theatre specifically for children, in the same way that we design clothes that fit women better, that suit men better.

Q: *In story-telling you can adapt the story as you go along, whereas you're saying there's a gap in formal scriptwriting?*

A: That is the challenge, and I think it should be taken up. When I do story-telling, I'm alone on stage. I go to town. It's my stuff; I can close my eyes and eat it. But there's all kinds of dynamics in the theatre. If the script is not strong, the actors can play around with it. So the script has to be strong to make the actor feel responsible for the character and that's a skill that needs to be developed. Also for the lasting effect, I like things that last. How many people saw (Barney Simon's work-shopped play) *Black Dog* (in which Gcina Mhlophe performed)? I don't know if it will ever be performed again. But if it's something that's scripted, on paper, I could be dead and the script will still be there.

Q: *The other aspect you mentioned of children's theatre? How do you intend contributing to that?*

A: My starting point will be to stage *The Snake*. But I think there's room for children's plays that talk about general things as well. I hope I'll live long enough to develop that. I've explored all kinds of things. I've jumped into all kinds of situations. But I'm now at the point in my life where I want to concentrate on children's theatre or children's writing.

Q: *Another gap seems to be the lack of theatre in rural areas. How do you think our theatre can be strengthened and developed in those parts of the country?*

A: The rural areas are very deprived. We complain a lot that we don't have proper theatre structures in the townships. In the meantime we have the churches and the halls, but, in the rural areas, there's hardly anything of that nature. Very few people have ever seen a professional play in their lives. If we're thinking of getting into rural theatre, we should change the format. It should not be the same kind of plays we put up at the Market Theatre in Johannesburg. Such plays cannot easily be put up in rural areas. The subject matter should be different, for starters. And the way we portray theatre — with lights and a stage — they're not used to it. There needs to be something like open-air theatre. So you can have a huge truck and just show up at a place at certain times of the year. But I don't think rural theatre can be commercial; it should be for enjoyment, and that puts a big strain on those who decide to do it. Because you've got to have money to do it. I admire (Lesotho-based playwright) Zakes Mda a lot; he does a lot of rural theatre. He just arrives at a new place with his group (Marotholi Travelling Theatre Company). They talk to the people. They display something and ask the people: what would you have done? People start throwing around ideas, and a new play is born. Then the group moves the play to the next village and do the same thing. I think that's important work.

Q: *In the urban areas, would you say the kind of work playwright Gibson Kente is doing is helping to create popular theatre? Or do you think there are some unfortunate commercial considerations at work there?*

A: I have a certain respect for Gibson Kente. He's been our university. Very, very few black theatre people haven't worked with him. He has very good skills in terms of teaching people to act, to sing and dance. Okay, the story might not be strong enough, but the part, the character you are given, he wants you to give your soul to it. Even if you're going to do it for a whole year. But you have to give it everything you've got.

And I think he's got something there. Whether his plays are commercial or not, that's another story. I respect him for being able to train raw people. That's his contribution. He has also played a big role in creating an awareness in the townships of theatre. It's not even a question of affording his plays, because they are not cheap. It's just a question of accessibility. Around the corner, the church that you go to every Sunday, there's a play happening. That's accessibility. And he doesn't write big political plays. He makes social comment plays. And they have a place in our society. Divorce, wife-bashing, teenage pregnancy, that's the kind of subject matter he deals with. I don't think it's less important than blacks taking over the country!

Q: *I've touched on all the areas I wanted to. Do you have any final comments on local theatre?*

A: To a certain extent, a lot of plays being performed at the moment are talking about what we've heard before. I think it's up to us who have travelled that road before to explore new ground. It's time — now — to discover new things.

1993

Q: *Have you shifted from theatre to story-telling since our last interview?*

A: There has been a certain kind of shift. First of all, I got into story-telling thinking it would be a part-time thing. But when I got inside, I saw how vast it was. The fact that I am who I am, and having the skills of theatre, I found my audience was ripe. Then the phone wouldn't stop ringing. I performed in schools, youth centres, art galleries, universities and conferences. For nursery schools, for primary schools, high schools and for adults who came from different walks of life. The first thing that excited me was that people of different political persuasions could share in story-telling. And children of different financial standing could be reached very cheaply. That's important. It's very cost-effective. No props, no major costumes and lights and set changes. That meant I could perform anywhere. One of the frustrations in theatre is that the bright lights can make you unable to see your audience. And I love to see my audience, I gain strength from that. That is just one of the little attractions (of story-telling). But something else was happening in South Africa. I was feeling the glaring demand to do specific kinds of theatre. And I don't know if I was in the minority, but I felt that political messages could also be put across through story-telling, without being party political.

Q: *Have you started using English less since you shifted to story-telling?*

A: It has not meant using less English. I ask my audience if I'm not sure what language they want. I speak three African languages and English. It's a big advantage, because language is a tool for a story-teller. There's a poem I wrote early last year, called 'In the company of words'. In the different art forms that I use, whether I'm acting or directing or telling stories, or being a writer, I use words. So I think that poem was inspired by being a story-teller. I was very aware of how much I was in the company of words.

Q: *Do you find languages such as Zulu and Xhosa more expressive?*

A: Certain languages are more expressive for what I want to say. For example, there are certain emotions and exclamations that you can drive home easier in Zulu than you can in English. There are expressions in the face, and also terms like 'Nx!' (indicating irritation or anger). That's all (you say. But) it has such an impact, combined with the expression I have on my face. So I don't even have to translate that into English.

Q: *Are the sources of your stories still primarily traditional folk tales?*

A: No. The sources of my stories have changed. Definitely still keeping the traditional folk tales as a solid basis (because they are) tried and tested. But now we create new stories.

Q: *We?*

A: The way I am working now has demanded that I train other story-tellers. I don't want something that's so wonderful to die. Also, I think if I see story-telling move on with me reversing, I can come back into theatre, and participate more than I am now. I had to put a hold on theatre because it was not possible to put as much into theatre at the same time as doing story-telling. There are now fifteen of us involved in the story-telling group *Zanendaba* (Bring me a story). We perform in different places, new stories that are contemporary and very recognisable for children that are growing up now, and relevant to certain situations that they have experienced. We are collecting stories from all over the African continent and abroad. My travels over the years have given me a wide range of contacts. And they are coming in very handy now. People who I've told about *Zanendaba* are sending me material in the form of books, audio-tapes and magazines. That is so useful.

Q: *Do these stories from different parts of the world have anything in common?*

A: A story well told is enjoyable to people of that culture as well as to any other listeners. Also, there are specific things that you find from culture to culture. The differences are the beauty and the colour of these stories. But some stories that come from another culture, like (that of) the native Americans, do have certain things that are very common to our story-telling even though the characters are different. In Africa, the tortoise, the rabbit and the spider are three common characters. This is part of story-telling all over the continent. Native Americans have the coyote and the turtle and the eagle. Japanese story-tellers will tell you again about the turtle, about the crane. (Those similarities are) exciting to me. Story-telling is a world of its own.

Q: *Apart from characters, do these stories from different parts of the world have any themes in common?*

A: Definitely. Take African stories about a woman who didn't fall pregnant. (She) tried this and that. Finally, a different force brings her a child, but that child somehow seems to wrap himself or herself around that woman's heart. That you find in African folklore as well as that of native Americans, aborigines and Japanese. I am particularly drawn to indigenous peoples of different parts of the world. I find their stories and cultures resonant and homely, welcoming to my culture. I don't feel any competition, of trying to be the best.

Q: *What are the themes or concerns of your stories?*

A: I am quite open. I find new stories exciting. I think the possibilities are so endless that it would be a shame if I stuck to the same stories. I also like looking at new things, like environmental stories, water stories, war stories, love stories. But there are particular stories that come from when I started doing story-telling that seem to work for some particular occasion.

Q: *What plays have you written since the last interview?*

A: *Love Child*, in July 1991. It was about a person who is born between two language groups. A person who believes that art can be a healing force. I used a traditional folk tale to start with, that talks about two villages that were fighting, but the chiefs were cousins. A young girl called Nomlambo came into one of the villages and fell in love with Mthunzi, the young man who was looking after the chief because he was not well. She took him to a deep pool in a river. They found a drum with magic powers, took it to the battlefield and, because of its music, the warriors forgot their spears and shields and held hands, dancing to the rhythm of the drum. It carried on to talk about the violence on the Reef, and how the press had labelled it as a Zulu-Xhosa war. Me, being a Zulu-Xhosa, I know that it was not the case. I saw myself as proof that Zulu-Xhosa people love one another still. And so do other people who belong to different language groups.

Q: *Do you still feel any party political pressure on your writing?*

A: Maybe people are weary of doing that, but I think I made my point clear to whoever felt like bothering me. I will never be an artist who doesn't work with people from various communities. I think that's enough freedom fighting for me. Also children are a major interest to me. When I look at our education system, and the problems that particularly African children are facing, I get worried about the future. I wish I could be among those who can help children in whatever way.

Q: *Why?*

A: I can't imagine this new South Africa we keep talking about if our children are not happy. We have had our pain, but the instincts of an adult — whether you have a child or not — are, and should be, to protect children from the pains that you know, and learn from them.

Q: *To return to theatre. How did you feel about the reception of your play* Somdaka *at the end of 1989?*

A: There were two things that went with *Somdaka*. One is that I don't think I put everything I felt into the script. I hope I'll have a chance to do it again, that's why I haven't published it yet. Number two: Being a woman telling a man's story isn't easy but it's possible, especially if you care for that man.

Q: *Do you have any other plays planned for the immediate future?*

A: I'm sitting on a script because I want to see *Zanendaba* on its feet first. It's a story about a person who is on death row. It's a true story. If I can leave it at that for now ...

Q: *What are your comments on post-1990 theatre?*

A: I think there has been some exciting stuff. But I miss the variety we used to have. And I'm to blame as well (even though I reversed from theatre for a good reason). We are in a very difficult transitional period. (For example) imported scripts don't seem to touch local audiences. Adaptation is important. Maybe the adaptation didn't work, or maybe the audiences weren't ready. I don't know.

Q: *What did you think about the Nokwe family's musical play* Singing the Times? *Was it doing anything different, or saying something different?*

A: I liked the closeness that their singing lent to each other and to the audience. It's very rare in South Africa that you find women playing instruments. But the story-telling was pretty straightforward. It could have been more theatrical.

Q: *Do you think that the fact that a work like* Singing the Times *is directed by a man (Barney Simon) affects the end product?*

A: It definitely affects the end product, no matter how sensitive the male director is. (Directing) is something that women have to learn; necessity should drive us to a point where black women know they've got to get in there and do it themselves rather than criticising that the man didn't do it this way or that way.

Q: *Is there any particular reason why this is not happening?*
A: I can't truthfully say I know for sure. I know that women sometimes get very nervous just to write a script, never mind to direct it. But I think that one of the things that those of us should do who have gotten to that stage is empower others. Maybe I could write a script and ask a sister who has the knowledge and experience in theatre to co-direct it with me. Once you've done it half-way, you can do it all the way.

INDEX

Natal.